LEGAL ASPECTS OF RADIOGRAPHY AND RADIOLOGY

BRIDGIT C. DIMOND

MA, LLB, DSA, AHSM, Barrister-at-law,
Emeritus Professor of the University of Glamorgan

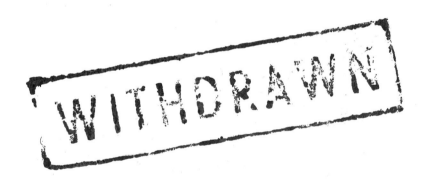

Blackwell
Science

© 2002 by Bridgit C. Dimond

Blackwell Science Ltd,
a Blackwell Publishing Company
Editorial Offices:
Osney Mead, Oxford OX2 0EL, UK
  Tel: +44 (0)1865 206206
Blackwell Science, Inc., 350 Main Street,
Malden, MA 02148-5018, USA
  Tel: +1 781 388 8250
Iowa State Press, a Blackwell Publishing
Company, 2121 State Avenue, Ames, Iowa
50014-8300, USA
  Tel: +1 515 292 0140
Blackwell Science Asia Pty, 54 University
Street, Carlton, Victoria 3053, Australia
  Tel: +61 (0)3 9347 0300
Blackwell Wissenschafts Verlag,
Kurfürstendamm 57, 10707 Berlin, Germany
  Tel: +49 (0)30 32 79 060

First published 2002 by Blackwell Science Ltd

Library of Congress
Cataloging-in-Publication Data
is available

ISBN 0–632-05502-2

A catalogue record for this title is available from
the British Library

Set in 10/12pt Century
by DP Photosetting, Aylesbury, Bucks
Printed and bound in Great Britain by
MPG Books Ltd, Bodmin, Cornwall

For further information on
Blackwell Science, visit our website:
www.blackwell-science.com

Contents

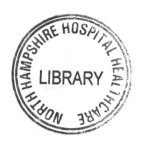

Foreword

The modernisation of the Health Service is dependent upon the ability of the workforce to deliver care to the patients in a manner which is sensitive to their needs and expectations. Clinicians in both the diagnostic and radiotherapy services are key members of the health care team and recent government policies and their supporting legislation have identified areas of priority and the skills necessary to deliver these priorities effectively.

It is therefore essential that those providing the service understand the important concepts, issues and strategies related to these developments and the many changes which have taken place associated with legal and clinical governance issues. In particular the new roles being advocated for radiographers mean that the practitioners will require to develop a high knowledge and expertise in all aspects of governance, professional leadership and service development.

The public and society at large must have confidence in the health care professionals and be assured of their competence, accountability and responsibilities. These responsibilities are especially applicable when the practitioner is in contact either directly or indirectly with patients, clients, carers or fellow professionals. Where healthcare is concerned statements of conduct, clinical competence and ethics are now increasingly under scrutiny and ever increasing expectations are held by the government and public alike.

Without a doubt the prime duty of these professionals remains that of having proper regard to the welfare of those using their services, thus safeguarding their health and wellbeing. The training and education of radiographers and radiologists has therefore quite rightly concentrated on the clinical and technological processes involved in this care. However in recent years the needs of both groups, whether in the diagnostic or the therapeutic disciplines, have increasingly involved issues relating to law and its relevance to themselves and to patients.

The advent of clinical governance has also added a further dimension to the practice of radiology and in particular it is important to understand the legal implications and challenges of implementing a 'no-blame' culture. This must be difficult to come to terms with in the light of advice given relating to 'whistleblowing'. This advice states that, 'Registrants must act to protect patients when there is reason to believe that they are threatened by a colleague's conduct, performance or health. The safety of the patient comes first at all times and should over-ride personal and professional loyalties'. Practitioners must therefore be aware of and act within the limits of their experience and knowledge and be able to judge their own performance. To do this they must have an understanding of the legal framework within which they practise.

Radiographers and radiologists have an increasing need to work as part of a multidisciplinary team and it is therefore becoming ever more important that practitioners not only update their knowledge related to clinical and technical skills but also in areas linked to relevant law and good practice.

Many books have been written about legal issues but this book is unique in that it concentrates on the topics relating to diagnostic and therapeutic radiography and radiology in a manner which can readily be understood by the reader. In addition the author has identified many areas which will help to develop the necessary skills and knowledge of practitioners in both diagnostic and radiotherapy departments and enable them to take a proactive as well as a reactive approach to issues arising from recent legislation.

Essential areas covered include professional registration, standards and misconduct , negligence, and record keeping. In addition to the valuable information provided by the author many related practical situations are discussed in detail. Very importantly the rights of the patient have not been neglected. It is extremely important that practitioners are aware of, understand and are able to communicate these rights to the patient. These rights, in the areas such as informed consent, confidentiality, access to records, and death and dying are quite rightly emphasised and explained in easy to understand language.

This excellent book is key reading for all those professionals who are involved with the diagnosis or treatment of patients and also those who have to make use of these services. It contains comprehensive information, reference and guidance in specific areas of legal requirements and will prove to be an excellent platform for further reading and research. It provides substantial benefits to the reader by clarifying many points, highlighting recent legislation and identifying future developments. Very significantly the knowledge it imparts will help to ensure that the confidence the government, patients and public require to have in the health care practitioner is justified and enhanced.

Sandy Yule, OBE
DSc, MSc, DMS, FCR, HDRC
Chair of the Conduct and Competence Committee of the Shadow Health Professions Council, of the Radiographers' Board of the CPSM, and Member of the Board of Management for the International Society of Radiographers and Radiological Technologists.

Preface

As explained in Chapter 1 this was not an easy book to write and I hope that the result is not too confusing. My aim is always to clarify the law for the practitioner, to break down the barriers created by law and its language and to give practitioners working in radiography and radiology an understanding of the legal framework within which they practise. What makes this book different from other health law books is the concentration on the legal issues which affect X-ray and radiotherapy departments and patients, the fact that simple situations with potential legal complexities are taken from these areas and the fact that many practitioners working in these fields have been consulted in order to ensure that as many relevant topics as possible have been included.

Because of the different people who work in this field I have used the term 'practitioner' to cover both therapeutic and diagnostic radiographers and radiologists, and also oncologists and any others who consider the chapters are relevant. There are always problems in the use of personal pronouns and for convenience and to avoid 'he/she' and 'his/her' usage practitioners have somewhat unusually been referred to as 'she' or 'her' since the majority of radiographers are women and the numbers of women in radiology are increasing. For clarity the patient is denoted by 'he' and 'him' although, of course, many are female. The reader should interpret 'she' and 'her' as including 'he' and 'him' and *vice versa*.

Clearly one of the most important areas of law is that related to radiation protection and the many regulations which apply in this field. I have not attempted to rewrite the excellent guidance which exists, such as the *Medical and Dental Guidance Notes* prepared by the Institute of Physics and Engineering in Medicine in association with the National Radiological Protection Board, Health and Safety Executive and Department of Health[1]. Nor have I attempted to reproduce the many statutory documents which are to be found in the NRPB's volumes of documents. I have, where appropriate, referred to these documents and set out the main principles relating to radiation regulation and protection, but this book endeavours to cover many other areas of law relevant to this practice. The result is I hope a useful and readable guide on the extensive legal framework within which the practitioner works.

References

1   Institute of Physics and Engineering in Medicine (2001) *Medical and Dental Guidance notes: A good practice guide to implement ionising radiation protection legislation in the clinical environment*, IPEM, London.

Acknowledgements

A work of this nature cannot be written without the generous help of many people. In some ways it is invidious to pick out the names of the many professionals who have given me advice and suggested some of the legal situations which should be covered. Special mention must be made however of Dr Ness Evans, who provided invaluable assistance in enabling me to have access to her library of useful publications and guidance from professional bodies, and who also gave me extremely useful advice on some of the technical aspects; Richard Price, who started my interest in the legal issues arising in radiography and has provided invaluable assistance, and Dr Absi, whose assistance is acknowledged in Chapter 26.

I would also like to thank the many radiographers – therapeutic and diagnostic – who have raised specific concerns on legal issues which I have attempted to address in this book: in particular Elizabeth Hunter, Michaela Davis, Trish Chudleigh, Susan D'Arcy, Neil Prime and Jane Arnett. I appreciate too being able to quote from the statutes and statutory instruments printed by the Stationery Office and from the law reports of decided cases produced by many different publishers. I thank my copy editor Tamsin Bacchus for her patience and hard work and my publisher Antonia Seymour for her belief in the importance of this book and her encouragement. I give my sincere thanks to my family for their constant support.

Finally I am extremely grateful to Bette for her considerable assistance and her diligent work in preparing the index and tables and reading the proofs.

I thank you all.

Abbreviations

ACAS   Advisory, Conciliation and Arbitration Service
ACPC   Area Child Protection Committee:
BCMA   British Complementary Medicine Association
BFCR   Board of Faculty of Clinical Radiology
BNF   British National Formulary
BPA   British Paediatric Association
CAR   Congenital Anomalies Register
CHC   Community Health Council
CHI   Commission for Health Improvement
CNST   Clinical Negligence Scheme for Trusts
COPE   Committee on Publication Ethics
CoR   College of Radiographers
COSHH   Control of Substances Hazardous to Health
CPD   Continuing Professional Development
CPR   Civil Procedure Rules
CPS   Crown Prosecution Service
CR   Computed Radiology (where image is converted in a digitised form
            through an intermediate process – contrast with DR)
CRD   Centre for Reviews and Dissemination
CRE   Commission for Racial Equality
DGH   District General Hospital
DHA   District Health Authority (abolished April 1996)
DR   Direct Radiology (where the image is created in a digitised format
            from its inception – contrast with CR)
DRL   Diagnostic Reference Levels
EHR   Electronic Health Record
EOC   Equal Opportunities Commission
EPR   Electronic Patient Record
ERA   Employment Rights Act (1996 and 1999)
Euratom   European Atomic Energy Community
FHSA   Family Health Services Authority (abolished April 1996)
HAI   Hospital Acquired Infection
HASAW   Health and Safety at Work Act 1974
HIS   Hospital Information System
HPC   Health Professions Council
HSC   Health Services Commissioner (ombudsman)
IAEA   International Atomic Energy Agency

HSE	Health and Safety Executive
IOS	Imaging and Oncology Science
IPEM	Institute of Physics and Engineering in Medicine
IRR	Ionising Radiation Regulations 1999 (SI 1999/3232)
IR(ME)R	Ionising Radiation (Medical Exposure) Regulations 2000
IVP	Intravenous pyelogram
LOLER	Lifting Operations and Lifting Equipment Regulations
LREC	Local Research Ethics Committee
MCREC	Multi-Centre Research Ethics Committee
MHRT	Mental Health Review Tribunal
MRI	Magnetic Resonance Imaging
NAD	Nothing Abnormal Discovered
NAI	Non-accidental Injury
NAO	National Audit Office
NDC	National Disability Council
NHSBSP	National Health Service Breast Screening Programme
NHSLA	National Health Service Litigation Authority
NICE	National Institute of Clinical Effectiveness
NRPB	National Radiological Protection Board
NSF	National Service Framework
PACS	Picture archiving and communication systems
PALS	Patient Advocacy and Liaison Service
PCG	Primary Care Group
PCT	Primary Care Trust
PD	Practice Direction (supplemented to CPR)
PSIG	Paediatric Special Interest Group
PUWER	Provision and Use of Work Equipment Regulations
RAID	Redundant Array of Inexpensive Devices
RCPCH	Royal College of Paediatrics and Child Health
RCR	Royal College of Radiologists
RIDDOR 95	Reporting of Injuries, Diseases and Dangerous Occurrences (Regs) 1995
RIS	Radiology Information System
RPA	Radiation Protection Adviser
RSA	Radioactive Substances Act 1993
RSI	Repetitive strain injury
SCoR	Society and College of Radiographers
SRSC	Safety Representatives and Safety Committees (Regs)
UKCCSG	United Kingdom Children's Cancer Study Group
UVR	Ultraviolet Radiation

A useful directory of terms used in MR is provided by Bryant and Blease (1997) *The A thru' Z of MR* Clinical Press Ltd, Bristol.

Section A
The Legal Context

Chapter 1
Introduction

The justification for this book is to provide practitioners (by which term is meant the diagnostic and therapeutic radiographer, the radiologist and the oncologist) with an understanding of the context within which they work.

Law can be perplexing to those who have never studied it. The jargon and the complexity of a lawyer's answer to the simplest question can place a significant barrier between the ordinary health professional and the lawyer. However every health professional or health service manager has to work within the context of the law and therefore has to know the basic legal principles which constrain or empower them and also have a clear understanding of when it becomes essential to bring in legal advice and support.

The aim is not to make lawyers of the health practitioners for whom this is written, but to provide them with an understanding of the context within which they practise so that they can, by their knowledge of the law, ensure that they, their patients and their colleagues are protected. Ignorance of the law is no defence to either criminal or civil actions and professional practice requires that practitioners have a good understanding of the way in which the law both restricts and enables them to perform safely and professionally. Programmes for professional development recognise the importance of a knowledge of the law. In their review, *Reflections on radiography*[1], Mary Hall and Michaela Davis emphasise that health care professionals have a legal obligation to their patients to provide a high standard of care and to act in the patients' best interests and that this requires law and ethics to be included in the curriculum of professional development.

Scope and coverage

The book is divided into six Sections the first five of which cover the basic principles of the legal system, the rights of the patient, professional issues of registration and professional conduct, accountability and management. These set the framework of the law which applies to practice and consider in particular the implications of the Human Rights Act 1998 and the Data Protection Act 1998 and other major changes to the legal powers of the patient. Also discussed are the ways in which practitioners are accountable for their actions and the organisation and management of the NHS. The final Section covers specialist topics of relevance to different practitioners being PACS, teleradiology and communications, dental X-rays, complementary therapies, the expanded role of the practitioner and legal aspects of research.

Scotland and Northern Ireland

This book describes the law which applies to England and Wales. This for the most part also applies to Scotland and Northern Ireland, but there are some differences since there are specific statutory provisions for these countries. Following the establishment of the Scottish Parliament, there are likely to be greater differences between the law for Scotland and that for England and Wales.

Different practitioner and client groups

Initially the book was planned for the radiographer and the radiologist covering the legal aspects of both the medical and the technical role. However as soon as one explores the legal dimensions of radiography one is faced with two extremely different professions: diagnostic and therapeutic. And if one is exploring the legal issues relating to radiology should one not also be considering the legal issues of oncology and so the field spreads into palliative care, pain management, euthanasia, letting die, suicide and a world away from diagnostic legal issues. There may have been advantages in writing four books instead of one. However in the end the decision was made to proceed with the one: there are sufficient commonalties of law across all these diverse professions and individual practitioners can, with a good index, pick those legal topics relevant to them. The different needs of the specialist practitioners have not been separated into different chapters, as there is so much common to them all. However, where appropriate, examples have been given of the different situations which can arise.

Specific client groups such as children and pregnant women have been considered separately in order that the relevant law and professional guidance could be brought together.

The law has been discussed in the context of the policy changes which are taking place within the NHS and the role of the new quangos and statutory bodies.

How to use the book

It is not recommended that the book should be read at a sitting, but that it should be used as a source of reference, following up specific topics as required.

References

1   Hall, M. & Davis, M. (1999) Reflections on radiography *Radiography*, **5**, 165–73

Chapter 2
The Legal System

This chapter is aimed at providing an introduction to the basic terms which are used and a description of the framework within which the law is implemented. A glossary provides an explanation of some of the technical terms which are used in this book.

Sources of law

Law derives from two main sources, statute law and the common law, both of which should now be interpreted in the light of the Human Rights Act 1998. The derivation and sources of law in the UK is illustrated in Figure 2.1.

Statute law

Statute law is based on legislation passed through the agreed constitutional process. Since signing the Treaty of Rome, the UK has accepted that it is bound by the legislation of the European Community, Regulations and Directives. The Regulations have direct application to Member States, whereas Directives must

---

Figure 2.1 Derivation and sources of law.

Statute Law	Common Law
EC Regulations	**EC Court rulings**
Acts of Parliament/Statutes made by House of Commons House of Lords Royal Assent	**House of Lords** – cases on important points of law **Court of Appeal** **High Court/Crown Court**
Statutory Instruments made by relevant Ministry laid before Parliament	Decisions binding on basis of rules of precedent and hierarchy

Statutes and statutory instruments as well as previous cases are interpreted by judges and the decisions become part of the common law and all law now has to be interpreted in the light of the Human Rights Act (see Chapter 3)

be incorporated into UK law to be effective, although this does not apply to their application to state authorities.

Legislation in the UK is formed by the introduction of a Bill into either the House of Lords or House of Commons (or into the Assemblies of Scotland and Northern Ireland) usually by the Government but sometimes by a private member. Each Bill follows through a recognised procedure by way of hearings, committee stages and report stage and eventually, following agreement by both Houses and the signature of the Queen, becomes an Act of Parliament. The actual date an Act comes into force will either be set out in the Act itself or will be determined at a later date by statutory instrument. An Act of Parliament may provide for powers to be delegated to Ministers or others for enacting detailed rules to supplement the Act. These are statutory instruments and the process is known as 'secondary legislation'. Statutory instruments must be placed before Parliament before coming into effect.

Since devolution the Scottish Parliament has the right to enact legislation within specified parameters, but the Welsh Assembly has more limited powers and can only pass secondary legislation.

Common law

Decisions by judges in court create what is known as the common law, case law or judge-made law. A recognised hierarchy of the courts determines which previous decisions are binding on courts hearing similar issues. The European Court of Justice in Luxembourg can hear cases between Member States on European law, or applications by the domestic courts for a ruling on a point of law.

A recognised system of reporting of judges' decisions ensures certainty over what was stated and the facts of the cases. The main principles which are set out in a case are known as the *ratio decidendi* (reasons for the decision). Other parts of a judge's speech which are not considered to be part of the *ratio decidendi* are known as *obiter dicta* (things said by the way). Only the *ratio decidendi* is directly binding on lower courts, but the *obiter dicta* may influence the decision of judges in later court cases. It may be possible for judges to 'distinguish' previous cases and not follow them on the grounds that the facts of the case in issue are significantly different. For example before the Occupier's Liability Act 1984 was passed which defined the liability of the occupier towards various types of trespasser, the liability was based on decisions made by judges on particular facts. Cases which involved harm to children where the occupier had been held liable were held not to be binding on judges hearing cases involving adults, so that the occupier was held not to be liable to an adult trespasser. The earlier cases relating to children were 'distinguished'.

Judges are however bound by statute and if case law results in an unsatisfactory situation, then this may be remedied by new amending legislation. Nevertheless statutes have to be interpreted by judges in court cases if disputes arise in relation to what the statute means. Thus law develops through a mix of statutory promulgation and common law decision making. The Human Rights Act 1998 (see below) takes precedence over other legislation, since a judge can refer back to Parliament for reconsideration statutes which appear to infringe the articles set out in the European Convention on Human Rights.

Procedure for judicial review

The decisions of judicial and administrative bodies can be challenged by an application to the Queen's Bench Division for the decision or adjudication to be reviewed. Thus if a person detained under the Mental Health Act 1983 were to appeal unsuccessfully to a Mental Health Review Tribunal (MHRT) and considered that the decision not to discharge him was based upon a failure to apply the correct law or because the principles of natural justice were infringed (e.g. the chairman was prejudiced against him personally), he could apply to the High Court, Queen's Bench Division for the decision of the MHRT to be reviewed[1]. However this procedure is not recommended where an Act of Parliament lays down a procedure for challenging the decision of a statutory body. For example in *Gossington* v. *Ealing Borough Council*[2], Mr Gossington applied for judicial review of the decision of London Borough of Ealing to provide him with five hours of home help per week instead of the original ten hours. The judge held that, since the Act provided for an application to the Secretary of State if a local authority fails to carry out its statutory functions, the applicant had not exhausted the other available routes open to him to remedy the wrong he felt he had suffered, and therefore the application for judicial review was refused.

The Human Rights Act 1998

The European Convention for the Protection of Human Rights and Fundamental Freedoms (1950) provides protection for the fundamental rights and freedoms of all people[3]. The UK is a signatory as are many European Countries which are not members of the European Community. Thus Norway is a signatory to the European Convention on Human Rights but not a member of the European Community. The Convention is enforced through the European Court of Human Rights which sits in Strasbourg. However following the passing of the Human Rights Act 1998 most of the articles are directly enforceable in the UK courts in relation to public authorities. This is considered further in Chapter 3.

Other international charters relating to health

The UK is also a signatory to, or has recognised, many other International Charters concerning rights in a variety of fields. These include the UN Convention on the Rights of the Child, the UN Convention on the Elimination of All Forms of Discrimination against Women, the Universal Declaration of Human Rights. There is also the Declaration of Helsinki developed by the World Health Organisation in 1964 and recently amended in 2000. This relates to research practice (see Chapter 27). These Charters are not directly enforceable in this country, though some of their principles may be contained in statutory or common law, and reflected in guidance provided by the Department of Health and professional bodies and organisations.

Civil and criminal law

The civil law covers the law which governs disputes between citizens (including corporate bodies) or between citizens and the state. Thus contract law and the law of torts (civil wrongs excluding breach of contract), rights over property, marital disputes and wrongful exercise of power by a statutory authority all come under the civil law.

Criminal law relates to proceedings in which an accused is prosecuted by the state (or rarely by a private individual) rather than sued by the victim. The sources of criminal law are varied: thus the definition of murder derives from a decision of the courts in the seventeenth century whereas theft is defined by an Act of Parliament of 1967 as amended by subsequent legislation.

Standard of proof

A prosecution is brought in relation to a charge of a criminal offence and heard in the criminal courts where the standard of proof is beyond reasonable doubt.

An action is brought in the civil courts in relation to an alleged civil wrong by a claimant who sues a defendant. The claimant has only to satisfy the lesser burden of proving his case on 'the balance of probabilities'.

Overlap

There is an overlap between civil and criminal wrongs. Touching a person without his consent may be a civil wrong – trespass to the person. It may also be a crime, i.e. a criminal assault or battery. Similarly driving a car carelessly may lead to criminal proceedings for driving without due care and attention and also lead to civil proceedings for negligence if there was an accident and it can be established that the driver was in breach of a duty of care owed a person injured as a result. In one case where a patient alleged that an unregistered physiotherapist had raped and indecently assaulted her, the police decided not to prosecute. However the patient brought a civil action for assault and obtained compensation of over £25 000, including an amount representing aggravated damages because the defendant put her through a harrowing ordeal by having to appear in court[4].

Criminal negligence

Gross negligence in professional practice causing death may amount to the crime of manslaughter. For example an anaesthetist who failed to realise that during an operation a tube had become disconnected (as a result of which the patient died) was prosecuted in the criminal courts and convicted of manslaughter[5]. The Law Commission[6] has recommended that the law should be changed to enable it to be made easier for corporations and statutory bodies to be prosecuted for manslaughter and this may lead to more charges being brought in connection with deaths which arise from gross negligence.

Types of civil action

Figure 2.2 illustrates some of the kinds of civil action which may be brought. In this book we are principally concerned with the law relating to negligence, breach of statutory duty and trespass to the person, but the practitioner should also be aware of the civil law relating to defamation and nuisance.

Figure 2.2   **Civil actions.**

- Negligence
- Breach of statutory duty
- Defamation
- Nuisance

- Trespass (to the person, goods or land)
- Breach of contract

Public and private law

Another distinction in the classification of laws is that of public and private law. Public law relates to a matter which is a subject of public concern such as protection of children, public nuisance, the carrying out of statutory duties. Private law relates to matters arising between individuals and/or organisations, such as purchasing a house, claiming damages for personal injury or suing for breach of contract. Public law deals with those areas of law where society intervenes in the actions of individuals. In contrast private law is concerned with the behaviour of individuals or corporate bodies to each other.

The Children Act 1989 covers both private law and public law relating to children: care proceedings, protection orders, child assessment orders are part of the public law while orders in relation to children made following divorce or nullity (such as with whom the child is to live) are part of the private law. Thus the *Cleveland Report* was concerned with the public law, the duty of Social Services Departments to take action to protect children. In contrast a dispute over whether or not consent has been given for a child to have treatment would be part of private law.

Legal personnel

If a patient believes that he has a claim for compensation because of the actions or omissions of health professionals, after possibly seeking advice from a Citizen's Advice Bureau, he would ask a solicitor to take his case. A solicitor is a professionally qualified person (usually a law degree followed by completion of the Law Society's professional examinations and completion of a set time in supervised practice) who tends to have direct contact with the client. The solicitor may seek the opinion of a barrister (known as counsel) on liability and the amount of compensation. A barrister will usually have a law degree and must complete the examinations set by the Council for Legal Education. The barrister must be a member of an Inn of Court and complete a term of apprenticeship known as pupillage.

Traditionally the barrister has had the role of conducting the case in court and preparing the documents which are exchanged between the parties in the run up to the court hearing (known as the pleadings). However, recent changes enable either of the professions to represent clients in court, subject only to their having the requisite training. Many would see the final result of this development as being a single legal profession. It was announced in June 2000 that the Inns of Court, the governing body for barristers, were to allow solicitors on to its Board.

New Civil Procedure Rules (the Woolf Reforms)

Failures in the old system of civil procedure were notorious and in the early 1990s Lord Woolf was invited to examine the deficiencies and make recommendations for reform. In June 1995 he issued an interim report *Access to Justice*[7], which noted the many hindrances to justice facing litigants. This reported on recommendations to change our system of civil litigation including obtaining compensation for personal injuries. It was followed in January 1996 by a consultation document[8] with papers covering the following issues:

- Fast track
- Housing
- Multi-party actions
- Medical negligent
- Expert evidence
- Costs.

The consultation paper on medical negligence cases considered that there could be considerable benefits from the proposed reforms[9].

Lord Woolf's specific proposals on medical negligence included:

- Training health professionals in negligence claims
- The GMC and other regulatory bodies to consider the need to clarify their professional conduct responsibilities in relation to negligence actions
- Improvement of record systems to trace former staff
- The use of alternative dispute mechanisms
- A separate medical negligence list for the High Court and county courts;
- Specially designated court centres outside London for handling medical negligence cases
- Reducing delays by improving arrangements for case listing
- Investigation of improved training for judges in medical negligence
- Standard tables to be used where possible to determine quantum
- Practice guide on the new case management
- A pilot study to consider medical negligence claims below £10 000.

The Final Report was published in July 1996[10] and led to the implementation of a new procedure for civil claims in April 1999. The general rules form the core of a single, simpler procedural code which applies to civil litigation in both the High Court and county courts.

Features of the scheme include:

- A system of case management with the courts rather than the parties taking the main responsibility for the progress of cases.

- Defended cases being allocated for the purposes of case management by the courts to one of three tracks:
  - ○ *Small claims* (up to £5000). This provides a procedure for straightforward claims which do not exceed £5000 in value, without the need for substantial pre-hearing preparation and the formalities of a traditional trial, and where costs are kept low.
  - ○ A *fast track* with limited procedures and reduced costs (up to £10 000). Factors deciding whether a case is allocated to the fast track include the limits likely to be placed on disclosure, the extent to which expert evidence may be necessary and whether the trial will last longer than a day.
  - ○ A *multi-track* (for more complex cases over £10 000), and recommended exceptions to the fast track such as medical negligence cases, even when the value is less than £10 000.

The court allocates each case to one of these three tracks on the basis of information provided by the claimant on the statement of case. If it does not have enough information to allocate the claim then it will make an order requiring one or more parties to provide further information on an Allocation Questionnaire within 14 days.

Case management (see below) directions are given at the allocation stage or at the listing stage. (The procedures relating to expert witnesses are discussed in Chapter 18.)

Mediation

One of the results of the Woolf Reforms in civil justice is that the parties are encouraged to resolve the dispute before going to court using mediation or other forms of 'Alternative Dispute Resolution'. Often such processes can be built in to the complaints procedure (see Chapter 19) to avoid litigation. In mediation an independent mediator attempts to assist the parties to bring about an agreement to resolve the dispute but unlike arbitration, the parties are under no compulsion to accept any ruling by that independent person. The Annual Report for 2000 of the NHS Litigation Authority points out the low uptake of mediation:

> 'Virtually everyone engaged in civil litigation pays lip service to the benefits of mediation, but in practice it is proving extremely difficult to persuade the parties to put their words into practice.'

Case management

The overriding principle enshrined in the new Civil Procedure Rules[11] (see Figure 2.3) is that all cases should be dealt with justly. The parties have a duty to help the court to further this overriding objective and the court must seek to give effect to this overriding principle when it exercises any powers under the Rules and when it interprets any rule. The court in furthering this principle of dealing justly must actively manage the cases before it. Active management includes:

Figure 2.3   **Overriding objective of the CPR.**

(1)   These Rules are a new procedural code with the overriding objective of enabling the court to deal with cases justly.

(2)   Dealing with a case justly includes, so far as is practicable –
    (a)   ensuring that the parties are on an equal footing;
    (b)   saving expense;
    (c)   dealing with the case in ways which are proportionate –
        (i)   to the amount of money involved;
        (ii)   to the importance of the case;
        (iii)   to the complexity of the issues; and
        (iv)   to the financial position of each party;
    (d)   ensuring that it is dealt with expeditiously and fairly; and
    (e)   allotting to it an appropriate share of the court's resources, while taking into account the need to allot resources to other cases. (CPR 1.1)

- Encouraging the parties to co-operate with each other in the conduct of the proceedings.
- Identifying the issues at an early stage.
- Deciding promptly which issues need full investigation at trial and accordingly disposing summarily of the others.
- Deciding the order in which the issues are to be resolved.
- Encouraging the parties to use Alternative Dispute Resolution procedures if it is considered appropriate and facilitating the use of any such procedure.
- Helping the parties to settle the whole or part of the case.
- Fixing timetables or otherwise controlling the progress of the case.
- Considering whether the likely benefits of taking a particular step justify the cost of taking it (proportionality).
- Dealing with as many aspects of the case as it can on the same occasion.
- Dealing with the case without the parties needing to attend court.
- Making use of technology.
- Giving directions to ensure that the trial of a case proceeds quickly and efficiently.

Clinical negligence pre-action protocol

As a consequence of the Woolf Reforms and the work of the Clinical Disputes Forum (a multi-disciplinary group formed in 1997 as a result of the Woolf recommendations) a clinical negligence pre-action protocol was drawn up which is now part of the Practice Directions and so part of the Civil Procedure Rules. This protocol requires parties to follow specific steps at the beginning of an action and they are penalised if they fail. Times are set for the response to requests for records etc.

Course of an action

Claim form is issued

This marks the beginning of the case. There are important time limits (see Chapter 14) within which the claim form (originally known as a writ) has to be issued. The claim form indicates that legal action is now being commenced. In medical negligence cases the claim form usually names the NHS trust as the defendant, but it is possible for an individual employee to be named as a party and more than one defendant can be named.

Service of the claim form

This must be sent to the defendant within four months of its issue. (The regulations on how service is to be effected have been relaxed. The papers can be sent by post or fax as well as being delivered personally or through solicitors.) The defendant must then respond by filing a defence or an admission on the acknowledgement of service form. If the defendant fails to respond then the claimant may be able to obtain judgment in default.

The drafting of the documents or statements of case (once known as pleadings) is arranged by the respective parties' solicitors who often instruct counsel (i.e. barristers). A litigant may, however, represent himself personally. Strict time limits are laid down for the service and response to documents. Under the Woolf reforms the documents exchanged between the parties should be simpler and have to be verified by the party who signs a 'statement of truth'. If there are uncertainties, the court can require these to be clarified.

Pre-trial review

There may be an assessment of the situation by the parties, together with a district judge or judge, to take account of the number of witnesses to attend and matters such as the exchange of any experts' medical reports. However, in the small claims and fast tracks automatic directions apply and even in more complex cases it is possible to agree such matters without the need to attend court for discussion. If the parties cannot agree the court will of its own power impose an order taking into account the overriding objective of the CPR (see Figure 2.3). Generally, the judge ensures that a strict timetable is adhered to and can himself make orders for a speedy but fair disposition of the issues without waiting for one or other of the parties to apply for what is required. Finally, the case will be set down for hearing.

Hearing

If a civil case proceeds to a hearing the stages set out in Figure 2.4 will take place.

If no appeal is lodged, and the claimant has won, judgment will be enforced against the defendant.

Payment into court/Part 36 offers

Rules about offers to settle and payments into court are set out in Parts 36 and 37 of the Civil Procedure Rules. In some cases where there is dispute over the amount of compensation but liability is accepted, the defendant will probably be advised to pay a sum in settlement of the case in to court. If the claimant

Figure 2.4 **A hearing in the civil courts.**

- Opening speeches
- Case for the claimant:
  - examination in chief
  - cross examination
  - re-examination
- Case for the defendant:
  - examination in chief
  - cross examination
  - re-examination
- Closing summaries
- Decision by judge

accepts this payment in then the court will be notified that there has been a settlement of the case and the defendant will be liable for the claimant's costs up to that point. A payment in may also be made where the defendant does not accept liability but he is not confident of winning the case and, rather than risk losing and having to pay the costs of both sides, he offers a sum in full and final settlement.

If the claimant decides that the payment in is not acceptable, the case will continue. In these circumstances the judge is not told that there has been a payment in. He will not therefore be influenced by that in determining the case and deciding what compensation to award. If he decides there is no liability by the defendant or even if he agrees with the claimant on the issue of liability but awards less than the payment in, then the claimant will have to pay both the defendant's costs from the time of the payment in as well as his own, since, of course, had the claimant accepted that sum at the outset (deemed reasonable in comparision with the judge's award) there would have been no time-consuming and costly court hearing. These costs may well exceed the amount of the award. The judge has a discretion over whether to award the defendant costs in these circumstances, but the claimant is at risk as to costs from the moment his time (21 days) expires for acceptance of the payment in.

For the first time under Part 36 of the CPR the claimant can give a formal indication of a figure he would be prepared to accept should the defendant make an offer.'

Conditional fees

Legal aid is being phased out from personal injury litigation. The Government has approved the system of conditional fees being introduced into this country. The plaintiff is able to negotiate, with a solicitor, payment on a 'no win – no fee' basis, i.e. if the claimant loses his solicitor does not charge any fees. Costs of the successful defendant would still be owing, and insurance protection is taken out to meet these and other costs not covered by the agreement with the solicitor. Recent statutory changes enable a successful party to claim the enhanced fees agreed with lawyers under the conditional fee agreement from the unsuccessful party. The impact of these charges on cases involving claims against NHS organisations is not yet clear.

Procedure in criminal courts

The magistrates are either lay people known as justices of the peace (JPs) tending to sit in threes ('the bench') or legally qualified persons known as stipendiary magistrates, who sit alone. Summary offences are heard in the magistrates court and indictable offences (the more serious offences) in the crown court, before a judge and jury. Many offences are triable either way and the accused can opt for trial by jury if he wishes.

In the magistrates court, the magistrates decide if, on the facts, guilt has been established and, if so, sentence the accused. Their powers of sentencing are limited but they have the power to remit an accused to the crown court for heavier sentencing by the crown court judge. In the crown court the jury (a panel of twelve members of the public) decide if the accused is guilty and, if so, the judge sentences the person so convicted. The magistrates have a gate-keeping role in relation to the more serious offences and oversee committal proceedings where they decide whether there is a case to answer and, if so, 'commit' it to the crown court for the trial to take place.

In criminal cases, the Crown Prosecution Service has the responsibility for preparing the case, including statements, witnesses etc.

Figure 2.5 shows the principal differences between a civil case and a criminal case.

Figure 2.5   Differences between civil and criminal hearings.

	Criminal hearings	**Civil hearings**
basis of action	a charge of a criminal offence	an alleged wrong by one person against another
action brought by	Crown Prosecution Service (CPS) – occasionally a private prosecution	the person wronged (the Claimant) or if a child, a person on his/her behalf
standard of proof	beyond reasonable doubt	balance of probabilities
facts decided by	Magistrates Courts – the magistrate(s) Crown Court – the jury	the judge
law applied by	Magistrates Courts – the magistrate(s) (lay magistrates advised by legally qualified clerk) Crown Court – the judge	the judge(s)

Accusatorial system

A feature of the legal system in this country is that it consists of one side with the responsibility of proving that the other side is at fault, guilty, or liable, of the wrong or crime alleged. This is known as an accusatorial or adversarial system and it applies to both civil and criminal proceedings. In criminal cases the prosecution attempts to show beyond all reasonable doubt that the accused is guilty of the offence with which he is charged. The magistrates, or the jury in the crown court, decide whether the prosecution has succeeded in this, the accused being presumed innocent until proved guilty. In civil proceedings the person bringing the action (known as the claimant or, formerly, plaintiff) has to establish on a balance of probability that there was negligence, trespass, nuisance or whatever civil wrong is alleged. The role of the judge or magistrate is to chair the proceedings, intervening where necessary in the interests of justice, and advising on points of law and procedure. In civil cases (apart from defamation) there is no jury and the judge also has the responsibility of determining whether the claimant has succeeded in establishing the civil wrong and deciding the amount of compensation.

The accusatorial system contrasts with a system of law which is known as 'inquisitorial' where the judge plays a far more active role in determining the outcome. An example of an inquisitorial system in this country is the coroner's court. Here the coroner is responsible for deciding which witnesses are needed to answer the questions placed before him by statute (i.e. the identity of the deceased and how, when and where he came to die) and it is he who examines the witnesses in court and decides who else can ask questions and what they can ask. As a result of this 'inquisition' he, or a jury if one is used, determine the cause of death.

As a result of the proposals put forward by Lord Woolf, a case management approach to civil claims has been introduced. This is in order to speed their progress and reduce the costs. The adversarial system is kept but judges are encouraged to take a more interventionist role and in certain cases it is envisaged that expert witnesses would be agreed by the parties or appointed by the court. These proposals are considered above and in Chapter 18 (expert witnesses).

Law and ethics

Law is both wider and narrower than the field of ethics. On the one hand, the law covers areas of practice which may not be considered to give rise to any ethical issue, other than the one as to whether or not the law should be obeyed. For example, to park in a no-parking area would not appear to raise any ethical issues other than deciding to obey or ignore the law. On the other hand there are major areas of health care which raise significant ethical questions where there appears to be little law. For example elective ventilation of a corpse in order to keep the organs alive for transplant purposes, raises considerable ethical issues for health professionals and relatives but, provided the requirements of the Human Tissue Act and the Transplant Act are satisfied, and there is no breach of Human Rights as set out in the European Convention on Human Rights, there is no legal issue. At any time, of course, a practice which is considered to be contrary to ethical principles can be challenged in court and the judge will determine the legal position on the basis of any existing statute law or decided cases.

Situations may arise where a health professional considers the law to be wrong and contrary to her own ethical principles. In certain cases the law itself provides for conscientious objection. Thus no one can be compelled to participate in a termination of pregnancy unless it is an emergency situation to save the life of the mother (Abortion Act 1967 (see Chapter 9)). Similar provisions apply to activities in relation to human fertilisation and embryology where the

Human Fertilisation and Embryology Act 1990 provides a statutory protection clause.

The Law Commission in its report on Mental Incapacity[12] drafted legislation to cover advance refusals of treatment but considered it would be inappropriate to have a conscientious objection clause for a health professional to ignore the existence of the previously declared wishes of the patient. A health professional may have strong ethical views about the need to save the life of a mentally competent adult who is refusing a life saving blood transfusion, but the law does not permit the refusal to be overruled, provided that it was expressed when the adult was mentally competent. In such a case she has to decide personally what action to take, in full awareness that she could face the effects of the criminal law, civil action, disciplinary procedure by her employer and professional proceedings by the registration body.

It is inevitable that any discussion of the function of the work of health professionals would be concerned with the ethical or philosophical beliefs of the therapist who is providing the treatment and it is essential that the practitioner understands the extent to which the law is in harmony with her ethical beliefs and values.

Ethics in training

An understanding of the rights of the patient requires not just consideration of the legal rights which are considered in Chapter 3 and throughout this book, but also consideration of the ethical dimensions. It is increasingly accepted that courses for continuing professional development requires an ethical content. How ethical issues could be included in the curricula is described by Alison Pettigrew[13]. She emphasises the importance, not of creating more additional modules, but of ensuring that the ethical issues are integrated with the core knowledge.

'Underpinning this more integrated approach is the need to define "ethics" and then to provide undergraduate and postgraduate students with the tools for ethical reasoning and problem solving, to ensure that they are able to manage a dynamic curriculum.'

Rules of professional conduct

Professional Associations such as the Society of Radiographers and the Royal College of Radiologists have issued Rules governing professional practice. These are not in themselves directly enforceable in a court of law, but could be used as evidence in civil or criminal proceedings that their reasonable professional standards of practice have not been followed. An allegation of a breach of the Rules could also be used as a basis for professional conduct proceedings, for which the ultimate sanction is removal from the Register. This is discussed in Chapter 12.

Other guidance

Many other organisations and public bodies issue guidance for professional conduct and procedures for the provision of health care. The National Health Service Executive and Department of Health issue circulars and executive letters providing advice for health and social services organisations and staff. These do not have the direct force of law, but the Department of Health would expect them to be followed. Thus on 11 July 1997 the High Court ruled against North Derbyshire Health Authority which had refused to fund the purchase of beta-interferon in the treatment of multiple sclerosis[14]. The judge found that the health authority had knowingly failed to apply national guidance in a NHS circular. It cannot be assumed however that the guidance is always correct in law, and in one case[15] the court held that ministerial guidance was incorrect.

Directions issued by the Secretary of State under statutory powers, e.g. under the National Health Service and Community Care Act 1990, are directly enforceable against health authorities through the default mechanisms provided for in the legislation.

Conclusions

The variety of sources of law and perplexity as to what a law is can be very confusing, but it is helpful for professionals, if they are confronted with a statement that 'the law says ...', to seek an explanation as to whether the basis for the assertion is a statute or the decision of a court, or derived from a Charter or Professional Code of Practice (which usually do not have the force of law) or, as may often be the case, is totally incorrect because there is no such law.

 ## Questions and exercises

1 A patient has consulted you about the possibility of bringing a claim for compensation. What advice would you give her on the procedure which would be followed and the steps which she should take?
2 Draw up a diagram which illustrates the difference between civil and criminal procedure.
3 Turn to the glossary and study the definitions of legal terms included there.
4 In what ways do you consider that a conflict between an ethical belief and the law should be resolved?

References

1 *R* v. *Hallstrom, ex parte W, R* v. *Gardener, ex parte L* [1986] 2 All ER 306
2 *Gossington* v. *Ealing Borough Council* (CA) 18 November 1985, Lexis transcript
3 See briefing note prepared by the Children's Legal Centre, 20 Compton Terrace, London. N1 2UN
4 *Miles* v. *Cain* 25 November 1988, Lexis transcript
5 *R* v. *Adomako* (HL) The Times Law Report, 4 July 1994, [1994] 3 All ER 79
6 Law Commission Report on Criminal prosecutions (March 1996) HMSO, London
7 Lord Woolf (June 1995) *Interim Report: Access to Justice.* HMSO, London

8 Lord Woolf (January 1996) *Access to Civil Justice Inquiry: Consultation Papers.* HMSO, London

9 Lord Woolf (July 1996) *Final Report: Access to Justice* (Paragraph 13: Medical negligence in the new system). HMSO, London

10 Lord Woolf (July 1996) *Final Report: Access to Justice* HMSO, London

11 I. Grainger & M. Fealy (1999) *Introduction to the new Civil Procedure Rules* Cavendish, London

12 Law Commission (1995) Report No 231 *Mental Incapacity* HMSO, London

13 A. Pettigrew (2000) Ethical Issues in Medical Imaging: Implications for the Curricula. *Radiographer*, **6**, 293–8 (No. 3, Nov. 2000)

14 M. Horsnell (1997) Refusal to give MS victim new drug was illegal. *The Times* 12 July; *R* v *North Derbyshire Health Authority* [1997] 8 Med LR 327

15 *R* v. *Wandsworth Borough Council, ex parte Beckwith* [1996] 1 All ER 129

Section B
Patient-centred Care

Chapter 3
Rights of the Patient

Introduction

This chapter aims to identify the rights of the patient and place them in the context of the work of the radiographer, radiologist and oncologist. The word 'right' is used in the sense of a legal right, i.e. one which can be the basis of an action in a court of law to compel a specific person (or organisation) who appears to be denying or refusing recognition of that right, to recognise its existence. There are, of course, ethical rights which would be recognised by many patients and health professionals but if they do not have a basis in law then they are not covered in this chapter. The list of recommended further reading includes books which consider ethical issues in health care.

Other rights of the patient which are considered later in the book include:

- the right to give or withhold consent and to receive information (Chapter 4)
- the right to confidentiality (Chapter 5)
- the right to access health information (Chapter 6)
- the right to complain (Chapter 19)
- the right to a reasonable standard of care as enforced through the laws of negligence (Chapter 14).

The practitioner's right of conscientious objection is considered in Chapter 9.

The Human Rights Act 1998

This long awaited Act came into force in England and Wales on 2 October 2000 (earlier in Scotland on devolution) and enables citizens in this country to bring an action in the courts to enforce their rights set out in the European Convention on Human Rights. Previously, those who felt that rights set out in the convention had been breached had to take a case to the European Court of Human Rights in Strasbourg, which could take several years with considerable cost. The Human Rights Act also requires judges to refer any legislation back to Parliament if they consider that it is in conflict with the rights set out in the Convention.

Who can be sued?

The Human Rights Act permits an action to be brought by a person who claims that a public authority has acted (or proposes to act) in a way which is incompatible with a Convention right. The definition of public authority includes a court or tribunal or any 'person certain', i.e. an organisation, with functions of a public nature. Public authorities include NHS trusts and hospitals case and law will develop on how organisations with functions of a public nature are defined. It is highly likely, for example, that this definition will include bodies (private or charitable) which care for persons in residential care or nursing homes paid for by statutory authorities. In addition private hospitals may be covered even though the costs are met through insurance or by patients personally.

The Convention

The Convention is set out in Schedule 2 of the Human Rights Act 1998 and can be found on various websites. Probably the most significant rights in terms of health care will be Articles 2, 3, 5, 6 and 8. These will be considered below.

Article 2

Everyone's right to life shall be protected by law. No one shall be deprived of his life intentionally save in the execution of a sentence of a court following his conviction of a crime for which this penalty is provided by law.

Recent decisions of the courts show how this right is being strictly interpreted. For example in a recent case[1], parents lost their attempt to ensure that a severely handicapped baby, born prematurely, was to be resuscitated if necessary. The judge ruled that the hospital should provide him with palliative care to ease his suffering, but should not try to revive him as that would cause unnecessary pain. (The case is considered in Chapter 10.)

In another case, the President of the Family Division, Dame Elizabeth Butler-Sloss, held that the withdrawal of life sustaining medical treatment where the patient was in a persistent vegetative state was not contrary to Article 2 of the Human Rights Convention and the right to life. The ruling was made on 25 October 2000 in cases involving Mrs M, aged 49 years who suffered brain damage during an operation abroad in 1997 and was diagnosed as being in a persistent vegetative state (PVS) in October 1998, and Mrs H, 36, who fell ill in America as a result of pancreatitis at Christmas 1999[2].

Article 2 was also invoked in the much publicised case involving the separation of Siamese twins[3], in which the Court of Appeal decided that they could be separated even though this would undoubtedly lead to the death of the one who depended upon the heart and the lungs of the other. (The case is considered in Chapter 8.)

Nevertheless more cases are likely to be heard on the issue as to whether there has been an infringement of the Article 2 right to life. For example, it might be used if a person is marked down as NFR and the relatives disagree with the clinicians. In addition, the Article could potentially be relied upon where a patient alleges that failure to provide health services is infringing her right to life. The courts have exhibited a cautious approach so far but each such case will be decided on its own facts and merits.

Article 3

No one shall be subjected to torture or to inhuman or degrading treatment or punishment.

Whilst it is hoped that torture does not take place in health-care, there are evident examples of degrading and inhuman treatment. The patient who is left on a stretcher outside the accident and emergency department whilst waiting for a bed could be said to be the victim of inhuman or degrading treatment and perhaps some of the treatments and investigations carried out in X-ray or Radiotherapy Departments are not always sensitive to the need to treat patients with dignity and mitigate their discomfort and distress. An instance of a pregnant prisoner being handcuffed to the bed during her labour would appear to be a *prima facie* breach of this right.

It remains to be seen the extent to which there are allegations of breach of this Article. A case heard by the European Court of Human Rights has ruled that severe corporal punishment by parents to discipline their children was a breach of Article 3[4]. A step father had beaten on several occasions a nine year old boy with a garden cane, had been prosecuted for assault occasioning actual bodily harm, but had been acquitted by the jury who had accepted his defence that the caning had been necessary and reasonable to discipline the boy. In a civil claim against the UK government the European Court of Human Rights held that ill-treatment must attain a minimum level of severity if it is to fall within the scope of Article 3 and this depended on all the circumstances of the case, such as the nature and context of the treatment, its duration, its physical and mental effects and in some instances, the sex, age, and state of health of the victim. In finding that in this instance there had been a breach of Article 3 it awarded the boy £10 000 against the UK government and costs. The UK government acknowledged that the UK law failed to provide adequate protection to children and should be amended. Subsequently guidance was issued by the Government on the use of corporal punishment against children.

However the House of Lords has held that illegal action to alleviate pain and suffering is not sanctioned by the Act. Diane Pretty could not obtain advance immunity from prosecution for her husband if he were to help her commit suicide as an escape from her pain (see Chapter 10).

Article 5

Everyone has the right to liberty and security of person. No-one shall be deprived of his liberty save in the following cases and in accordance with a procedure prescribed by law.

Many exceptions are then given including: 'the lawful detention of persons for the prevention of the spreading of infectious diseases, or persons of unsound mind, alcoholics or drug addicts or vagrants.'.

The House of Lords had decided in the Bournewood case[5] that a person who lacked the mental capacity to consent to admission to psychiatric hospital could be detained there in his best interests without necessarily being detained under the provisions of the Mental Health Act 1983. Although such detention is justified under common law (i.e. judge-made law), statutory provision to ensure that such *de facto* detentions are not contrary to Article 5 is now essential. Nevertheless the Court of Appeal has held that in the absence of statutory provision for mentally incapacitated adults, the court does have an inherent power to hear issues involved in the day to day care of such persons and to grant declarations in the best interests of mentally incapable persons[6]. (See Chapter 7 for the care of the mentally incapacitated and Chapter 4 for the common law power to act out of necessity.)

Article 6

Everyone has the right to a fair trial.

This right will have significant implications since it applies not just to criminal charges but also to the determination of civil rights and obligations. It would therefore apply to disciplinary actions and other such forums where at present employees may not have representation and so could be in a very weak situation compared with the employer. The new professional conduct and registration machinery for health professions has been drafted with the rights set out in this Article in mind (see Chapters 11 and 12).

Article 8

Everyone has the right to respect for private and family life, his home and his correspondence.

There shall be no interference by a public authority with the exercise of the right except such as is in accordance with the law and is necessary in a democratic society in the interests of national security, public safety or the economic well-being of the country, for the prevention of disorder or crime, for the protection of health or morals, or for the protection of the rights and freedoms of others.

This right will require greater sensitivity about patient privacy than has been shown in the past within healthcare. It may be necessary to review the traditional ward round, where a curtain is seen as a sound proof barrier and all those on the ward can hear the intimate details of a patient's diagnosis, prognosis and treatment. Other steps may also have to be taken in order to ensure that this right of the patient is recognised and protected. The Caldicott Guardians, whose role is considered in Chapter 5, could take on the responsibility for ensuring that there is no breach of Article 8.

Article 8 will have to be interpreted in relation to Article 10 which recognises a right to freedom of expression. Both Articles 8 and 10 are qualified by specified circumstances in which the right is limited, and the courts will balance the one against the other in determining whether there has been a breach of either. Total privacy for the individual and total freedom of expression in the public interest are mutually exclusive and in all such cases there will be a balance to be struck.

Other significant articles

Whilst these Articles have been looked at in some detail there are others which have considerable significance for healthcare. Article 14, for example, prohibits discrimination in the application of the articles of the European Convention. Article 2 of the First Protocol recognises a right to education which may be significant for staff who are caring for children with long-term illnesses. Parents also have the right to ensure that such education and teaching is in conformity with their own religious and philosophical convictions.

Defences

Many articles have their own specific defences as can be seen from the text of the Act. Some rights are absolute, others qualified. With absolute rights (such as Article 3) there can be no interference. Where rights are qualified (such as Article 8) interference is permitted provided that it is justified. Where there is an apparent conflict the Courts will have to balance the rights of the individual with the broader interests of society as a whole in order to determine the level of justification. Following the Woolf reforms the courts also have to apply the concept of proportionality in interpreting the application of those articles which are absolute, and a major action for a minor breach of even an absolute right is a waste of precious court resources and time – a matter that could be reflected in any order on costs.

Rights of staff

It should not be forgotten that the Human Rights Act 1998 applies not only to patients but also to staff. When they are employed by a public authority or an organisation exercising public functions, then staff are entitled to have their rights set out in Schedule 1 to the Act respected. Article 6 and the right to a fair hearing is particularly relevant as is Article 14 which prohibits discrimination and is considered in Chapter 22 on employment. In addition of course, staff can use other statutes and the rights recognised in civil and criminal laws to protect themselves. For example in Chapter 15 the risks to staff of violence, bullying and harassment are considered. The extent to which staff are entitled to regard patients as having responsibilities for themselves and towards health professionals is considered in the author's book, which though written for nurses would apply to all health professions[7].

Action

There are considerable advantages in each Department in an NHS trust or hospital carrying out an audit to ascertain the extent to which it is human rights compliant. Changes may be required, but these could simply be of a procedural kind rather than ones which require expenditure or building work.

Charters and conventions

There are, in addition to the European Convention on Human Rights, many other international, national, professional and other Charters, Declarations and Statements of Rights of varying legal weight. The United Nations Convention on the Rights of the Child has been adopted by this Country but unlike the European Convention on Human Rights has not yet been brought into the legislative framework. Unlike the European Convention on Human Rights with its court in Strasbourg, there is no judicial machinery to enforce the UN convention. The UN does however report to those national governments who signed the Convention on the extent to which they are fulfilling their obligations under it. The UK government has recommended to those who commission children's health services that they should take into account the UN Convention on the Rights of the Child[8]. Similar Charters include the Resolution of the European Parliament on a Charter for Children in Hospital (1986), the European Charter for Children in Hospital, the Charter of the National Association for the Welfare of Children in Hospital (now Action for Sick Children).

In general it can be said that, unless a Charter repeats the provisions of a statute or a precedent laid down by the courts, it is not enforceable in the UK courts. This is certainly true of the Citizen's Charter and the Patient's Charter which were published in the UK in the early 1990s. Although time limits within which a patient should be seen in out-patients and then attend for treatment were set in various Patient's Charters, failure to meet these targets could not be used as the basis of a legal action in court. There were other ways of taking action of course. A complaint can be made to the Trust about failure to meet the Patient's Charter criteria, or alternatively a complaint can be made to the commissioning Health Authority, which in its agreement with the Trust would require it to comply with these standards. However compensation for failure to achieve the standard would not be payable. In extreme circumstances, of course, failure could amount to inhuman and degrading treatment in which case action in the UK courts is now be available under the Human Rights Act 1998.

The European Community is at the present time developing its own Declaration on Human Rights to be observed by all member states.

The Declaration of Helsinki relates to research and is accepted by all health professional organisations as applying to healthcare research on patients and others. It has not been incorporated directly into the law of this country, but many of its provisions are already part of statutory regulation of research.

In general it could be said that charters may identify good practice and may lay down standards which eventually become recognised under the Bolam test as the reasonable standard of care (see Chapter 14). They also provide useful tools for audit and monitoring. The work of the National Institute of Clinical Excellence (NICE) and the Commission for Health Improvement (CHI) may also find charters useful in their work in ensuring that health-care achieves reasonable standards of performance. (See Chapter 21 for further discussion of these organisations.)

The right to obtain NHS services

The Secretary of State has a statutory duty under NHS legislation to provide a comprehensive National Health Service to meet all reasonable requirements. This covers both prevention and treatment and specifically requires a number of services to be provided. The details of the legislation are set out in Chapter 21. These duties have been considered by the courts in a number of different cases and the general consensus is that the statute does not give an absolute right to obtain services, and that, provided there is no obvious evidence of irrational or unreasonable setting of priorities, the courts will not be involved in the determination of the allocation of resources. Thus in the inevitable situation where resources are finite and demand outmatches supply providers and commissioners of services have to weigh priorities.

Examples of when individual patients have sought to enforce the statutory duty to provide services and the courts have refused to intervene include the following cases.

- In 1979 patients brought an action for breach of statutory duty against the Secretary of State for Health and the Regional and Area Health Authorities concerned on the grounds that they had waited too long for hip operations but failed in their claim[9]. The court held it could only interfere if the Secretary of State acted so as to frustrate the policy of the Act or as no reasonable minister could have acted.
- In 1987 Mrs Walker failed to obtain a declaration that heart surgery should be carried out on her child[10]. The court held that it was not for the court to substitute its own judgment for that of those responsible for the allocation of resources. It would only interfere if there had been a failure to allocate funds in a way which was unreasonable or where there had been breaches of public duties. Mrs Walker's application was refused.
- In 1995 Jamie Bowen, a child suffering from leukaemia, was refused a course of chemotherapy and a second bone marrow transplant on the grounds that there was only a very small chance of the treatment succeeding and therefore it would not be in her best interests for the treatment to proceed. The Court of Appeal upheld the decision of the health authority[11], being unable to fault its reasoning process. The Master of the Rolls (Sir Thomas Bingham) stated that

  'while I have every sympathy with B, I feel bound to regard this as an attempt – wholly understandable, but nevertheless misguided – to involve the court in a field of activity where it is not fitted to make any decision favourable to the patient.'
  (An anonymous donor then came forward and paid for further treatment for the child but she died a year later.)

More recently however there have been several cases where the courts have upheld the right of an individual patient to access services, but always on the basis of a flaw in the health authority's reasoning or procedures, never on clinical judgment. The first was in relation to the failure of a health authority to permit a drug for multiple sclerosis to be prescribed in its catchment area[12]. The health authority decided that it would not enable beta-interferon to be prescribed for patients in its catchment area on the basis that it was not yet proved to be clinically effective for the treatment of multiple sclerosis. A sufferer from multiple sclerosis challenged this refusal and succeeded on the grounds that the health authority had failed to follow the guidance issued by the Department of Health[13]. A declaration was granted that the policy adopted by the health authority was unlawful and it was required to formulate and implement a policy which took full and proper account of national policy as stated in the circular.

In the second case a health authority refused to fund treatment for three transsexuals who wished to undergo gender reassignment[14]. This was on the grounds that such treatment had been assigned a low priority, being in the authority's list of procedures considered to be clinically ineffective in terms of health gain. Under this policy gender reassignment surgery was, amongst other procedures, listed as a procedure for which no treatment (apart from that provided by the authority's general psychiatric and psychology services) would be commissioned, save in the event of overriding clinical need or exceptional circumstances. The transsexuals sought judicial review of the health authority's refusal and the judge granted an order quashing the authority's decision and the policy on which it was based. The health authority then took the case to the Court of Appeal but lost its appeal. The Court of Appeal held as follows:

- Whilst the precise allocation and weighting of priorities is a matter for the judgment of the authority and not for the court, it is vital for an authority:
  - to asses accurately the nature and seriousness of each type of illness; and
  - to determine the effectiveness of various forms of treatment for it; and
  - to give proper effect to that assessment and that determination in the formulation and individual application of its policy.
- The authority's policy was flawed in two respects:
  - it did not treat transsexualism as an illness, but as an attitude of mind which did not warrant medical treatment; and
  - the ostensible provision that it made for exceptions in individual cases and its manner of considering them amounted to the operation of a 'blanket policy' against funding treatment for the condition because it did not believe in such treatment.
- The authority were not genuinely applying the policy to the individual exceptions.

Nevertheless:

- Article 3 and Article 8 of the European Convention on Human Rights (see above) did not give a right to free health care and did not apply to this situation where the challenge is to a health authority's allocation of finite funds.
- The patients were not victims of discrimination on the grounds of sex.

In spite of the decision of the Court of Appeal in this case that the Articles of the European Convention of Human Rights did not apply to the allocation of resources, there are undoubtedly likely to be cases in the future where claimants will seek to utilise the Human Rights Act 1998 if facilities and services have not been made available and, as a consequence, a person has been subjected to inhuman or degrading treatment. Such actions might be assisted where NICE, CHI and National Standards Frameworks publish guidance on what they consider to be minimal standards of care (see Chapter 21). Such guidance will have to take into account technological developments in medicine, including PACS and telemedicine (which are considered in Chapter 24). It may be that eventually reasonable standards of care will require the availability of tele-medicine across the country and that legal action could be brought if such equipment were not made available.

NHS Plan

The NHS Plan[15] was published in July 2000 and is a strategy prepared by the Department of Health for investment and reorganisation of the NHS over five years. In this additional powers for patients are envisaged. Chapter 10 proposes:

- Greater information being made available to patients (see Chapter 24 of this book)
- Greater patient choice
- Patient advocates and advisers in every hospital
- Redress over cancelled operations
- Patients' forums and citizens' panels in every area
- A new national panel to advise on major reorganisations of hospitals
- Stronger regulation of professional standards (see Chapters 11 and 12 of this book).

At the time of writing these initiatives have not been fully implemented. Clause 20 of the NHS Reform and Healthcare Bill 2002 abolishes Community Health Councils (see Chapter 19 of this book). The extent to which these initiatives reduce the increase and level of litigation and lead to higher standards within healthcare remains to be seen.

Conclusions

Patient care and an awareness of the rights of the patient are essential to the carrying out of any diagnostic or therapeutic procedures. *Patient Care* by Erica Koch Williams[16], whilst written for an American audience in a programmed learning style, explains many of the procedures which a practitioner might be required to carry out and provides useful checklists for many different activities. The Human Rights Act 1998 may be seen in future years as a watershed in the laws of this country and could become the focal point for ensuring that reasonable standards of care are maintained across all areas in health care.

 Questions and exercises _____

1 Do you consider that patients could ever have an absolute right to healthcare which is legally enforceable? What are the obstacles to such a legal right?
2 To what extent do you consider that your department is 'human rights compliant'?
3 Obtain a copy of any of the Charters relevant to healthcare and analyse the

clauses in order to decide which are already legally enforceable on the basis of existing statute or common law.

References

1   O. Wright & L. Peek (2000) Judge rules boy must be left to die. *The Times* 13 July; *A National Health Service Trust* v. *D*, The Times Law Report, 19 July 2000
2   F. Gibb (2000) Rights Act does not bar mercy killing. *The Times* 26 October, *NHS Trust A* v. *Mrs M* and *NHS Trust B* v. *Mrs H* [2001] Lloyds Rep Med 27
3   R Jenkins (2000) Coroner records rare verdict on Siamese twin. *The Times* 16 December
4   *A* v. *The United Kingdom* (100/1997/884/1096) judgment on 23 September 1998
5   *R* v. *Bournewood Community and Mental Health NHS Trust, ex parte L* [1998] 3 All ER 289
6   *Re F (Adult: Court's Jurisdiction)* (CA) (2000) 2 FLR 512
7   B. Dimond (1999) *Patients' Rights, Responsibilities and the Nurse*, 2nd edn. Quay Publishing Mark Allen Publishing
8   Department of Health (1995) *Child Health in the Community: A guide to Good Practice* HMSO, London
9   *R* v. *Secretary of State for Social Services, ex parte Hincks and others.* (1979) Solicitors' Journal **123**, 436
10 *R* v. *Central Birmingham Health Authority, ex parte Walker* (1987) 3 BMLR 32, *The Times*, 26 November 1987
11 *R* v. *Cambridge HA, ex parte B* [1995] 2 All ER 129
12 *R* v. *North Derbyshire Health Authority* [1997] 8 Med LR 327
13 Department of Health (1997) NHS Executive Letter: EL (95)97
14 *North West Lancashire Health Authority* v. *A, D & G* [1999] Lloyds Rep Med 399
15 Department of Health (2000) *NHS Plan: a plan for investment, a plan for reform* DoH London; also www.nhs.uk/nhsplan/contentspdf.htm
16 E.Koch Williams (1999) *Patient Care*, McGraw Hill, New York

Chapter 4
Consent and Information Giving

This chapter covers the legal issues relating to consent to treatment. It will be concerned with issues which arise in relation to the mentally competent adult. The laws relating to consent in the case of children and mentally incapacitated adults are covered in the specialist chapters dealing with those client groups (Chapters 8 and 7 respectively). Reference should also be made to the guidance issued by the Department of Health in 2001[1]. The topic of disclosure is considered in the Chapter 5 on confidentiality.

Basic principles

There are two distinct aspects of the law relating to consent to treatment. One is the actual giving of consent by the patient which acts as a defence to an action for trespass to the person. The other is the duty on the practitioner to give information to the patient prior to the giving of consent. The absence of consent could result in the patient suing for trespass to the person. The failure to provide sufficient relevant information could result in an action for negligence. These two different legal actions will be considered separately.

Trespass to the person

A trespass to the person occurs when an individual has not given consent and either apprehends a touching of his person (this is technically known as an assault) or is actually touched (this is known as a battery).

The person who has suffered the trespass can sue for compensation in the civil courts (and in certain cases a criminal prosecution could also be brought). In the civil cases, the victim has to prove:

- the touching or the apprehension of the touching; and
- that it was a (potentially) direct intentional interference with his person.

The victim does not have to show that harm has occurred. This is in contrast with an action for negligence in which the victim must show that harm has resulted from the breach of the duty of care (see below and Chapter 14).

Defences to an action for trespass to the person

The main defence to an action for trespass to the person is that consent was given by a mentally competent person. In addition there are two other defences in law which are:

- statutory authorisation, e.g. under the Mental Health Act 1983
- the common law power to act out of necessity.

Consent

There are two key factors for consent to treatment to be valid:

- the person giving it must be mentally competent (a child of 16 or 17 has a statutory right to give consent and a child below 16, if 'Gillick competent,' (see Chapter 8) may also give consent, and
- the consent must be given without any duress or force or deceit.

It can be given by word of mouth, in writing or can be implied, i.e. the non-verbal conduct or body language of the person may indicate that he is giving consent. All these forms of giving consent are valid, but where procedures entail risk and/or where there may be a dispute on the issue, it is advisable to obtain consent in writing, since it is then easier to establish in court that consent had been given.

The consent form

Examples of consent forms are given in the Department of Health's guidance on consent to examination and treatment[2]. These include forms to be used by health professionals generally and could be used by a practitioner for treatments and investigations.

The Department of Health has published a Guide to Consent for Examination or Treatment which is available from the DoH website. It is a comprehensive document covering a wide range of situations with appendices which set out the principles to be followed in applications to court when there is doubt as to the patient's capacity to consent and which provide for further reading and the legal references. It is intended that the Reference Guide will be regularly updated. It was followed by a document providing a guide to implementation. This latter guide includes suggested forms which can be used as evidence that consent has been given. The Department of Health has also provided individual guides on seeking consent for children, older people and people with learning difficulties.

There are clear advantages in obtaining the patient's consent in writing if there are any risks inherent in the treatment or investigation or if there is likely to be a dispute later as to whether consent was actually given. Completing the form should ensure that all the requisite information is recorded. The guidance also recommends a form to be completed when an adult who lacks mental capacity to give consent to treatment is provided with care in the absence of consent (see below). This form could be adapted for completion by the different practitioners.

Treatment plan

There are clear advantages for the practitioner to obtain consent in writing from the patient at the beginning of any treatment plan. At this time the practitioner can explain to the patient the nature and extent of the treatment, its likely effects, any side effects or inherent risks. If at any time, the treatment plan is significantly changed, this may be reflected in a new written consent by the patient.

Withdrawal of consent and self-discharge

It is a principle of consent that a person who has given consent can withdraw it at any time, unless there is a contractual reason why this is not so. This means that, if a person wishes to leave hospital contrary to his best interests then, unless he lacks the capacity to make a valid decision, he is free to go. Clearly there are advantages in obtaining the signature of the patient that the self-discharge or refusal to accept treatment was contrary to clinical advice. Nevertheless, if the patient refuses to sign a form that he is taking discharge contrary to clinical advice, that refusal must still be accepted. It would be advisable in such a case to ensure that there is another professional who is a witness to this and that a careful record is made by both professionals. Where there could be serious danger to the patient by withdrawing in the middle of a treatment plan, this should be carefully explained to the patient but, unless the patient lacks the mental capacity to make their own decision or is under 18 years, his refusal must be accepted. A young person who is 'Gillick competent' (see Chapter 8) or over 16 can *give* consent in their own right to treatment but, if under 18, cannot *refuse* consent to life-saving care.

Refusal to consent

The Court of Appeal set out the basic principles of self-determination of the mentally competent adult in the case of *Re T*[3]. However it also emphasised the importance of the health professional ensuring that any refusal to give consent to life saving treatment and care was valid.

Case *Re T(refusal of blood transfusion)*

> A woman had made it clear that she would not wish to have a blood transfusion. She was very much under the influence of her mother a Jehovah's Witness. When it became evident that she would need blood to stay alive, the Court allowed the cohabitee's and father's application for the blood to be given on the grounds that her refusal was not valid. This decision was confirmed by the Court of Appeal.

The Court of Appeal laid down the following propositions

- *Prima facie* every adult has the right and capacity to decide whether or not he will accept medical treatment, even if a refusal may risk permanent injury to his health or even lead to premature death. It matters not whether the reasons for the refusal were rational or irrational, unknown or even non-existent.
- The presumption of capacity is rebuttable. An adult may be deprived of his capacity to decide either by long-term mental incapacity or retarded development, or by temporary factors such as unconsciousness or confusion or the effects of fatigue, shock pain or drugs.
- If an adult patient did not have the capacity to decide at the time of purported

refusal and still does not have that capacity, it is the duty of the doctors to treat him in whatever way, in the exercise of their clinical judgment, they consider to be in his best interests.

- Doctors faced with a refusal of consent have to give very careful and detailed consideration to the patient's capacity to decide at the time when the decision was made.
- Doctors must also consider if the refusal has been vitiated because of the will of others who have sought to persuade the patient to refuse. If his will has been overborne, the refusal will not represent the true decision (as was the case in *Re T*).
- In all cases doctors will need to consider what is the true scope and basis of the refusal.
- Forms of refusal should be redesigned to bring the consequences of a refusal forcibly to the attention of patients.
- In cases of doubt as to the effect of a purported refusal of treatment, where failure to treat threatens the patient's life, doctors and health authorities should not hesitate to apply to the courts for assistance.

The right of the adult mentally competent person to refuse food was upheld in the case of a prisoner who had gone on hunger strike. Although the prisoner was diagnosed as suffering from a personality disorder he was held to be of sound mind so that the law required the Home Office, prison officers and doctors to accept his refusal to take food or drink[4]. This case overruled an early case where suffragettes who went on hunger strike were force-fed[5], where the defence of acting out of necessity was applied. It is now clear that this defence is only available when the adult is mentally incompetent (see below).

The principle of the right of self-determination if the adult is mentally competent has subsequently been considered by the Court of Appeal in two cases where a compulsory caesarean had been carried out. In the first case[6], where the pregnant woman suffered from needle phobia and would not agree to an injection preceding the caesarean, the court held the needle phobia rendered her mentally incapable and therefore it declared that doctors performing a caesarean, acting in her best interests, would not be acting illegally. (For the common law power to act in the best interests of the patient out of necessity see below.) The Court of Appeal laid down principles to assist clinicians in treating a pregnant woman.

- In cases where the competence of the mother to make a decision is in issue, the doctors are advised to seek a ruling from the High Court on the point.
- Those involved with the pregnancy should identify a potential problem as early as possible so that both hospital and patient can seek legal advice.
- As far as is possible the need for an emergency application to court should be avoided.
- Both parties should be represented, unless the mother refuses. An unconscious mother should be represented by the guardian *ad litem*.
- The Official Solicitor should be notified of all applications.
- There should be some evidence of the lack of competence of the patient (not necessarily from a psychiatrist.)

In the second case[7], the Court of Appeal held that the detention of a woman under the Mental Health Act 1983 following her refusal to accept treatment for hypertension was invalid and she should not have been compelled to have a caesarean.

The difference between the two cases is that in the first case the woman was held, as a result of the extreme needle phobia, to be mentally incompetent, and therefore the caesarean could be carried out in her best interests without her consent. Whereas in the second case the woman was held not to be mentally incompetent and therefore the compulsory caesarean was a trespass to her person. In neither case did the Court consider that the rights of the foetus could influence the decision making. The fetus is not regarded in law as a legal personality until birth. Until then the wishes of a mentally competent pregnant woman will prevail whatever the effect on the fetus.

Determining capacity

In 1995 the Law Commission in its *Report Mental Incapacity*[8] (see below) used the following definition of mental incapacity:

'A person is without capacity if at the material time he or she is:
1. Unable by reason of mental disability to make a decision on the matter in question, or
2. Unable to communicate a decision on that matter, because he or she is unconscious or for any other reason.

The existence of a mental illness will not automatically mean that a person is incapable of giving a valid refusal of treatment in his best interests as in the case of *Re C*[9], where a patient in Broadmoor was considered to have the capacity to refuse an amputation of the leg which doctors had advised him was indicated as a life saving measure. An injunction (see glossary) was ordered against any doctors carrying out an amputation on him without his consent.

The principles established by the court for consent to be seen as competent were:

*   Could the patient comprehend and retain the necessary information?
*   Was he able to believe it?
*   Was he able to weigh the information, balancing risks, and needs, so as to arrive at a choice?

In applying this test to C the judge was completely satisfied that the presumption that C had the right of self-determination had not been replaced. Although his general capacity had been impaired by schizophrenia, he had understood and retained the treatment information, and believed it and had arrived at a clear choice.

Mental Health Act 1983

Part IV of the Mental Health Act 1983 enables treatment for mental disorder to be given to a detained patient in certain specified situations. Compliance with such statutory requirements would constitute a defence to an action for trespass to the person brought by a person detained under the Mental Health Act 1983 (see Chapter 7).

Common law power to act out of necessity

Where, but only where, the patient lacks the capacity to give consent to treatment, treatment can proceed on the basis that it is in the best interests of that individual and is given according to the reasonable standard of the profession. This is known as the right at common law (i.e. judge-made law) to act out of necessity in the best interests of a mentally incompetent person. In such circumstances, the health professional would not be committing a trespass to the person. This was the ruling in the House of Lords in the case of *Re F*[10]. In that case the House of Lords declared that it was lawful for doctors to sterilise a mentally handicapped young woman who lacked the capacity to give a valid consent provided that they acted in her best interests. The court did however require a reference to the court to be made in future cases, and a Practice Direction[11] was issued setting out appropriate guidance. Under the principle established in *Re F* many health professionals provide care to persons who are unable to give consent to treatment. (This is further discussed in Chapter 7.)

The House of Lords, in the case of *R* v. *Bournewood Community and Mental Health NHS Trust*[12], held that the common law power to act out of necessity in the best interests of the patient also included the right to admit adult mentally incapacitated patients to psychiatric hospital. In a subsequent case the Court of Appeal has ruled that there was an inherent power for the court to grant declarations for decisions to be made in the best interests of mentally incapable adults[13] (see Chapter 3).

Relatives do not have the power to consent on behalf of the mentally incompetent adult, although their views should be ascertained (see Chapter 7).

Proposals for reform

At present there is a vacuum in the law. If a mentally incapacitated adult is unable to make their own decisions, no relative can give or withhold consent on their behalf. The only sure option is recourse to the court which is costly, time consuming and traumatic for all involved. The Law Commission has made recommendations on how this vacuum should be filled[8] and this was followed by a consultation paper issued by the Lord Chancellor's Office in 1997[14]. The Government's response[15] to the consultation was published in 1999 but at the time of writing a Bill to enact its recommendations is still awaited (see further Chapter 7).

Duty to inform

As part of the duty of care owed in the law of negligence the professional has a duty to inform the patient about the significant risks of substantial harm which could occur if treatment were to proceed.

If the harm has not been explained to the patient, and the harm then occurs, the patient can claim that had he known of this possibility he would not have agreed to undergo the treatment. He could then bring an action in negligence. To succeed the patient would have to show:

- that there was a duty of care to give specific information;
- the defendant failed to give this information and in so doing was therefore in breach of the reasonable standard of care which should have been provided;
- as a result of this failure to inform, the patient agreed to the treatment; and
- subsequently suffered the harm.

The leading case is that of *Sidaway*[16] where the House of Lords stated that the professional was required in law to provide information to the patient according to the Bolam test (i.e. the standard of the reasonable practitioner following the accepted approved standard of care (see Chapter 14)).

To ensure that the patient understands the information which is given, there are considerable advantages in a leaflet being provided (checking of course that the patient is literate). This would also assist if there were any dispute over the information having been given.

The *Sidaway* case also recognised that, in exceptional circumstances, a practitioner could withhold information from a person if that information would have a deleterious effect. This is known as therapeutic privilege. The GMC recommends that the view that information should be withheld and the reasons for it should be recorded in the patient's notes[17]. The author is not however aware of any case which has been brought by a patient because too much information was given.

Application to the practice of radiography and radiology

Trespass to the person

An example of a trespass to the person would be where a patient gave consent to a chest X-ray but an X-ray examination was carried out on other parts of his body without his consent. In practice there are many radiographic investigations and treatments which cannot proceed without the co-operation of the patient and consent to the involvement is often implied from the patient's non-verbal communication. In such cases therefore, trespass to the person actions are unlikely. Therefore the focus is more likely to be on the nature of the information which is given (see below). Care should however be taken if it is necessary to examine a patient or have physical contact with him or her to ensure that the patient is consenting to this contact, arranging where appropriate a chaperone of the same sex.

Competence

It has been emphasised that a patient must have the competence to give a valid consent and that it is the duty of the health professional to ensure that a person who was refusing a necessary treatment had the capacity to do so. Where there is any doubt about the competence of an individual to give a valid consent or their capacity to refuse treatment there are considerable advantages if this could be checked by a person who is not involved in the treatment which is being recommended. This person should record her actions and observations.

Informing the client

The duty placed upon the practitioner is that she should ensure that the patient is given information about the significant risks of substantial harm which could arise from treatment or investigation. The practitioner would be judged by the Bolam test, the standard of the reasonable practitioner in that situation with that specific patient (this is further discussed in Chapter 14 on negligence) and the practitioner needs to ensure that she maintains her competence and knowledge about current issues and research. On each occasion the practitioner should make an assessment of the competence of the client to understand what he is being told, and use language which conveys the necessary information accurately and effectively. In difficult situations it would be advisable for a practitioner to ask a colleague, possibly a psychologist to provide an independent assessment of the mental competence of the patient.

The fact that there has been a failure in informing a patient of the risks of an investigation or treatment, may nevertheless not lead to a successful action for compensation if the patient would still have agreed to the investigation or treatment had he known of the risks. For example, in the Canadian case of case of *Meyer* v. *Rogers*[18] there was a breach of the duty to inform the patient about possible reactions from an IVP (intravenous pyelogram). She signed the consent form and died from an allergic reaction. Her estate failed to obtain compensation for her death because the evidence was that she would have gone ahead with the IVP even had she known of the risk factor of 1 in 100 000 deaths. (The case is discussed in Chapter 14.)

Guidance from the NRPB and RCR

The National Radiological Protection Board has issued guidance for the general public on the safety of X-rays in a leaflet[19] which seeks to put the risks into perspective. (See also Chapter 16.)

Professional guidance has been given on consent by the Royal College of Radiologists in the light of the General Medical Council booklet, *Seeking Patients' Consent: the ethical considerations*. This RCR leaflet[20] quotes from the GMC advice and applies this to radiology in the areas of:

- providing information;
- communication;
- withholding information;
- presenting information to patients;
- risks of ionising radiation;
- obtaining consent; and
- obtaining consent in emergencies.

It also covers the special categories of children, the disabled and other groups. Forms of consent, including express and implied consent and consent to screening programmes and research are also explained. The leaflet cites the fundamental principle of consent as being that

'Patients should be provided with sufficient information to allow informed decisions about their investigation and treatment.'

It also emphasises that, if information is deliberately withheld from patients,

'this should be entered into the notes together with the reasons behind the decision as you may have to justify this in law. It is expected that this would only occur in exceptional circumstances.'

The Department of Health[21] has issued the following advice:

'Since the Sidaway case, judgments in a number of negligence cases (relating both to the provision of information and to the standard of treatment given) have shown that courts are willing to be critical of a 'responsible body' of medical opinion. It is now clear that the courts will be the final arbiter of what constitutes responsible practice, although the standards set by the health professions for their members will still be influential.'

The Department of Health quotes the case of *Pearce* v. *United Bristol Healthcare NHS Trust*[22] where the Court of Appeal stated that it will normally be the responsibility of the doctor to inform a patient of 'a significant risk which would affect the judgment of a reasonable patient'. 'Significant' is not defined by the courts numerically.

The practitioner must accept that the law recognises the autonomy of the mentally competent patient to decide whether or not to participate in treatment activities. The onus is on the health professional to inform the patient fully about the benefits and risks of the treatment.

Recent research

Disease-oriented information
An investigation was carried out in the Netherlands into giving information to radiotherapy patients and whether the information supplied met their needs[23]. The authors reviewed patients' information needs and what was provided in 1993 and, in the light of the results, modified the information leaflets and information given to patients. They then carried out further research to assess the level of patient satisfaction with the changes. The conclusion was that the majority of the patients were satisfied with the information in the booklet but a substantial minority (17.2%) suggested that the booklet should be more disease-oriented. The authors point out that written information and information by word of mouth are supplementary; there are advantages in using the same wording. As a result of the findings in the 1996 data collection, the authors of the study took steps to give more detailed information to patients on personal needs, tailored to patients' disease and treatment and planned the development of a treatment-oriented patient booklet linked with the departmental Automated Radiation Therapy (ART) information system, giving more information on the disease, such as relevant instructions, target-specific side-effects and care needs.

An active role for patients

These findings on the value of specific information to patients are supported by earlier research carried out by Gomez[24]. Gomez had prepared a teaching booklet for patients undergoing Mantle-Field irradiation in order to prepare patients more effectively for the side effects of radiation treatment and any possible acute and long-term sequelae. It proved to be an effective tool as patients now had a strategy to manage their side effects. Other research[25] by Van den Borne quoted by the Dutch study also showed the advantages of giving patients more specific information:

> 'When patients have an active role, its gives them a feeling of being more in control of their disease and its treatment, which gives a positive effect on recovery.'

Patient information leaflets are considered by Linda Tutty and Geraldine O'Connor[26] with the aim of establishing a set of guidelines for the design of patient information leaflets for diagnostic imaging procedures. Tutty and O'Connor provide guidance on comprehensibility, layout, terminology, illustrations and how patients' fears can be allayed and they emphasise the need for constant reappraisal of existing leaflets.

Computers as a tool

Peter Hogg and others have evaluated a computer-based information system for patients and members of the public[27]. A computer-based information system for obstetric ultrasound patients, their partners and accompanying persons was set up and evaluated in a 22 month clinical trial. The researchers found that the target population liked the system and found it easy to use. It provided them with useful information. They also indicated that it should be located at a range of health-care and non-healthcare sites. Personal contact with a health care professional was still considered essential; the computer was viewed as an additional but not exclusive source of information. The interactive nature of the system was valued. The on-line questionnaires provided useful data which was automatically recorded to disc. The feedback was also of use in highlighting deficiencies in the information provided. The study concluded that computer-based information systems are a valuable method of informing people about health care, but not as a replacement for personal contact.

Use of video

Communication does not of course have to take part in the department or on the ward and, in oncology, experiments have taken place in using video cassettes which patients can see at home. Dr Robert Thomas reviewed the work of the Information for Patients Research Group at the Addenbrookes Hospital, Cambridge and the Primrose Oncology Centre, Bedford[28]. A video film titled *Chemotherapy and Radiotherapy* was made and given to patients before treatment. It sets out a description of the therapy with a clear idea of the risk of various treatment options using patients who describe their experiences. There were two phases to the study. In the first the film was given to the patients after diagnosis of cancer but before their treatment and 87% felt that the video was helpful or very helpful. In the second phase patients were randomly given either conventional hospital-based support by radiographers, nurses and written material or the same plus the video. The results showed that there was a significant reduction in both treatment-associated anxiety and depression compared to the control group and satisfaction with the information received was 55% higher. However, as with the computer-based system (above), the technology is a supplement to human contact and interaction, not a replacement for it.

Mammography

An example of the importance of sensitive communication when mammography is undertaken is seen in research conducted by B Hafslund[29]. It was concluded that the study showed the importance of the radiographer giving time and information to all women, whatever their educational or socio-economic background. Certain words were found to be very useful in explaining the procedure such as 'pressing, tiring, pinching and unpleasant'. It was also suggested there should be more research on pain in a radiographic examination.

Withholding information from the patient

Policy has changed on how much information should be given to a patient. Thus Peter Morris in a case study on a cancer patient's experience of diagnostic imaging[30], quotes from Guex[31] who stated that prior to the 1970s doctors tended to withhold the true nature of a terminal cancer, instead informing close relatives so that they could decide how much the patient needed to be told. In more recent times, a more frank approach has been adopted and research into patients' own preferences indicates that they feel that they have the right to know the truth concerning their condition. In law, however, there is no absolute right of the patient (either by statute or common law) to obtain all the available information, nor an absolute right to see his health records. The statutory right of access is subject to several exceptions (see Chapter 6).

Communication

At the heart of good patient/professional relationships lie the skills of communication. Radiographers, radiologists and oncologists spend many hours of their work talking to patients in very distressing circumstances. The law requires that those who are receiving information from or giving information to patients follow a reasonable standard of care, such that would be supported by a competent body of professional opinion[16]. The standard of care would take into account any limitations on the patient's ability to absorb and understand the information being imparted. This would obviously include emotional barriers such as fear, distress, and tension as well as physical obstacles to understanding including pain, hearing disabilities, language barriers etc. All these would have to be taken into account by the practitioners.

Information on clinical radiology

A Clinical Radiology Patients' Liaison Group (CRPLG) has been set up by the Royal College of Radiologists with six lay members, three clinical radiologists, a radiographer and the President and Dean of the Faculty of Clinical Radiology[32]. It held its first meeting on 7 May 1998. It aims are:

- to improve public understanding of the role of the clinical radiologist
- to inform the Clinical Radiology Board of concerns
- to improve the dialogue between clinical radiologists and patients and
- for issues of concern to both doctors and patients to be discussed in an atmosphere of trust.

Leaflets have been prepared by the British Society of Interventional Radiology (BSIR) and CRPLG. They are intended as information leaflets for patients who are recommended to have any one of sixteen specific interventional radiology procedures and each can be a starting point to aid discussion prior to obtaining informed consent. Departments are invited to use the leaflets as they stand or include the text in other information provided to patients in advance of their appointments, subject to the appropriate acknowledgement. Each leaflet is provided in HTML and Word format for viewing or downloading on the Royal College of Radiologists (RCR) website[33] alternatively individual leaflets can be ordered from the website or the RCR.

The CRPLG has developed advice for radiology departments on patient friendliness called *Making your Radiology Services more Patient-Friendly*[34] which was published in December 2000.

Audits of patient care – feedback

In an article on patient care during barium enemas, Geraldine O'Connor and Geraldine Butler[35] identify factors which could be used in any audit. Questions were asked on the clarity of instructions given in preparation for the procedure and during it; on how the patients were greeted at reception and on entering the room, and whether they had been treated better than they expected. (One finding of concern in this study was that over 50% of the patients were not told when or from whom they would receive the results of their examination.) The authors concluded that satisfaction with information, humaneness and overall satisfaction could be measured effectively. They recommended that:

- patient satisfaction would be improved by making comment cards available to patients so that their perceptions of staff could be recorded;
- that management needed to foster good patient/staff interaction by providing feedback to staff and by providing them with opportunities for improvement in social skills; and
- that some reward system should be put in place both to motivate staff and to bring about a greater identity of staff with their department.

This article was written before the Human Rights Act 1998 (see Chapter 3 and Appendix 1) came into force, but the recommendations for regular audit on the lines suggested should ensure that departments are proactive in preventing a breach of Article 3.

Conclusion

The law on consent and the duty of care to provide information is fundamental to the responsible care of the patient and is at issue in a significant number of cases brought against health service professionals. Guidance has been issued by the Medical Protection Society which is available to non-members[36]. The training resource pack includes guidance on obtaining consent; who can take consent; presenting information to patients; implied, express, verbal and written consent; competency to give consent; the right time to obtain consent and the legal and statutory framework.

 Questions and exercises _____

1 Analyse your practice in relation to obtaining consent from the patient and decide if it could be improved.
2 Draw up a form for consent to different radiographic investigations.
3 Prepare a handout for the client/patient giving information about the nature of any specific treatment which you provide, setting out any inherent risks.
4 In what circumstances could a person other than the individual who is to carry out the treatment obtain consent from the patient and what specific precautions should be taken?

References

1 Department of Health (2001) *Reference Guide to Consent for Examination or Treatment*, D H, London
2 Department of Health (2001) *Good Practice in Consent: Implementation Guide*, D H, London
3 *Re T (Adult: Refusal of Medical Treatment)* [1992] 4 All ER 649
4 *Secretary of State for the Home Department* v. *Orb* [1995] 1 All ER 677
5 *Leigh* v. *Gladstone* (1909) 25 TLR 139
6 *In re M B (Caesarean Section)* The Times Law Report 18 April 1997; *Re MB (Adult: Medical Treatment)* [1997] 2 FLR 426
7 *St George's Healthcare National Health Service Trust* v. *S* The Times Law Report 3 August 1998: [1998] 3 All ER 673
8 Law Commission (1995) *Mental Incapacity* Report No 231. HMSO, London
9 *Re C (Adult: Refusal of Medical Treatment)* [1994] 1 All ER 819
10 *F* v. *West Berkshire Health Authority and another (Re F)* [1989] 2 All ER 545
11 Practice Note [1993] 3 All ER 222 (replaces previous Practice Note issued 1989)
12 *R* v. *Bournewood Community and Mental Health NHS Trust, ex parte L* [1998] 1 All ER 634
13 *Re F (Adult: Court's Jurisdiction)* 2000 2 FLR 512
14 Lord Chancellor's Office (1997) *Who Cares?* HMSO, London
15 Lord Chancellor's Office (1999) *Making Decisions* HMSO, London
16 *Sidaway* v. *Bethlem Royal Hospital Governors* [1985] 1 All ER 643
17 General Medical Council (1998) *Seeking Patients' Consent: the ethical considerations* GMC, London
18 *Meyer* v. *Rogers* [1991] 2 Med LR 370

19 National Radiological Protection Board (May 2001) *X-rays: How safe are they?* NRPB, London
20 Royal College of Radiologists (1999) *Guidance on Consent by patients to examination or treatment in Departments of Clinical Radiology* (BFCR(99)8), RCR, London
21 Department of Health (2001) *Reference Guide to Consent for Examination or Treatment* (paragraphs 5.2 and 5.3)
22 *Pearce* v. *United Bristol Healthcare NHS Trust* (1999) 48 BMLR 118
23 M. Bakker, D. Weug, M. Crommelin & M. Lybeert (1999) Information for the radiotherapy patient *Radiography* (May 1999) Vol. **5**, pages 99–106
24 E.A. Gomez (1999) Teaching booklet for patients receiving Mantle-Field Irradiation *Oncology Nursing Forum* 1995, Vol. 22, pages 121–6
25 H.W. Van den Borne (1997) *Patient education. The patient from information receiver to an informed decider*, University of Maastricht, 2–36
26 L. Tutty & G. O'Connor (1999) Patient information leaflets: some pertinent guidelines *Radiography*, (February 1999) Vol 5, pages 11–14
27 P. Hogg, T. Boyle, C. Henressy, S. Cossidy, J. Dodgeon, J. Hindle, D. Hogg & J. Priestley (2000) Evaluation a computer-based information system for patients and members of the public *Radiography* (May 2000) Vol 6, pages 89–100
28 R. Thomas (1999) Seeing is believing, *Synergy* (May 1999) page 4
29 B. Hafslund (2000) Mammography and the experience of pain and anxiety *Radiographer* (November 2000) Vol 6, No 3 pages 269–272
30 P. Morris (1999) A Cancer patient's experience of diagnostic imaging *Synergy* (May 1999) pages 12–15
31 P. Guex (1994) *An introduction to Psycho-oncology*, Routledge
32 P. Wilkie (1998) *Clinical Radiology Patients Liaison Group* RCR (Summer 1998) Issue No 54 page 17
33 Royal College of Radiologists www.rcr.ac.uk/colstruct
34 RCR (2000) *Making your Radiology services more Patient-Friendly*, RCR, London (see also www.rcr.ac.uk)
35 G. O'Connor & G. Butler (1999) Aspects of patient care during a barium enema identified as potential factors for audit *Radiography* (February 1999) Vol 5, pages 15–22
36 e-mail *keith.haynes@mps.org.uk*

Chapter 5
The Duty of Confidentiality

All practitioners, whether working in the public or the private sector, have a duty to maintain the confidentiality of information obtained from or about the patient. This chapter explores the source of this obligation and the exceptions recognised in law to that duty[1]. The most significant legislation in this field is the Data Protection Act 1998 and the general effect this Act is mentioned in this chapter. However the specific provisions of the 1998 Act and its regulations on access by persons to their health records will be considered in the Chapter 6.

The nature of the duty of confidentiality

The duty to respect confidentiality arises from a variety of sources which are set out in Figure 5.1.

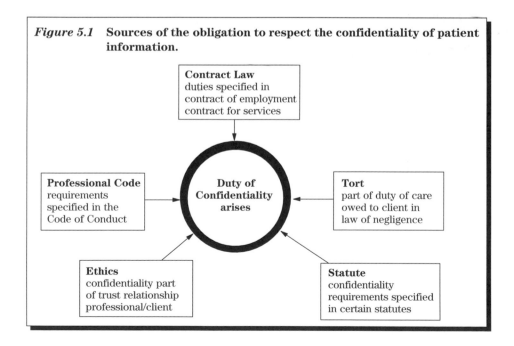

Figure 5.1 **Sources of the obligation to respect the confidentiality of patient information.**

Contract Law
duties specified in
contract of employment
contract for services

Professional Code
requirements
specified in the
Code of Conduct

**Duty of
Confidentiality
arises**

Tort
part of duty of care
owed to client in
law of negligence

Ethics
confidentiality part
of trust relationship
professional/client

Statute
confidentiality
requirements specified
in certain statutes

The code of professional conduct

Each registered professional has certain professional obligations which are enforceable through the professional conduct machinery set up by the GMC and under the Health Professions Council.

The contract of employment/contract for services

The employed health professional also has an obligation, enforceable by the employer and which derives from the contract of employment, to observe the confidentiality of patient information. This will usually be set out expressly in the contract of employment but, even if the contract is silent on the topic, the courts may imply into it such a term. Should the health professional be in breach of this express or implied term, then the employer can take appropriate action through the disciplinary machinery. This may be simply counselling or an oral warning, or any of the stages in the disciplinary procedure may be invoked, depending on the circumstances. In serious cases, the employer may even be justified in dismissing the employee (see Chapter 22).

Those who work as self-employed professionals do not have an obligation to an employer but they do have a contract for services with their patients which may impose conditions relating to confidentiality. Should the health professional be in breach of these contractual conditions, then the patient could bring an action in the civil courts and have the usual remedies for breach of contract.

The duty of care owed in the law of negligence

The health professional owes a duty to the patient to retain information given to her in confidence. Should the health professional be in breach of this duty, then the patient could bring an action against the employer of the health professional on the basis of its vicarious liability for the actions of an employee acting in course of employment.

Case: *Furniss* v. *Fitchett*[2]

> In this New Zealand case the court upheld an action for damages in the tort of negligence for breach of confidence. A doctor treating the plaintiff had given to the patient's husband a letter about the patient's mental state which was used by the husband's solicitor in matrimonial proceedings.

The doctor was held to be in breach of the duty of care which he owed to the patient. The court did not express an opinion on whether such disclosure would always be a breach of the duty of care.

One weakness with the patient's right of action in the law of negligence is that the patient has to prove harm. Harm may eventually arise following unauthorised disclosure, but, until it does so, the patient cannot obtain compensation. He might however obtain an injunction to prevent the disclosure.

Case: X v. Y^3

Two general practitioners were diagnosed as having contracted AIDS. They received counselling in a local hospital, but continued their medical practice. A journalist heard of the situation from an employee of the health authority and wrote an article for a national newspaper. The health authority sought an injunction to prevent any further disclosure of the information obtained from the patients' records.

The judge granted the injunction on the grounds that the records of hospital patients, particularly those suffering from this appalling condition should be as confidential as the courts could properly make them. He rejected the defendant's argument that it was in the public interest for the public to know the identity of these doctors, and ordered an injunction to be issued to prevent the disclosure by the press of the identity of doctors suffering from AIDS.

The judge did not however agree to the health authority's application for disclosure of the name of the employee who had disclosed the information to the journalist. He held that the exceptions under section 10 of the Contempt of Court Act 1981 to the principle that the court cannot require disclosure from a journalist did not apply to the situation and the journalist was entitled to protect his source.

Duty set out in specific statutes

Figure 5.2 identifies the statutes which make it an offence to disclose specified information.

Figure 5.2 **Statutory prohibition against disclosure.**

- Abortion Regulations 1991 (made under the Abortion Act 1967)
- NHS (Venereal Disease) Regulations 1974
- Human Fertilisation and Embryology Act 1990 (as amended by the Human Fertilisation and Embryology (Disclosure of Information) Act 1992)
- Data Protection Act 1998
- Human Rights Act 1998 (Article 8)

Article 8 of the Human Rights Act 1998 states that everyone 'has the right to respect for his private and family life, his home and his correspondence'. This came into effect on 2 October 2000 in terms of enforcement in England and Wales and in Scotland on devolution. Before then any violation of the European Convention on Human Rights had to be taken to European Court of Human Rights in Strasbourg (see Chapter 3). It is too early to determine how this right to privacy will strengthen the duty of confidentiality.

Where information is disclosed in breach of these statutory provisions, the holder of the records or the patient can initiate the appropriate enforcement machinery. In the case of unauthorised disclosure of information by a person or organisation registered (or who should be registered) under the Data Protection Act 1998, the Data Protection Commissioner can remove from a data controller his right to be registered under the Act and to hold personal information in computerised form (see Chapter 6).

The trust obligation between health professional and patient

This duty was acknowledged by the House of Lords[4] in the case known as 'the Spycatcher' case. It was accepted that as a broad principle a duty of confidence arises:

- if information is confidential; and
- comes to the knowledge of a person where he or she has notice or is held to have agreed, that the information is confidential, with the effect that it would be just that he or she should be precluded from disclosing the information; and
- it is in the public interest that the confidentiality should be protected.

Clearly these principles would apply to information which a practitioner is given by or about a patient. The principles were applied in the case of *Stephens* v. *Avery*[5].

Case: *Stephens* v. *Avery*

In this case concerning unconscionable disclosure the plaintiff and first defendant were close friends who freely discussed matters of a personal and private nature on the express basis that what the plaintiff told the first defendant was secret and disclosed in confidence. The first defendant passed on to the second and third defendants, who were the editor and publisher of a newspaper, details of the plaintiff's sexual conduct, including details of the plaintiff's lesbian relationship with a woman who had been killed by her husband. The plaintiff brought an action against the defendants claiming damages on the grounds that the information was confidential and was knowingly published by the newspaper in breach of the duty of confidence owed by the first defendant to the plaintiff.

In an action by the defendants to strike out the claim as disclosing no reasonable cause of action, the defendants failed and appealed to the Chancery Division. They lost this appeal on the grounds that, although the courts would not enforce a duty of confidence relating to matters which had a grossly immoral tendency, information relating to sexual conduct could be the subject of a legally enforceable duty of confidence if it would be unconscionable for the person who had received information on the express basis that it was confidential subsequently to reveal that information to another.

Exceptions to the duty of confidentiality

All the sources of law which recognise that there is a duty of confidentiality also recognise that there will be exceptions where it is lawful to disclose confidential information.

The main exceptions to the duty of confidentiality are shown in Figure 5.3

Consent of the patient

The duty of confidentiality is in the interest of the patient and the patient therefore can give consent to disclosure which without that consent would be unlawful. The patient should be competent to give consent. In the case of a mentally incompetent adult, consent to disclosure could be given on the patient's

---

Figure 5.3   Exceptions to the duty of confidentiality.

- Consent of the patient
- Disclosure in the clinical care or in the interests of the patient
- Court order or pre-trial disclosure
- Statutory duty to disclose
- Disclosure in the public interest

---

behalf in the patient's best interests by a representative guardian or carer of the patient. Where the patient is a child under 16 years, then the principles of the Gillick case would apply (see Chapter 8) and a mature competent child under 16 could give consent to disclosure of confidential information.

The consent of the patient or his representative would be a defence against any potential proceedings being brought against the health professional. It is essential that evidence is available that consent has been given. There are therefore considerable advantages in obtaining this consent in writing.

The patient has the right to withdraw consent unless the terms of the disclosure are contrary to this. For example a patient may agree that a video could be made about his care and treatment. Considerable expense may then be incurred for the video to be produced. The patient may then decide that he does not wish the video to be shown. Whether or not this can then be prevented will depend upon the terms on which his agreement to the disclosure was obtained.

Where the patient specifically refuses to give his consent to the disclosure of his diagnosis to others, such as his relatives, this request should as far as possible be respected under the duty of confidentiality and only if a specific exception to the duty applies could the information be passed on.

For clinical care or in the interests of the patient

Health professionals, working in a multi-disciplinary setting, need to share information about the patient in order to fulfil their duty of care to the patient. Indeed it could be said that if relevant information were not passed to other professionals caring for the patient and harm were to occur to the patient as a result of that failure, then the professional and her employer could be answerable to the patient in a negligence action.

Situation: Justifiable disclosure

A diagnostic radiographer who is carrying out an X-ray of a suspected fracture is told by the patient that he has suffered from unexplained bouts of feeling faint. However he did not want any fuss made. The radiographer informed the casualty doctor who had requested the X-ray. The patient's complaint about this disclosure was defended as a justifiable disclosure in the best interests of the patient. Without this significant information, the doctor might have recommended an incorrect treatment.

Where information is disclosed to colleagues as part of the duty of care to the patient, care should be taken to ensure that it is relevant to and necessary for their responsibilities, and documented.

Court order

Subpoena

The court has the right to require that information, relevant to an issue being decided at the hearing, is made available to the court in the interests of justice. Both criminal and civil courts therefore have the right to issue a subpoena (see glossary) for the necessary information to be produced before them. Other quasi-judicial proceedings such as inquiries may also have a right to subpoena information depending upon the statutory provisions under which they are established.

Where a court requires information, a health professional cannot refuse to comply on the grounds that the information was received in professional confidence. The courts do not recognise any privilege from disclosure attaching to the doctor or other health professional, or even a priest. The only exceptions recognised by the courts to their right to order disclosure are: legal professional privilege and privilege on grounds of the public interest (e.g. national security). If a health professional refuses to answer questions in court on the grounds that this would lead to a breach of confidentiality, the judge has the power to send her to prison for contempt of court.

Disclosure of documents relevant to matters in issue can also be ordered under the Civil Procedure Rules, either in advance of litigation where they are held by a body potentially involved in the case (e.g. the NHS trust in a clinical negligence claim) or after the claim form has been issued if held by a third party.

Legal professional privilege

This covers communications between clients and their legal advisers. The judge cannot order disclosure of such communications. The reason is that it is in the interests of justice for a client to be able to confide fully with legal advisers without fear that such communications would be ordered to be disclosed in court. Reports to legal advisers used also to be privileged from disclosure if the principal purpose for which they were written was in contemplation of litigation[6]. However, since the Woolf reforms bringing more open justice, the preliminary report might now be disclosable if the health professional writing it is later instructed to give expert evidence in the case. Anyone in this position should ensure that she clarifies matters with the lawyers concerned and request very clear instructions.

Public interest immunity

The other exception to the right of the judge to order disclosure of any document relevant to an issue before it, is that of public interest immunity. This covers such interests as the national security. The privilege from disclosure is given under the sworn affidavit of a Minister and can nevertheless be overruled by the judge. Public interest immunity was considered by the Scott inquiry which recommended that immunity certificates should not be issued in criminal proceedings if the liberty of the subject was at stake.

Statutory duty to disclose

Several statues require disclosure to be made, whether or not the patient gives consent. They are shown in Figure 5.4.

Figure 5.4   **Statutory provisions requiring disclosure to be made.**

Notifications of Communicable Diseases
Public Health Act 1936
Public Health (Infectious Diseases) Regulations 1988 (SI 1988 No. 1546)
Public Health (Control of Disease) Act 1984
Public Health (Aircraft) Regulations 1979 (SI 1979 No. 1434)
Public Health (Ships) Regulations 1979 (SI 1979 No. 1435)

Notifications of Abortions
Abortion Act 1967, section 2
Abortion Regulations 1991 (SI 1991 No. 499)

Notification of Births and Deaths
National Health Service Act 1977, section 124
National Health Service (Notification of Births and Deaths) Regulations 1982 (SI 1982 No. 286)

Notification of poisonings and health and safety matters
Health and Safety at Work etc. Act 1974 (see Chapter 15)
Reporting of Injuries, Diseases and Dangerous Occurrences Regulations 1995 (SI 1995 No. 3163)

Disclosure for civil justice
The Civil Procedure Rules

Disclosure for criminal justice
Police and Criminal Evidence Act 1984
The Prevention of Terrorism Acts
Road Traffic Act 1988, section 172

Where these Acts are relevant to the work of the practitioner she should ensure that she is fully conversant with the statutory requirements on disclosure and ensure that any disclosure which is made can be justified in law.

Under section 60(1) of the Health and Social Care Act 2001 the Secretary of State has power to make regulations to require or regulate the processing of prescribed patient information for medical purposes as he considers necessary or expedient in the interests of improving patient care, or in the public interest.

Sub-sections 2 and 3 of section 60 set out details and these regulations may include enabling health service bodies to disclose patient information. Specific restrictions on these powers include prohibiting such processing if it would be reasonably practicable to achieve that purpose by other means. Under Section 61 the Secretary of State must establish a Patient Information Advisory Group whose advice must be sought before any regulations are laid before Parliament. Sections 60 and 61 came into force on the passing of the Act (11 May 2001).

A White Paper on the reform of the Mental Health Act has also been published[7]. This envisages that there will be a new statutory duty of disclosure of information about patients suffering from mental disorder between health and social services agencies and other bodies, for example housing agencies or those concerned with criminal justice.

Disclosure in the public interest

This is the most difficult exception to the duty of confidentiality. Professional registration bodies all recognise that in certain circumstances, disclosure without the patient's consent and contrary to his wishes may be justified. Disclosure in the 'public interest' would include situations where there were reasonable fears to the safety of the patient or of other persons. The most obvious example would be concern about child abuse. This is considered in Chapter 8.

In one decided case[8] on the issue of disclosure in the public interest, the Court of Appeal held that it was permissible for a psychiatrist (who had been asked for a report by a patient who was seeking his discharge from detention under the Mental Health Act 1983) to send his report warning how dangerous the patient was to the Mental Health Review Tribunal and the hospital to be held permanently on file, despite the express prohibition of the patient.

Other situations where disclosure in the public interest would be justified would include a situation where harm is occurring or likely to occur to a child or another person.

Situation: Disclosure in the public interest

> A mother, who has undergone a course of radiotherapy and is very weak, is refusing care for herself when she needs it to look after the child appropriately. She forbids the practitioner to discuss her needs with colleagues.

In this situation, in the interests of the child, the mother must accept that the child's interests require information to be made available about the mother's needs. It could be pointed out to the mother sensitively that if, because of her own needs, she is unable to give the necessary care to the child, then action may have to be taken under the Children Act 1989 to secure the well-being of the child.

Implications for the practitioner

A procedure is necessary for the practitioner to ensure that the confidential nature of information about the patient is preserved. This would also include safe storage of the records which she keeps and should also cover any sharing of records on a multi-disciplinary team basis. In addition the exceptions to the duty should be clarified so that the practitioner can be confident that she is acting within the law and retains the trust of the patient.

Figure 5.5 shows a checklist for ensuring that precautions are taken against any unauthorised disclosure.

Figure 5.5 **Checklist for good practice in maintaining confidentiality.**

- Are the records securely stored with restricted access?
- If access to the records or information is requested, who is making the request?
- What are their reasons for the request?
- What relationship do they have with the patient?
- Has the patient given consent?
- If not, why not?
- Is the patient under the care of a consultant?
- Has the consultant been asked to permit disclosure?
- Is there a duty in law to disclose?
- If so, under what category does the duty arise?
- What part, if any, of the information should be released to the person making the request?
- What should be recorded about the request and the response?

Caldicott guardians

The Government appointed a committee chaired by Dame Fiona Caldicott to make recommendations on how to improve the way in which the NHS managed patient confidentiality. It reported in December 1997[9] and included in its recommendations the need to raise awareness of confidentiality requirements, and specifically recommended the establishment of a network of 'Caldicott Guardians' of patient information throughout the NHS. Subsequently a steering group was set up to oversee the implementation of the Report's recommendations. Following a consultation period the NHS executive issued a circular on the establishment of Caldicott Guardians[10], giving advice on the appointment of the Guardians, a twelve month programme of work for improving the way each organisation handles confidential patient information and identifying resources, training and other support for the Guardians.

Each health authority, special health authority, NHS trust and Primary Care Group was required to appoint a Caldicott Guardian by 31 March 1999. Ideally the Guardian should be at Board level, be a senior health professional and have responsibility for promoting clinical governance within the organisation. The name and address of the Guardian is to be notified to the NHS Executive[11]. The Guardian is expected to liaise closely with others involved in patient information such as IM&T security officers and Data Protection Officers. In making the appointment and defining the role of the Guardian, the duties which are not to be delegated should be clarified. Guardians are responsible for agreeing and reviewing internal protocols governing the protection and use of patient-identifiable information by the staff of their organisation and must be satisfied that these proposals address the requirements of national guidance, policy and law. The operation of these policies must also be monitored. Policies for inter-agency disclosure of patient information to facilitate cross boundary working must also be agreed and reviewed.

In 2000 the Department of Health issued guidance to Caldicott Guardians on the method by which information flows should be reviewed in NHS organisations[12]. It provided a manual which covers the mapping of information flows, the prioritising of mapped flows for review purposes and a rolling programme of review. The specific areas which are considered include: commissioning flows, clinical audit, coding, medical records and patient care services.

If issues on confidentiality arise a healthcare practitioner can raise these with the Caldicott Guardian, who in turn can access the legal advisers to the Trust.

Conclusion

The Data Protection Act 1998 has strengthened provisions on access to and disclosure of personal information putting more pressure on the decisions of the individual practitioner. However the absence of a statutory definition of 'the public interest' makes it difficult to determine whether the exception applies. Each individual practitioner is personally and professionally accountable for any disclosure. The Human Rights Act, in enabling persons to bring actions against public authorities who have failed to uphold a person's right to respect for privacy set out in Article 8, is likely to lead to more litigation where patients claim that their right to confidentiality has not been respected. It is too early to evaluate the effect of the powers given to the Secretary of State under section 60 of the Health and Social Care Act 2001 and the influence of the Patient Information Advisory Group, but there is every possibility that excessive orders for disclosure of confidential information for the purposes of section 60 will lead to challenges based on the Data Protection Act 1998 and Article 8 of the Human Rights Act 1998.

 Questions and exercises _____

1 Examine your practice in relation to passing on confidential information. What faults would you see in it?
2 To what extent can an employer enforce the duty of confidentiality amongst employees? Prepare a procedure for this.
3 What exceptions have you relied upon in passing on confidential information?

References

1 For further information see B. Darley, A. Griew, K. McLoughlin & J. Williams (1994) *How to Keep a Clinical Confidence.* HMSO, London
2 *Furniss* v. *Fitchett* [1958] NZLR 396
3 *X* v. *Y* [1988] 2 All ER 648
4 *Attorney General* v. *Guardian Newspaper Ltd (No 2)* [1988] 3 All ER 545
5 *Stephens* v. *Avery and others* [1988] 2 All ER 477
6 *Waugh* v. *British Railway Board* [1980] AC 521
7 Department of Health (2000) *Reforming the Mental Health Act* The Stationery Office, London
8 *W* v. *Edgell* [1989] 1 All ER 1089
9 The Caldicott Report 1997, Department of Health, London

10   NHS Executive (1999) *Caldicott Guardians* (HSC 1999/012) 31 January 1999
11   NHS Executive 3E58, Quarry House, Leeds. LS2 7UE (Fax 0113 254 6114)
12   Department of Health (2000) *Protection and using patient information: A Manual for Caldicott Guardians* DoH, London

Chapter 6
Data Protection and Access to Records

Introduction

The Data Protection Act 1998 enables access to both computerised and manually held records to take place following the same procedure. Previously access to computerised records was possible under Data Protection Act 1984 provisions and, to address the anomaly of computerised health records being available but not manual ones, from 1991 access to manually held personal health records was allowed under the Access to Health Records Act 1990. The Access to Health Records Act 1990 has now been repealed except the provisions relating to the records of deceased persons. There has never been an absolute right to access healthcare records. Access can be withheld in certain defined circumstances. This chapter considers the 1998 Data Protection Act in general and explains the right of access to health records and the exceptions to it. It also looks at some cases involving X-rays and records.

Data protection legislation

The European Directive on Data Protection (1995)[1] was implemented in this country by the Data Protection Act 1998 which amended and extended the Data Protection Act 1984, bringing it into line with the Directive. Member States were required to comply by 24 October 1998 although the UK did not meet this target since the Act did not come into force until after the following year. Under the legislation members had to establish a set of 'principles' with which users of 'personal information' must comply. The legislation also gives individuals the right to gain access to information held about them and provides for a supervisory authority to oversee and enforce the law. NHS guidance on the Act was provided by a circular in March 2000[2] and the NHS Information Authority action plan for the NHS is available on its website to ensure the processing of personal data within the organisation is in compliance with the Act[3]. The main provisions of the Act are shown in Figure 6.1.

There are some significant differences between the Data Protection Act 1984 and the Data Protection Act 1998 as follows:

- The 1998 Act applies to certain manual records (if they form part of a relevant filing system) as well as to computerised records.
- Some terms are defined differently, such as 'personal data', 'processing', etc.
- There are tighter provisions on the processing of sensitive personal data.
- The fundamental rights are amended.

Figure 6.1 **Data Protection Act 1988 – main provisions.**

Part I Preliminary: basic interpretative provisions; sensitive personal data; the special purposes; data protection principles; application of Act; the Commissioner and Tribunal.

Part II Rights of Data subjects and others:
- right of access to personal data
- right to prevent processing likely to cause damage or distress
- right to prevent processing for direct marketing
- rights in relation to automated decision-taking
- compensation for failure to comply with certain requirements
- rectification, blocking, erasure and destruction

Part III Notification by Data Controllers: duty to notify; register of notifications; offences; preliminary assessment by Commissioner; power to make provision for appointment of data protection supervisors; duty of certain data controllers to make certain information available; notification regulations; fees regulations.

Part IV Exemptions:
- national security
- crime and taxation
- health, education and social work
- regulatory activity
- journalism, literature and art
- research, history and statistics
- information available to the public by or under enactment
- disclosure required by law or made in connection with legal proceedings
- domestic purposes
- powers to make further exemptions by order

Part V Enforcement: notices; rights of appeal; powers of entry and inspection.

Part VI Miscellaneous and General

Schedules
- (1) Data protection principles
- (2) Conditions for processing any personal data
- (3) Conditions for processing sensitive personal data
- (4) Cases where the eighth principle does not apply (restriction on data transfer outside EEA)
- (5) Data Protection Commissioner and Data Protection Tribunal
- (6) Appeal proceedings
- (7) Miscellaneous exemptions
- (8) Transitional Relief
- (9) Powers of entry and inspection
- (10) Assistance under section 53 (in cases involving special purposes)
- (11) Educational records
- (12) Accessible public records

- There are new rules for the transfer of personal data outside the European Community.

Other changes are more procedural:

- There are changes to the system for registration.
- The person in charge is now known as the Data Protection Commissioner.

The Data Protection Act 1998 must be read in conjunction with the Human Rights Act 1998 (see Chapter 3) since Article 8 of the European Convention of Human Rights recognises an individual's right to privacy, subject to specific qualifications.

Computerised and manually held records

The Data Protection Act 1984 applied only to computerised records but, since the passing of the Data Protection Act 1998, patient records held in a manual form may come under the same rules as those held on a computer. 'Data' now includes manually held records if they form part of a relevant filing system. A possible example of manual records not coming under data protection provisions would be clinical supervision records in which specific patients are named. These may not come under the provisions of the Data Protection Act since they may not form part of a relevant filing system. However a court decision on the interpretation of 'relevant filing system' is required to clarify the point.

Terminology

Some of the terms used in the Data Protection Act 1998 are given different definitions from those used in the 1984 Act.

- The 'data subject' is 'the individual who is the subject of personal data', but under the 1998 provisions the law applies only to living people. Also if the information is anonymous then the person will not be considered to be identifiable, unless it is possible to link together separate items of information in order to identify an individual. If that is possible, the Act would then apply.
- Processing under the 1998 Act includes any operation involving personal data including the holding of the information.
- The term 'data user' (from the 1984 Act) is replaced by the term 'data controller' and is the person who determines the purposes for which and the manner in which any personal data are to be processed.
- 'Computer bureau' is replaced by 'processor'.
- The Data Protection Registrar, who is the national officer responsible for the oversight of the implementation of the law, is now to be known as the Commissioner.

Data protection principles

The 1998 Act slightly amends the Data Protection Principles and the new wording is shown in Figure 6.2. Interpretation of these principles is provided in Part II of Schedule 1 of the 1998 Act.

Figure 6.2 **Data Protection Principles (Schedule 1 Part I).**

(1) Personal data shall be processed fairly and lawfully and, in particular, shall not be processed unless –
   (a) at least one of the conditions in Schedule 2 is met, and
   (b) in the case of sensitive personal data, at least one of the conditions in Schedule 3 is also met.

(2) Personal data shall be obtained only for one or more specified and lawful purposes, and shall not be further processed in any manner incompatible with that purpose or those purposes.

(3) Personal data shall be adequate, relevant and not excessive in relation to the purpose or purposes for which they are processed.

(4) Personal data shall be accurrate and, where necessary, kept up to date.

(5) Personal data processed for any purpose or purposes shall not be kept for longer than is necessary for that purpose or those purposes.

(6) Personal data shall be processed in accordance with the rights of data subjects under this Act.

(7) Appropriate technical and organisational measures shall be taken against unauthorised or unlawful processing of personal data and against accidental loss or destruction of, or damage to, personal data.

(8) Personal data shall not be transferred to a country or territory outside the European Economic Area unless that country or territory ensures an adequate level of protection for the rights and freedoms of data subjects in relation to the processing of personal data.

Pre-conditions for processing data

Principle 1 refers to 'Schedule 2' conditions and these include:

- the consent of the data subject
- that the processing is necessary
  - for the performance of a contract to which the data subject is a party
  - for taking steps, at the request of the data subject, to enter a contract
- that the processing is necessary for compliance with a legal obligation of the data subject
- that the processing is necessary to protect the vital interests of the data subject
- that the processing is necessary
  - for the administration of justice
  - the exercise of functions conferred by any enactment
  - the exercise of functions of the Crown, Minister or government department or
  - for the exercise of other functions of a public nature
- that the processing is necessary to meet the legitimate interests of the data controller or a third party

Clearly patient records are covered by several of these conditions only one of which is needed to legitimise the basic processing. However records relating to physical or mental health come within the definition of sensitive personal data (see Figure 6.3) and further compliance with one of the Schedule 3 conditions for the processing of such information is required.

***Figure 6.3* Sensitive personal data.**

Personal data consisting of information as to:

- the racial or ethnic origin of a data subject
- their political opinions
- their religious beliefs or other beliefs of a similar nature
- whether they are a member of a Trade Union
- their physical or mental health or condition
- their sexual life
- the (alleged) commission of any offence by them or
- any proceedings for any (alleged) offence, disposal of such or sentence

---

These Schedule 3 Conditions for disclosure of sensitive personal data specifically include that:

'8.   (1) The processing is necessary for medical purposes and is undertaken by —
    (a)   a health professional, or
    (b)   a person who in the circumstances owes a duty of confidentiality which is equivalent to that which would arise if that person were a health professional.

(2) In this paragraph 'medical purposes' includes the purposes of preventative medicine, medical diagnosis, medical research, the provision of care and treatment and the management of healthcare services.'

Satisfaction of this condition would obviate the need to obtain the explicit consent of every patient, in order for their health records to be processed.

Consent

The consent of the data subject or, in the case of sensitive personal data, their explicit consent is one of the other conditions that enables processing to be carried on. Moreover special provision is made for where processing is necessary to protect the data subject's vital interests but consent cannot be given by him or on his behalf or the data controller cannot be reasonably expected to obtain that consent. Schedule 3 gives as an alternative condition that:

3.   The processing is necessary—
    (a)   to protect the vital interests of the data subject or another person, in a case where—
        (i)   consent cannot be given by or on behalf of the data subject, or
        (ii)   the data controller cannot reasonably be expected to obtain the consent of the data subject, or

(b) in order to protect the vital interests of another person, in a case where consent by or on behalf of the data subject has been unreasonably withheld

This situation would obviously cover records relating to mentally incapacitated adults and also children.

Rights of the data subject

The rights of the individual under the Data Protection Act 1998 are as follows:

- of subject access (sections 7 to 9)
- to prevent processing likely to cause damage or distress (section 10)
- to prevent processing for the purposes of direct marketing (section 11)
- in relation to automated decision taking (section 12)
- to take action for compensation if the individual suffers damage by any contravention of the Act by the data controller (section 13)
- to take action to rectify, block, erase or destroy inaccurate data (section 14)
- to make a request to the Commissioner for an assessment to be made as to whether any provision of the Act has been contravened (section 42).

Detailed consideration of these rights is outside the scope of this book but section 7, which enables an individual to be informed of data held about him and to access that data, is considered below.

Data protection commissioner

The Data Protection Commissioner has the responsibility for promoting good practice and observance of the laws, providing an information service and encouraging the development of Codes of Practice. He has considerable powers of enforcement under Parts III and V of the Act. These include the power to serve enforcement notices and powers of entry and inspection. Information is available from the Commissioner's office free of charge[4]. An explanatory guide to the new legislation is also available[5].

Offences under the Act are:

- Offences relating to failure to notify the Commissioner or comply with his requests
- Unlawfully obtaining personal data
- Unlawful selling of personal data
- Forcing a person to supply access
- Unlawful disclosure of information by the Commissioner his staff or agent.

Guidance from the NHS executive

The NHS Executive has published guidelines on the protection and use of patient information to support the implementation of the Data Protection Act[6]. It states that a Working Group at the Department of Health is developing national guidance to assist NHS bodies and local authorities on the principles and practical issues involved in sharing client/patient records for service delivery and of using such aggregated data for planning, commissioning, managing and monitoring.

Access to health records

Right under section 7 Data Protection Act 1998

Section 7 gives to a data subject a right of access to personal data. The request must be made in writing to the data controller with the appropriate fee (if any). Sufficient information must be given for the data controller to be satisfied about the identity of the person making the request and the location of the information. The data controller must comply with the request within 40 days or other prescribed period.

Under the access provisions of the 1998 Act, the data subject can have:

- a copy of the data
- a description of the data being processed
- a description of the purposes which it is being processed
- a description of any potential recipients of his data; and
- any information as to the source of his data where this is available and if the exceptions do not apply.

Under the 1984 Act, the data subject was only entitled to have a copy of any data processed with reference to him.

Qualifications on access to personal data provisions

Under section 30 of the DPA 1998 the Secretary of State is given the power to exempt personal data consisting of information as to the physical or mental health or condition of the data subject from the subject access information provisions.

The Data Protection (Subject Access Modification) (Health) Order (SI 2000 No. 413) modifies section 7 of the DPA 1998 which enables data subjects to access their records.

Serious harm
Personal data is exempted from the subject access provisions 'to the extent to which the application of [section 7] would be likely to cause serious harm to the physical or mental health or condition of the data subject or any other person'.

Duty to consult
A data controller who is not a health professional (as defined by section 69 of the Data Protection Act) can neither withhold nor communicate information until the appropriate health professional has been consulted on whether or not the exemption applies.

The appropriate health professional for this consultation is:

- the health professional who is currently or was most recently responsible for the clinical care of the data subject in connection with the matters to which the information which is the subject of the request relates; or
- where there is more than one such health professional, the one who is most suitable to advise on those matters; or

- where there is no-one falling within the above definitions (or the data controller is the Secretary of State in his functions under the child support or social security legislation) a health professional who has the necessary experience and qualification to advise on those matters.

This duty to consult does not apply where the data subject has already seen or knows about the information which is the subject of the request, nor in certain circumstances where consultation has been carried out prior to the request being made.

Requests on behalf of children or mentally incapacitated adults

Where a request is made on behalf of a child by a person with parental responsibility or on behalf of a person who is incapable of managing his own affairs by a person who has been appointed by a court to manage those affairs, then, even though such a person may have a right under any statute or rule of law to make the request, they cannot have access to:

- information provided by the data subject in the expectation that it would not be disclosed to the person making the request;
- information obtained as a result of any examination or investigation to which the data subject consented in the expectation that the information would not be so disclosed; or
- information which the data subject has expressly indicated should not be so disclosed.

The first two exceptions do not apply if the data subject has expressly indicated that he no longer has the expectation referred to.

Third party identification

Under the access provisions of section 7, access can be withheld if another individual would be identified by the information disclosed. This does not apply and access should be given where:

(1) the individual concerned has consented to the disclosure; or
(2) where it is reasonable in all the circumstances to comply with the request for access even without such consent; or
(3) where the other individual is a health professional who has contributed to the health record or has been involved in the care of the data subject in her capacity as a health professional.

Access would still be withheld if the health professional would suffer serious harm to her physical or mental health or condition by the giving of access. Such circumstances would be unusual, but are a possibility in the care of psychiatric patients.

The circumstances referred to in point (2) above would take into account:

- any duty of confidentiality owed to that individual;
- any steps taken by the data controller with a view to seeking the consent of the other individual;
- whether the other individual is capable of giving consent; and
- any express refusal of consent by the other individual.

Access in all those circumstances should be given to any other information which can be disclosed without identifying the third party.

Evidential reports

Exemptions from subject access also include information supplied in a report or other evidence given to a court by a statutory body (including an NHS trust), a probation officer, or other person in the course of any proceedings under specified legislation dealing with children.

Application

The Data Protection Act 1998 applies to both computerised records and also to manually held records held in a file, which clearly covers most health records. Application for access to these health records is now made under the DPA 1998 provisions and the Access to Health Records Act 1990 will only apply in relation to access to the records of patients who are deceased.

From 24 October 2001 patients have been able to apply for records containing information about them, whether or not they were created by a health professional and health bodies can only charge of £10 administration fee with no photocopying charges. Up to then they could charge up to £50 for administration and add on copying, including X-rays. As stated above, non health professionals cannot give access to records unless they have consulted the appropriate health professional to find if serious harm would be caused.

X-rays and the access provisions

In the case below the court considered the issue of whether X-rays were part of a patient's medical records.

Case: *Hammond* v. *West Lancashire HA*[7]

Following the death of his wife, Hammond (on behalf of her estate) brought a negligence action against West Lancashire Health Authority. The case was started more than three years after he came to know of the cause of action and so, strictly speaking, outside the limitation period (see glossary) (Limitation Act 1980 section 14(1)). However the judge exercised his discretion under section 33 of the Act and allowed the case to proceed. The judge expressed dissatisfaction with the health authority's practice of destroying patients' X-rays after three years, particularly as it knew that proceedings were being contemplated, because initial requests had been received from solicitors for the patient's notes.

The judge said that such a procedure was 'wholly unacceptable'. 'It shows a cavalier disregard for the rights of patients to have access to their records. How anyone could think that the X-rays are not part of the patient's medical records is beyond me. If the defendant is so remiss as to have such a system in place, then this court will pay little regard to any prejudice to their case that they may claim later.'

The Health Authority appealed against the decision of the judge but the Court of Appeal dismissed the appeal. It held that the judge was entitled to conclude that X-Rays formed part of a patient's notes and should be sent as a matter of course when notes were requested. A health authority which showed an obvious indifference to the rights of patients to access their medical records would encounter difficulties in pleading prejudice when defending an attempt by the claimant to allow the limitation period to be extended.

Conclusions

The fact that there is a statutory right of access does not of course mean that informal access cannot be permitted in healthcare. Provided there is no justification in preventing access to records because of a fear of serious harm to the physical or mental health of a person, or the possibility of identifying a third person who has asked not to be identified, a patient could have access to their records, without going through the formal system of applying under the Data Protection subject access regulations. Clear local procedures should be laid down to facilitate open access. The introduction of the electronic health record (which is considered in Chapter 18) should facilitate patient access to their health records and improve systems of communication.

Access by children to their records is considered in Chapter 8 and access on behalf of mentally incapacitated persons is considered briefly in Chapter 7, although the position here is not at all clear pending long-awaited legislation on consent and decision making on behalf of such people.

 Questions and exercises _____

1   How would you define the words 'serious harm to the physical or mental health or condition of the data subject or any other person'? Give examples of situations where this exception to the right of access would apply.
2   As a health professional working in X-Ray you have been intimidated by a patient and as a consequence have reported him to the police. You are now informed that the patient is seeking access to his medical records, and you fear that if he learnt that you were the informant your safety would be endangered. What action could you take?
3   Analyse your department's policy in relation to rights of access to records and consider any ways in which it could be improved.

References

1   European Directive on Data Protection Adopted by the Council of the European Union in October 1995 (1995 OLJ 281)
2   NHS Executive (2000) *Data Protection Act 1998* (HSC 2000/009)
3   http://www.standards.nhsia.nhs.uk/sdp
4   Data Protection Commissioner (Registrar), Wycliffe House, Water Lane, Wilmslow, Cheshire SK9 5AF. Information line: 01625 545745; Switchboard: 01625 545700; Fax 01625 524510
5   Data Protection Registrar (1998) *The Data Protection Act 1998: an introduction* Office of Data Protection Registrar, Wilmslow
6   NHS Executive (2000) *Data Protection Act: Protection and Use of Patient Information* (HSC 2000/009)
7   *Hammond* v. *West Lancashire HA* [1998] Lloyd's Rep. Med 146

Chapter 7
Mentally Incapacitated Adults

Introduction

This chapter considers the issues relating to the care, treatment and investigations carried out on mentally incapacitated adults. This term includes those over 18 years who are incapable of decision making and therefore would include adults suffering from Alzheimer's and those with learning disabilities. There is no separate chapter dealing with the law relating to the elderly, since they have the same legal rights as others. The main concerns relate to:

- giving or refusing consent
- understanding information
- standards in care and treatment
- future legislative changes.

Some clients with learning disabilities also suffer from a mental illness and may be sectioned under the Mental Health Act 1983. Reference should be made to specialist works on that topic[1].

Decision making and incapacity

Patients who have certain mental incapacities may, depending upon the nature of the matter in issue, still have the capacity to make certain decisions on their own account. Clearly the client's capacity must be related to the nature of the decision to be made. The client may be able to choose what food to eat, what clothes to wear or buy but might not have the capacity to decide whether or not to undergo radiotherapy, have an X-ray or agree to an operation. The basic principle of law is that a mentally competent adult has the right to give or refuse consent and cannot be compelled to have treatment even if it is life saving[2] (see Chapter 4). Whilst parents can make decisions for their children under 18 years, once a person is over 18 there is at present in the law no power for anyone to make treatment decisions for them. No person has the legal power to make such decisions in the name of a mentally incapacitated adult. (In Scotland an Adults with Incapacity (Scotland) Act 2000 came into force in April 2001.)

Determination of capacity

Crucial to any decision making is whether an individual can be deemed to have the necessary capacity to make a decision. This is discussed in Chapter 4 where the case[3] of a Broadmoor patient who refused an amputation of his leg was considered. The judge in that case held that the test of capacity for an adult was whether he was able to:

- comprehend and retain the necessary information;
- believe it; and
- weigh the information, balancing risks and needs, to arrive at a choice.

The Court of Appeal in the case of *Re MB*[2] stated that there was a presumption in law that an adult had the necessary capacity but this could be rebutted by evidence to the contrary.

The definition of capacity recommended for use by the government in its proposals for legislation on behalf of mentally incapacitated adults is that:

- A person is without capacity if, at the time that a decision needs to be taken, he is **'unable'** by reason of **mental disability to make a decision** on the matter in question; or unable to communicate a decision on that matter because he or she is unconscious or for any other reason'.
- Mental disability is 'any disability or disorder of the mind or brain, whether permanent or temporary, which results in an impairment or disturbance of mental functioning'.
- A person is to be regarded as unable to make a decision by reason of mental disability if the disability is such that, at the time when the decision needs to be made, the person is 'unable to understand or retain the information relevant to the decision or unable to make a decision based on that information'.

(Emphasis is in the Government document)

The government supports the Law Commission recommendation that a person should not be regarded as incapable of communicating decisions unless 'all practicable steps to enable him or her to do so have been taken without success', and accepts the principle that a decision should not be regarded as invalid merely because it would not be made by a 'person with ordinary prudence'.

The vacuum in the law

In a leading case, *Re F* (1989)[4], carers wanted a woman with learning disabilities to be sterilised in her best interests. Since no person had the legal right to give consent the issue was brought to court. The House of Lords recognised the vacuum in law but stated that a professional had the duty to act in the best interests of an adult person who lacked the necessary mental capacity, and follow the Bolam test (see glossary) in providing a reasonable standard of care. The House of Lords nevertheless recommended that any decision relating to an operation for sterilisation or similar treatment should be brought to the court and a Practice Direction was issued setting out details for this procedure[5].

The Law Commission, following an extended period of consultation on the issue of decision making and mental incapacity, had prepared draft legislation[6] which, if implemented, would have ensured that a statutory framework would be established for decisions to be made in accordance with their seriousness. Court approval would be required for decisions relating to sterilisations, abortions, etc.

but at the other end of the scale day to day decisions could be made by a carer or health professional who would have the necessary statutory power.

The Lord Chancellor issued a further consultation document in December 1997[7] *Who Decides*. In 1999 the government's proposals for legislation were published[8]. The recommendations include:

- provision for a statutory decision maker to be recognised
- for there to be continuing powers of attorney to include medical treatment
- for new courts to be established (possibly a revamped Court of Protection) where disputes could be resolved and decisions on what was in the best interests of a mentally incapacitated adult could be taken.

At the time of writing a Mental Incapacity Bill is awaited. In the meantime, carers and health professionals in giving treatment and care to those who do not have the capacity to give a valid consent are protected by the powers recognised at common law in the case of *Re F*[4], provided that they act in the best interests of the client and follow the reasonable standard of care.

A later House of Lords decision[9] has confirmed that the power of acting out of necessity in the best interests of a person who lacks mental capacity can also apply to the admission of such patients to psychiatric care. The House of Lords overruled the Court of Appeal decision which had held that any adult who lacked the mental capacity to give consent to voluntary admission to psychiatric care had to be examined with a view to detention under the provisions of the Mental Health Act 1983. Subsequently the Court of Appeal has held that there is inherent power for the court to grant declarations in the best interests of mentally incapacitated adult on day to day decisions[10].

Patients detained under the Mental Health Act 1983

Patients who are detained under the Mental Health Act 1983 would normally be escorted on a visit to X-ray or radiotherapy departments. The radiographers and radiologists should be able to look for assistance from the escort. In certain situations Part IV of the Mental Health Act 1983 enables treatment to be given without the consent of the detained patient, but this only applies to treatment for mental disorder. It is therefore unlikely that X-rays or radiotherapy treatment could be provided under the Part IV of the Act. If a patient makes it clear that they are unwilling to have the X-rays or treatment given, then the patient's refusal should be accepted. The only exception to this would be where the patient is lacking mental capacity and the diagnostic tests or radiotherapy treatment is in the patients best interests. Pending the major reforms to the Mental Health Act 1983 (see above) it may be necessary for the issue to be aired in court.

Specific care issues

Specific issues arise in in relation to the care and treatment of adults who are mentally incapacitated.

Direct patient contact

A client may be asked to remove his clothes. Those with learning disabilities and elderly infirm adults may be unable to give a valid consent to the treatments and removal of clothing.

Situation: Preparation for X-ray

A patient with learning disabilities requires an X-ray and is brought to the Department by an informal carer. The carer is asked to assist the patient in removing his clothes and putting on a gown. The patient is unable to understand what is happening to him and resists the removal of his clothing. What action should be taken and what is the law?

Every effort should be made to explain to the patient what the reason is for putting on a gown and what is about to happen to him. Where there is no carer, there would be strong reasons to ensure that the practitioner is chaperoned, both for her own protection and for that of the patient.

Restraint

Situation: Splints to prevent harm to the face

Rachel, a woman of 32 with severe disabilities, scratches her face and eyes and arm splints are used to protect her.

There would appear to be justification in the short term to prevent Rachel from harming herself, but long term methods of behavioural therapy and other treatments should be used to obtain a fundamental change in the patient's behaviour. Records should be kept of the use of the splints and regular monitoring should take place to identify alternative ways of preventing her harming herself, e.g. by staff being in attendance on her.

Any restriction on the liberty of a person is a false imprisonment, unless there is a lawful justification. Such justification could include a lawful arrest by a police constable or citizen exercising the right to arrest under the Police and Criminal Evidence Act 1984. Acting temporarily in the best interests of an adult who lacked mental capacity could also be lawful: thus to hold back a person with learning disabilities from running across the road, would be defensible under the doctrine of necessity, recognised at common law.

Situation: Restraint

John Turner has severe learning disabilities. His health necessitates intravenous treatment and therefore he has to have a cannula put in place in order to insert contrast material. He resists any attempt to get a needle into his arm. What action can lawfully be taken to ensure that the cannula is inserted?

In exceptional circumstances restraint may be justified as a temporary measure, but it must be in the best interests of the mentally incapacitated adult; it must be of short duration and the minimum necessary to protect the health and safety of the person. Extreme forms of restraint such as tying up a person into a chair would be an unlawful act; a false imprisonment, and also a breach of the Human Rights Act 1998 as degrading treatment under Article 3 and/or a loss of freedom under Article 5. Records should be kept and any restraint should be regularly monitored. In certain situations restraint may be required by law such as the wearing of seat belts. It may be that in the above circumstances, some form of sedation will be necessary to enable the patient to be cared for with minimum distress. Obviously the sedation should be the minimum necessary to achieve the outcome required.

Manual handling

Situation: Lifting a patient with cerebral palsy

Radiography staff who have had no training in lifting patients with severe physical disabilities ask if they can lawfully refuse to use manual handling on such patients.

The answer to this question is that all health professionals have a duty of care to a patient. The radiographers cannot refuse to care for a heavy person with learning disabilities. However their employer, in accordance with the Manual Handling Regulations, has to minimise their risk of injury and they are entitled in law to receive training in risk assessment, risk management and the appropriate lifting methods. Their employer should also supply the necessary equipment to ensure that such lifting can be undertaken safely by the staff (see Chapter 15).

Suspected abuse

Situation: Suspected Abuse

A radiographer cares for an elderly patient who lives with her daughter and son-in-law and suspects that she may be the victim of sexual abuse. What action should she take?

She has a duty of care to the patient and this would include taking appropriate action if she suspected physical or mental abuse. There is no clear mechanism for the protection of the mentally incapacitated adult as there is under the Children Act 1989, though some local authorities now have procedures for dealing with the abuse of the elderly. A vulnerable adult may have impaired mental capacity rather than being completely mentally incapacitated. The practitioner should discuss her concerns regarding possible abuse with the multi-disciplinary team and ensure that an appropriate report is made to social services. In some circumstances, it may become a police matter and lead to prosecution.

The practitioner should keep clear comprehensive documentation of her observations of the patient and any evidence of abuse, ensuring that the suggested procedure in dealing with suspected child abuse is followed as far as is possible.

Department policy

There is evidence of growing recognition that each department should have a clear policy for dealing with patients with physical and mental disabilities and this would apply equally to radiography and radiotherapy departments. Tony Browne explored the needs of learning disabled patients presenting for an X-ray in a small scale[11]. His conclusions were that providing the same service for learning disabled patients as provided for 'normal' patients does not meet their needs. The study highlighted the need for X-ray staff to adapt procedures and techniques to accommodate the special needs of the learning disabled patient. He gives various suggestions to ensure that identified needs would be addressed. These suggestions are set-out below.

- A radiographer should be appointed as an advocate to be known as the responsible radiographer.
- The responsible radiographer should identify any special needs that an LD patient might have and should ensure those needs are met.
- The responsible radiographer should ensure that procedures concerning LD patients are implemented and maintained.
- Adequate training and support should be made available to the responsible radiographer.
- All X-ray reception staff, radiographers and helpers should attend a study day or workshop to increase their awareness of LD needs.
- There should be positive discrimination when making up examination lists and appointment times that relate to the specific needs of LD patients.
- If required a room should be made available for the LD patient and his carer during waiting periods.
- The procedure should be explained to the patient and carer before the radiographer begins the examination, for any special needs of the patient or carer to be identified. If necessary a dummy run could be enacted so the patient is more fully aware of what is expected.
- The carer should be involved at all times and be treated as a member of the healthcare team. Physical breaks and refreshments should be ensured.
- All GP and ward appointments for an X-ray examination should be referred to the responsible radiographer.
- The responsible radiographer should informed of any casualty patient with LD before the patient is sent for the X-ray examination.
- An information booklet for all staff should be produced.
- Medical imaging undergraduate programmes should include a clinical placement element with establishments dedicated to the care of people with LD.

These excellent suggestions are also extremely useful for care of children and others who lack mental capacity.

A letter to *Radiography*[12] on the article by Tony Browne on the needs of learning disabled patients and the differences between those with learning disabilities emphasised that some have lived in institutions and have a natural suspicion of health professionals. Others may associate a visit to hospital with punishment. Carers also may be unfamiliar with hospitals and be apprehensive or embarrassed in a situation that they do not fully understand. The writers recommend that in the case of learning disabilities, additional information should be provided on referral including the name, address and telephone number of a key and trusted carer, and the most convenient times for the hospital visit, taking into account transport arrangements and staffing levels. They also suggest that advance warning should be given and an explanation of what procedures are involved, especially with CT and MRI scans.

> Sometimes there is a suggestion that the patient needs sedation in advance of an X-ray/scan. It is very hard to predict in advance what dose of medication is required successfully and safely to reduce arousal, enabling the examination to take place. People with a learning disability are generally more sensitive to neuroleptic side effects and, in the case of benzodiazepines, there is the added risk of respiratory depression.

The correspondents suggest that X-ray departments and learning disability services could create protocols for dealing with these situations to their mutual benefit.

The appropriate adult

It is a requirement that where a person with learning disabilities is involved in any police investigations or court proceedings an 'appropriate adult' should be appointed to protect the interests of the patient.

An appropriate adult could be a parent, relative, advocate or other person capable of safeguarding the best interests of the patient with learning disabilities.

Access to health information

Where a patient lacks the mental capacity to make their own decisions, carers or relatives may seek access to their medical records. The provisions of the Data Protection Act 1998 and the Regulations under it (see Chapter 6) are open to different interpretations in relation to an application on behalf of a mentally incapacitated adult[13]. One interpretation is that relatives could have access to the records of a mentally incapacitated adult providing that it would be reasonable to comply with the request without the patient's consent. However the information must not have been given in the expectation that it would not be disclosed to the relatives in question and there must be no express prohibition by the patient (before the onset of the incapacity) on disclosure (see Chapter 6).

Reform of mental health care

Following publication of a consultation on the reform of the Mental Health Act 1983, a White Paper was issued in December 2000[14]. This proposes a new legal framework for the mentally disordered and the second part makes provision for high risk patients. The new mental health legislation will provide a single framework for the application of compulsory powers for care and treatment. The White paper states that the new legislation will be compatible with the European Convention on Human Rights.

At the time of writing this significant legislation protecting the interests of those adults lacking mental capacity is awaited. Only when this is enacted and implemented, can it be said that the human rights of this group of people are properly respected.

✍ **Questions and exercises** _____

1 What actions would you take as the manager of an X-ray department in respect of the care of mentally incapacitated adults.

2 A mentally incapacitated adult is being treated for cancer and requires radiotherapy. In what circumstances do you consider that sedation by medication would be justified?

3 You and your colleagues are concerned at the apparent harsh treatment which a carer is giving a patient with learning disabilities. What action could you take and what is the law?

4 In what circumstances could a mentally incapacitated adult refuse to undergo diagnostic procedures or receive treatment?

References

1 B. Dimond & F. Barker (1996) *Mental Health Law for Nurses*, Blackwell Science, Oxford, (2001), R. Jones *Mental Health Law*, 7th edn. Sweet & Maxwell, London

2 *Re MB (Adult: Medical Treatment)* [1997] 2 FLR 426

3 *Re C (Adult: Refusal of Medical Treatment)* [1994] 1 All ER 819

4 *F* v. *West Berkshire Health Authority and Another (Re F)*[1989] 2 All ER 545

5 Practice Note [1993] 3 All ER 222 (replaces previous practice Note issued 1989)

6 Law Commission (1995) Report No 231 *Mental Incapacity* HMSO, London

7 Lord Chancellor's Office (1997) *Who Decides* Lord Chancellor's Office

8 Lord Chancellor's Office (1999) *Making Decisions* Lord Chancellor's Office

9 *R* v. *Bournewood Community and Mental Health NHS Trust, ex parte L* [1998] 3 WLR 107

10 *Re F (Adult: Court's Jurisdiction)* [2000] 2 FLR 512

11 T.A. Browne (1999) Small Scale Exploratory Study of the Needs of Learning Disabled Patients Presenting for an X-ray examination *Radiography* **5**, 89–97

12 B. Fitzgerald & R. Fitzgerald (1999) Letter to the editor The needs of learning disabled patients presenting for an X-ray examination *Radiography* (May 1999) **5**, 177–9

13 I. Kennedy & A. Grubb (2000) *Medical Law* 3rd edn. Butterworths, London

14 Department of Health (2000) *Reforming the Mental Health Act* White Paper December 2000

Chapter 8
Legal Issues Relating to Children

Introduction

This chapter sets out the law relating to the care and rights of children, considers some situations which could arise and identifies some of the special arrangements which could be made for children in both diagnostic and therapeutic departments. The BMA has recently published guidance on the rights of the child and young person, which considers both the legal and ethical issues[1]. The legal situation of the unborn child and the law relating to congenital disabilities are discussed in Chapter 9.

Children Act 1989

This Act set up a new framework for the protection and care of children and established clear principles to guide decision making in relation to their care. The principles which the court should take into account are shown in Figure 8.1. The overriding principle is that 'the child's welfare shall be the court's paramount consideration'.

The Act is detailed and prescriptive and section 1(3) sets out the considerations which the court should take into account in making certain orders.

'(a) the ascertainable wishes and feelings of the child concerned (considered in the light of his age and understanding);
(b) his physical, emotional and educational needs;
(c) the likely effect on him of any change in his circumstances;
(d) his age, sex, background and any characteristics of his which the court considers relevant;
(e) any harm which he has suffered or is at risk of suffering;
(f) how capable each of his parents, and any other person in relation to whom the court considers the question to be relevant, is of meeting his needs;
(g) the range of powers available to the court under this Act in the proceedings in question.'

Finally in deciding whether or not to make an order, the court 'shall not make the order or any of the orders unless it considers that doing so would be better for the child than making no order at all'.

Whilst the considerations set out above apply to specific decisions to be made

Figure 8.1 **Principles of the Children Act 1989.**

- The welfare of the child is the paramount consideration in court proceedings.
- Wherever possible children should be brought up and cared for in their own families.
- Courts should ensure that delay is avoided.
- Children should be kept informed about what happens to them, and should participate when decisions are made about their future.
- Parents continue to have parental responsibility for their children, even when their children are no longer living with them. They should be kept informed about their children and participate when decisions are made about their children's future.
- Parents with children in need should be helped to bring up their children themselves.
- This help should be provided as a service to the child and his family, and should:
  - be provided in partnership with parents,
  - meet each child's identified needs,
  - be appropriate to the child's race, culture, religion, and language,
  - be open to effective independent representations and complaints procedures, and
  - draw upon effective partnership between the local authority and other agencies including voluntary agencies.

under the Act they provide a convenient 'checklist' for practitioners in the care of any child.

Child protection

The College of Radiographers has provided guidance on the implications for radiographers of the Children Act[2].

The importance of the radiographer knowing child protection principles (see Figure 8.1) and practice is emphasised in a guest editorial to *Radiography*[3]. This states

'The child protection responsibilities of the radiographer are clearly defined. These responsibilities fall into two distinct categories: diagnostic imaging for clinical and evidential purposes – these have been well documented – and the protection of children. Protection of children, as part of the routine care given by radiographers, is an area of growing concern and interest. However radiographers' knowledge of child protection has previously been reported as inadequate.'

The editorial refers to a regional survey that found only 17% of radiographers knew their Trust had procedures for child protection[4].

Initial concerns

Guidance for radiographers on child abuse and child protection is provided by Peter Hogg and others[5]. This emphasises that radiographers must be trained to be aware of relevant radiographic signs as well as non-radiographic manifestations, and be familiar with local procedures for raising concerns. There are two situations where radiographers are likely to be involved.

● where the imaging is directly concerned with suspected abuse;
● where concerns are raised because of the words of a child, their behaviour, physical signs of observed or imaging; and there will be a proportion of children they see who are likely to be experiencing abuse, even though no one outside the family is aware of the fact.

It is therefore important that radiographers are able to access child protection training courses.

A review of major aspects of the radiology of Non-accidental Injury (NAI) is given by Rao and Carty[6]. This shows the types of injuries seen in NAI with reference to their underlying causes and their varied presentations. The authors state.

'It is incumbent upon us all to be alert to the possibility of NAI. The diagnosis of abuse is straightforward if characteristic visible signs exist but in more subtle atypical cases the diagnosis may be overlooked. The main aims of radiological imaging are to document injuries and detect unsuspected or occult injuries. In many cases initial imaging in the emergency situation may be performed by a general radiologist. If there is doubt about the significance or presence of a lesion a second opinion should be sought from a paediatric radiologist. A wrong diagnosis of NAI is as devastating as a missed diagnosis. A missed diagnosis may condemn the child to continued abuse, which may subsequently result in severe mental and physical impairment or even death.'

Many radiographers are apprehensive of initiating the child protection process[7], expecting A&E staff and social services to take the lead. When a child has aroused suspicions, these are not followed up nor are they documented, as the temptation is to think that the child will either tell his story in A&E or other members of staff will share any suspicions and take the appropriate action.

Where a practitioner is concerned that a child or the sibling or child of one of her patients, is being abused, whether physically, sexually or mentally, she should take immediate action to ensure that this is drawn to the attention of the appropriate persons. She should also make a detailed record. She may have to give evidence in later proceedings and so a detailed contemporaneous record of her observations and actions is essential.

The practitioner may notice bruising, signs suggesting cigarette burns or other scars. Alternatively she may see a parent inflicting severe corporal punishment on a child and consider that action should be taken. All this means that she must be familiar with the provisions for child protection and know who to contact.

It is not always easy to decide if action is necessary, but the practitioner should see as her main priority the safety of the child. As 1991 DoH the guidelines on the Act and inter-agency co-operation state[8]:

'The difficulties of assessing the risk of harm to a child should not be underestimated. It is imperative that everyone who deals with allegations and suspicions of abuse maintains an open and inquiring mind.' (Paragraph 1.13)

It is known that inappropriate intervention can be damaging, but the decision of whether or not the relevant agencies should be informed is to be made by the senior person in the hospital who has the contact with the Social Services Department.

Procedure for the management of child abuse

NH trusts and other bodies should have an agreed procedure for the management of child abuse cases which any practitioner working with them should know about. Such a procedure should ideally set out the role of the department if child abuse is suspected. This could require anyone working in the department who suspects that there is a possibility of ill-treatment, serious neglect, sexual or emotional abuse of a child to inform the senior practitioner in charge of the department who should contact a consultant paediatrician. If the paediatrician confirms the possibility of abuse, then the Social Services Department should be informed immediately.

What if the doctor disagrees with the practitioner?

If the consultant takes the view that there is no abuse, then the practitioner has to accept this but should remain vigilant about the safety of the child and continue to report any further concerns. Unfortunately insufficient attention is often given to the views and evidence of non-medical staff and particularly non-registered staff. Louis Blom-Cooper pointed out in his Report on the Investigation of Jason Mitchell[9] that vital information was ignored by the multi-disciplinary team because it was reported by an occupational therapy assistant. Assertion skills and determination are obviously essential if there is a conflict over suspected abuse but all concerned should work within any procedural framework that has been laid down.

What about the practitioner's duty of confidentiality?

Apparent breaches of confidentiality are justified by most health professional organisations where they are necessary to protect the welfare of the patient or prevent harm, or are justified in the public interest. If the practitioner is in doubt, she should seek advice. The lawyers to the NHS trust would be able to advise on the legality of breaching confidentiality in exceptional circumstances. Any reasonable suspicion of child abuse can be notified to the appropriate agencies without fear of a successful action for breach of confidentiality by the parents. If a suspected case is reported to the police, social services, or NSPCC and it turns out that the suspicions are unfounded, the parents have no right to be given the name of the person reporting them. The House of Lords has held that it is not in the public interest for such information to be disclosed to the parents[10].

What if abuse is not certain?

If the consultant is not able to confirm the suspected child abuse and there are no medical grounds for requiring the child to be detained in hospital, then a parent could not be stopped from taking the child home. However there should ideally be arrangements in place for all such concerns to be notified to the appropriate health visitor or school nurse and also to the appropriate general practitioner.

What if suspected child abuse is confirmed by the consultant paediatrician?

The agreed procedures and the inter-agency arrangements should be followed immediately. The provisions of the Children Act 1989 enable the following orders to be made:

- child assessment order (section 43)
- emergency protection order (section 44)
- removal and accommodation by police in emergency (section 46).

For further details of these sections and the other provisions of the Children Act 1989 reference should be made to the Department of Health guides[11].

Inter-agency co-operation

There should be in existence in each local authority area, a forum to ensure co-operation between all the agencies involved in the protection of children at risk. This forum is known as the Area Child Protection Committee (ACPC). On this forum there should be representatives of the medical and nursing services. There are also advantages in having representatives from professions allied to medicine. This representation should be at a senior level and there should be a designated senior professional for child protection within each hospital or community unit.

Child protection register

Each local authority must maintain a child protection register. This provides a record of all children in the area who are currently the subject of a Child Protection Plan and helps to ensure that the plans are formally reviewed at least every six months. The register also acts as a central point of speedy inquiry for professional staff who are worried about a child and want to know whether official note has already been taken of similar concerns.

Access to this register would be permitted to an agreed list of personnel including senior medical staff or paediatric social workers in the local hospital departments. Radiographers are unlikely to be included in this agreed list but those to whom they make their concerns known under any local procedure would have access. Difficulties can sometimes arise if there is not a 24 hour access service to the register. This is a matter that could be brought up at the ACPC for arrangements to be made for the register to be kept by the paediatric or A&E department or by the police either of which would provide a 24 hour service.

Updated guidance has been produced by the Department of Health.

Consent by the child

Chapter 4 covers the basic principles relating to trespass to the person and the importance of obtaining the consent of the patient. This section deals with the specific laws relating to consent by or on behalf of the child (i.e. a person under 18 years of age).

The child of 16 and 17

A child of 16 or 17 has a statutory right to give consent to treatment under section 8 of the Family Law Reform Act 1969.

'(1) The consent of a minor who has attained the age of sixteen years, to any surgical, medical or dental treatment, which in the absence of consent, would constitute a trespass to the person, shall be as effective as it would be if he were of full age; and where a minor has by virtue of this section given an effective consent to any treatment it shall not be necessary to obtain any consent for it from his parent or guardian.

(2) In the section "surgical, medical or dental treatment" includes any procedure undertaken for the purposes of diagnosis, and this section applies to any procedures (including, in particular, the administration of an anaesthetic) which is ancillary to any treatment as it applies to that treatment.

(3) Nothing in the section shall be construed as making ineffective any consent which would have been effective if this section had not been enacted.'

The definition of treatment under section 8(2) would probably cover most treatments given by a practitioner where these are under the aegis of a doctor. Diagnosis and care provided by diagnostic and therapeutic radiographers would be included.

Section 8(3) covers two situations: the giving of consent by a parent on behalf of the child of 16 or 17 and the giving of consent of a Gillick competent child (see below) under 16 years.

It does not therefore follow that a child of 16 or 17 cannot be compelled to have treatment and the Court of Appeal in the case of *Re W*[12] upheld the decision of the High Court judge to order a child of 16 years who was suffering from anorexia nervosa to undergo medical treatment against her will. Parents can give consent on behalf of a child under 18 years but, if the child refuses the proposed treatment an application should be made to the court to determine what is in the child's best interests.

The child under 16

The parent has a right at common law to give consent on behalf of the child. In addition, as a result of the House of Lords ruling in the Gillick case[13] a child under 16 years who has sufficient understanding and intelligence to be capable of making up his own mind can give a valid consent to treatment. As a result of this case we now have the term 'Gillick competent' for children who have the maturity and competence to make a decision in the specific circumstances arising.

In life saving situations however it is unlikely that the child under 16 years would be able to make a decision contrary to his or her best interests. Even where the child and parents both agree that treatment should not be given, as in the case of a Jehovah's Witness family, the court can order treatment to proceed if it is considered to be in the best interests of the child[14].

Disputes between parents

Even when parents are divorced or separated, under the Children Act 1989 section 2(1) both parents retain 'parental responsibility' for their children. Under section 2(7) where more than one person has parental responsibility for a child each of them may act alone and without the other (or others) in meeting that responsibility. Even where one parent has a residence order in their favour, the other still retains parental responsibility and can exercise this to the full. It also follows that one parent does not have the right of veto over the other's actions. If however there has been a specific order by the court relating to a decision affecting the care or treatment of the child, then a single parent cannot change this or take any action which is incompatible with this order unless the approval of the court is obtained.

It therefore follows that, if there is a dispute between parents over treatment decisions in respect of the child, the matter needs to be taken to court for a specific issue or prohibited steps order to be made.

Prohibited steps order

Where one parent wishes to prevent the other taking action he may seek a prohibited steps order. This is made under section 8 of the Children Act 1989 and means that no step which could be taken by a parent in meeting their parental responsibility for a child and which is of the kind specified in the order shall be taken without the consent of the court. It is usually used on matters of travel and contact but if one parent feared, for example, that the other was likely to agree to a mentally impaired daughter being sterilised or a younger child being given a controversial vaccine then that parent could obtain a prohibited steps order preventing that procedure without the consent of the court.

If the child is over 16 or considered to be 'Gillick competent' and disagreed with the actions which his parents were intending, he could also seek the leave of the court to obtain a prohibited steps order. The child would have to apply to the High Court and the court must be satisfied that the child has sufficient understanding to make the proposed application (section 10(8))[15].

Specific issue order

This is similar but applies where action is to be taken rather than prevented.

Parental refusal

Pursuing the best overall outcome

Doctors can obtain legal authority from the court to proceed in the best interests of the child even where the parents' consent is withheld. This can sometimes give rise to difficult legal and ethical issues. In a recent case[16] the Court of Appeal declared that it was lawful for Siamese twins to be separated, even though the operation would necessarily involve the death of the twin who was dependent upon the heart and the lungs of the other for survival.

Case: *Re A (minors) (conjoined twins: medical treatment)*

By international arrangements a Maltese woman, anticipating difficulties, came to Manchester where the Siamese twins were born by caesarean section on 8 August 2000. The bodies of the two girls were fused together at the base of their spines. The parents, both devout Roman Catholics, had refused consent to any operation to separate them. The doctors applied to the High Court for a declaration that it would be lawful to separate the twins. Medical evidence presented to the court suggested that one sister, Jodie, could have a reasonable chance of survival if they were to be separated, but such an operation would mean the death of the other, Mary. If no operation were performed, then there was a likelihood that Jodie would not survive for many months because of the additional strain placed upon her heart and Jodie's death would inevitably be followed by Mary's. The High Court judge issued a declaration that the operation should proceed. The parents appealed against this decision. The Court of Appeal asked for additional medical evidence, and also received a submission from the Catholic Archbishop of Westminster.

The Court of Appeal held it was lawful for doctors to carry out the operation to separate the twins. The crucial questions to be answered were:

(1) Was it in Jodie's best interests that she be separated from Mary?
(2) Was it in Mary's best interests that she be separated from Jodie?
(3) If those interests were in conflict was the court to balance the interests of one against the other and allow one to prevail against the other and how was that to be done?
(4) If the prevailing interest favoured the operation, could it be lawfully performed?

The Court concluded that the operation would give Jodie the prospects of a normal expectation of relatively normal life. The operation would shorten Mary's life but she would be likely to die in any event as she would survive only as long as Jodie survived and Jodie was unlikely to live very long if the operation did not proceed.

The operation could be carried out under the doctrine of necessity. The essential elements of that doctrine were all satisfied:

● the act was needed to avoid inevitable and irreparable harm
● no more would be done than was reasonably necessary for the purpose to be achieved
● the harm inflicted was not disproportionate to the harm avoided.

The court further held that its decision was not in conflict with Article 2 of the European Convention on Human Rights.

The parents were given leave to appeal to the House of Lords but decided not to do so. The operation was carried out: Mary died and Jodie survived. The extent of her disabilities are not known. At the Inquest a unique finding of death was made, the coroner resorting to a 'narrative verdict': 'Mary died after surgery to separate her from her conjoined twin, and that the surgery was permitted by order of the High Court, confirmed by the Court of Appeal'[17].

Diagnostic tests
What if the circumstances in which the parents refuse to consent to a diagnostic

test are not immediately life threatening, could the refusal be overruled? For example, parents may decide that a skeletal survey for NAI in a child should not be carried out, what is the legal position? In such a situation, it is probable that the local authority would be involved and therefore if it was considered to be in the best interests of the child, an application could be made to court under the Children Act 1989 for the necessary tests to be conducted. The parents' refusal could therefore be overruled. Evidence would be required on what was in the child's best interests.

In other situations, parents may consent to plain films, but not to magnetic resonance (MRI), or ultra-sound, or computerised tomography or radionuclide imaging (RNI). It may be that the more sophisticated tests are not absolutely essential and the parents' refusal can be accepted. If this is not so and the additional tests are necessary in the best interests of the child, then an application would have to be made to court for a declaration that they can be lawfully carried out. In such situations there will be examples where it is of life-saving necessity that certain tests or treatments are carried out, in which case the appropriate action will be taken and court authorisation obtained and at the other extreme there will be treatments and diagnostic tests which would have been helpful, but can be omitted without serious harm to the child. Between these two extremes there will be very difficult decisions to make.

Parents' refusal upheld by the courts

In the case of *Re T*[18] the court unusually upheld the parents' refusal to consent to liver transplant for their baby. The facts were unusual in that the parents lived outside the country and were health professionals. The Court of Appeal upheld the appeal of the parents against the High Court judge's order that the transplant should proceed. The paramount consideration was the welfare of the child and not the reasonableness of the parent's refusal of consent. It must be stressed that *Re T* is a very unusual case and there were very special circumstances which led to the court upholding the wishes of the parents over those of the doctors.

Right to insist on treatment

Parents do not have the right to insist upon care or treatment which the doctors consider is unjustified or not in the best interests of the child. As has been discussed in Chapter 3, the courts will not generally interfere in the allocation of resources or clinical judgment in individual cases (see the case of Jamie Bowen referred to in Chapter 3).

Confidentiality and health records

Confidentiality of child information

The same principles apply in relation to maintaining the confidentiality of information provided by the child patient (16 and 17 year olds and Gillick competent under 16s) as apply to information provided by the adult patient (see Chapter 5). However there may be situations where the interests of the child require confidential information to be passed on to an appropriate authority or their parents. If possible the consent of the child should be obtained to the disclosure. However where the child refuses consent, or where the child lacks the capacity to give consent, the practitioner should notify the child of her view that the information should be passed on in his best interests. A practitioner may learn, in confidence, from the mother that there is abuse by the stepfather. She should try to obtain consent to pass this information on, but it may be necessary to breach confidence in the interests of the child.

The practitioner should not make a commitment to the child or anyone else that the confidential information will never be passed on but she should also ensure that she takes advice before breaching confidentiality. She should record the action she has taken and the reasons for it, and be prepared to justify her actions if subsequently challenged.

Access to children's health records

Chapter 6 covers the basic principles which apply to access to health records. Here we are concerned with access to records about children.

Access by child to his health records
The Data Protection Act 1998 does not make express provision for access by a child but such an application would come under section 7. Where the child has the capacity he can apply under the Act for access to his personal health data kept in both computerised form and held manually. The data would include plain film images as a result of radiographic investigation. No definition of the capability of the child is given in the Act but it is submitted that the Gillick test of competence (see above) adapted to the specific conditions of access to records would be applied. It would also be good practice to follow the Department of Health recommendation[19] concerning the provisions of the 1984 Data Protection Act that a responsible adult should certify that the child understands the nature of the application.

Unlike the provisions under the Access to Health Records Act 1990 (where access to a child's records could be refused if it was not in the child's best interests), access can be refused only if serious harm to the physical or mental health or condition of the patient or another person would be caused, or where a third person who has asked not to be identified would be identified by the disclosure (see Chapter 6). It is a defect in the new legislation that the special case of children is not considered.

Rights of the parents
The exclusion of access provisions apply (see Chapter 6) and significantly a Gillick competent child or a 16 or 17 year old can state at the outset that their records are not to be disclosed to their parents.

Standards in the care of children

Chapter 14 sets out the principles of law which apply in ensuring that reasonable standards of professional care are provided. For children particularly this will include multi-disciplinary team working and the rational determination of priorities. Practitioners must ensure that they maintain their competence and that they keep up to date with developments in their field of specialisation. Multi-disciplinary care of the child may involve the use of unorthodox treatments and investigations. However the practitioner must be aware that there is no legal concept of team liability, and if she acts contrary to the standards of professional competence of a reasonable practitioner in her field, she could not use as a defence that she was carrying out the instructions of the team. If therefore a team member proposes an unorthodox treatment or investigation in the care of a child, she must be assured that this complies with the reasonable standards of care and that the parents/and or the child have given consent to the treatment, in the full knowledge that the proposed treatment is not of the usual kind, but is in the circumstances justifiable.

Roger Taylor writes about the importance of a specialist multi-disciplinary team working in the field of paediatric oncology and considers the *Guidelines for Services for Children and Young People with Brain and Spinal Tumours*[20], published by the United Kingdom Childrens' Cancer Study Group (UKCCSG) (a network of 22 Paediatric Oncology Centres). The guidelines describe the multi-disciplinary team and the support services required. They also include a series of clinical scenarios illustrating the varied diagnoses and problems which need to be tackled.

Guidelines on Best Practice in the X-Ray imaging of children[21] is a manual provided by the radiographers and radiologists at St George's Hospital, who used as their basis the European guidelines on Quality Criteria to Diagnostic Radiographic Images. Such works are of considerable value to other practitioners in other hospitals but it does not follow that the procedures recommended in it are necessarily the ones which all hospitals must follow. There may be professional differences of opinion over the most appropriate procedure in a given set of circumstances. National criteria based on research of clinically effective practice will always have to be updated in the light of changing developments.

Paediatric Special Interest Groups

The advantages of establishing a Paediatric Special Interest Group (PSIG) are spelt out by Melanie Drummond and Claire York[22] from their experience at Kettering General Hospital. The PSIG was established to evaluate paediatric practice in order to achieve consistently the highest possible standards of paediatric radiography. The PSIG was eventually composed of six radiographers plus a medical physicist, the radiology services manager and a consultant radiologist. It developed paediatric examination protocols (liasing with others such as paediatric, A&E and orthopaedic clinicians) took action to reduce exposure levels, established written policies (including consent and pregnancy policies) and carried out audits in specified areas.

A study by Maryann Hardy[23] highlights a need for paediatric imaging education at all levels, from interest-only study days and short courses designed for evidencing continuous professional development (CPD) to recognised postgraduate qualifications.

Occupier's liability and a child

Where a child is allowed onto premises the duty of the occupier to ensure that the visitor is reasonably safe takes into account the fact that children will require a higher standard of care than an adult. Thus the Occupier's Liability Act 1957 specifically states 'an occupier must be prepared for children to be less careful than adults' (section 2(3), see Figure 15.7 on p. 189).

Practitioners must therefore take into account any reasonably foreseeable harm which could arise if children come into their departments or onto their premises[24].

A duty of care may also be owed under the Occupier's Liability Act 1957 in respect of children who come onto hospital premises with their parents who are the patients. Unless their presence is expressly prohibited they would also come under the definition of visitors.

Case: *Glass door injuries*[25]

A 13 year old pupil was injured when she pushed open the right hand door of double doors comprising glass panes. Her hand slipped from the push plate onto the adjacent panel of glass. The glass shattered causing severe injuries to her right hand and wrist. The County Council was found liable under the Occupier's Liability Act 1957 and at common law in failing to fulfil its duty of care. It had failed to comply with the BS standards for glass in doors. There was no finding of contributory negligence

Appropriate precautions
Precautions therefore have to be taken to prevent children harming themselves in Radiology Departments. Doors into cupboards containing hazardous substances should be kept locked to prevent accidents. Special procedures should be in place if patients are accompanied by children.

Other examples of potential dangers include:

- Drugs on the cardiac arrest trolley. (This needs to be accessible in case of an emergency, but kept in a safe place away from children.)
- Syringes and needles on trolleys as above.
- Fingers sliced by rise and fall floating top tables.

Contributory negligence and the child

In Chapter 14 the defence of contributory negligence is discussed. This means that if the client is partly to blame for the harm which has occurred then there may still be liability on the part of the professional but the compensation payable might be reduced in proportion to the client's fault. However where a child has been harmed, any defence of contributory negligence must take into account the fact that a child is less capable than an adult of taking care of him or herself. The courts have been reluctant to find contributory negligence by a child where an adult is at fault, as the case of *Gough* v. *Thorne*[26] illustrates.

Control of the child

Corporal punishment of any kind is unacceptable and may be contrary to the rights of the child following a decision of the European Court of Human Rights in Strasbourg[27]. Even if corporal punishment is the parents' main form of control it is not open to the health practitioner to use it. However the borderline between restraint and physical control may not always be easy to discern. Difficult children can be extremely demanding and may require increased staffing. In certain circumstances, where it is vital to ensure that treatment or investigations are carried out, some sedation may be in the best interests of the child. Distraction techniques are described by Joanne Hodgson[28] in relation to carrying out a micturating cysto-urethrogram. Sedation is not routinely given in her department since it reduces the chance of the child voiding voluntarily. With older children it was found that a full explanation of the procedure usually achieved co-operation without resorting to play therapy.

Radiographic aides can be used to assist in the care of younger children and some departments employ play specialists[29]. There are clear advantages since they have the time to reassure children, pick up on any misconceptions and provide information. Feedback from the radiographer as to how the tactics worked can be useful in assisting other child patients.

The different uses of sedation and anaesthesia in Radiology are considered in a report prepared by a Joint Working party of the RCR and the Royal College of Anaesthetists[30] which states:

'Children often find simple radiological procedures frightening and painful. Young children may require sedation for any procedure where they are required to lie still. The presence of a parent with a child during a procedure may reduce the need for sedation and should be encouraged.'

The Human Rights Act (see Chapter 3) will have an impact on standards for the care of children and their rights, but at this early stage, before the cases are heard, it is difficult to estimate its effect.

The role of the expert witness in child abuse cases

Case: *Re AB (Child Abuse: Expert Witnesses)*[31]

In this case there was a dispute between experts over whether the medical conditions suffered by a child were the result of non-accidental injury. The facts were that a baby of 10 weeks suffered what the parents described as an apnoeic attack. After resuscitating him by allegedly shaking and smacking him, they called a doctor who sent him to hospital. There he was found to have multiple fractures and some brain damage. The evidence was that the fractures were recent and had occurred on two or three separate occasions and that the brain damage had occurred some days before admission. The three experts (a paediatric consultant and two consultant paediatric radiologists) called by the local authority and guardian ad litem were of the view that the injuries were non-accidental. The medical expert called by the parents considered that in the absence of bruising, and the fact that nothing untoward had been noticed by the health visitor, grandparents or others, the injuries were due to some form of brittle bone disease which, since the baby had never suffered from osteogenesis imperfecta, he categorised as 'temporary brittle bone disease'.

Judge Wall held that it was clear that the baby's injuries were entirely consistent with non-accidental injury and inconsistent with anything else. He discounted the evidence of the expert called by the parents since he had failed to take into account or to explain the brain damage, research showed that the absence of bruising did not have the significance which he had placed on it, and he had not only failed to disclose the controversial nature of his research into temporary brittle bone disease but appeared to have assumed the role of advocate to promote his belief in it. It was therefore held that the child had suffered multiple non-accidental injuries whilst in the care of his parents.

The judge emphasised that the duty of an expert witness in children's cases is to form an assessment and express his opinion within the particular area of his expertise. The judge, having no medical training, decides particular issues in individual cases on the basis of all the evidence. It follows that the dependence of the court on the skill, knowledge and, above all, the professional integrity of the expert witness cannot be overemphasised.

The following points for expert witnesses were laid down by the judge:

- Where an expert advances a hypothesis to explain a given set of facts, he owes a very heavy duty to explain to the court that what he is advancing is a hypothesis, that it is controversial (if it is) and to place before the court all the material which contradicts the hypothesis.
- The expert must also make all his material available to other experts in the case.
- Where the medical evidence points overwhelmingly to non-accidental injury, any expert who advises the parents and the court that the injury has an innocent explanation has a heavy duty to ensure that he has considered carefully the available material and is expressing an opinion that can be objectively justified.

The role of the expert witness following the Woolf Reforms in civil justice is discussed further in Chapter 18.

Conclusions

Paediatric care can present considerable challenges to the practitioner. Many lessons can be learnt from a clear and consistent monitoring of the service provided and a willingness to learn from weaknesses. Lynne Howard[32] writing in the occupational therapists' journal has researched multi-disciplinary quality assessment in relation to the child development team and concludes that quality assessment requires a judicious combination of both consumer satisfaction and professional standard setting and the biggest stumbling block is outcome assessment. This may also be true of many different specialities within radiography and oncology and must be remedied if the practitioner is to play his or her full role in the care of the child.

Questions and exercises _____

1 A parent brings to the department a child whom you suspect is subject to abuse. Outline the procedure which you would follow.

2 You are involved in the care of a girl with learning disabilities and learn that her mother wishes her to be sterilised. You are of the view that her disability is not severe. What action would you take? (See also Chapter 4.)

3 A child that you are caring for tells you in confidence that she is being abused by her father. She emphasises that she does not want you to take any action. What is the legal situation? Does the age of the child make any difference and if so how?

4 You were involved in the taking of X-ray images of a child who was subsequently the subject of child abuse investigations and a prosecution. You have been asked to attend as a witness at court. How would you prepare for giving evidence? (See also Chapter 18.)

References

1 British Medical Association (2001) *Consent, Rights and Choices in Health Care for Children and Young People* BMJ Books, London

2 College of Radiographers (1995) *The implications for radiographers of the Children Act* College of Radiographers, London

3 P. Hogg (1999) Guest Editorial *Radiography* (August 1999) **5**, 3, p. 127

4 J. Sudbery, C. Eaton, V. Hancock & P. Hogg (1997) Child Protection and radiography: social and emotional context, *Child Abuse Review* **6**, 283–90

5 P. Hogg, D. Hogg, J. Sudbery & C. Eaton (2000) Child abuse and child protection *Synergy* (October 2000) p. 17–19

6 P. Rao & H. Carty (1999) Non-accidental Injury: Review of the radiology *Clinical Radiology* (January 1999) **54**, p. 11–24

7 Michaela Davis PhD research – personal communication with the author

8 Home Office, Department of Health, Department of Education and Science, Welsh Office (1991) *Working Together Under the Children Act 1989: a guide to arrangements for inter-agency co-operation for the protection of children from abuse.* HMSO, London; and Department of Health, Home Office, Department for Education and Employment, National Assembly for Wales (1999) *Working together to safeguard children* Department of Health, London

9 L. Blom-Cooper *et al* (1996) *The case of Jason Mitchell: Report of the Independent Panel of Inquiry* Duckworth, London

10 *D* v. *National Society for the Prevention of Cruelty to Children* [1977] 1 All ER 589

11 Department of Health (1989) *An introductory guide to the Children Act for the NHS.* HMSO, London

12 *Re W (a minor) (Medical Treatment)* [1992] 4 All ER 627

13 *Gillick* v. *West Norfolk and Wisbech Area Health Authority* [1986] 1 AC 112

14 *Re E (a Minor) (Wardship: Medical Treatment)* [1993] 1 FLR 386

15 See further the rights of the child as applicant in: N. Wyld (1994) *When Parents Separate* Children's Legal Centre, 20 Compton Terrace, London. N1 2UN

16 *Re A (Minors) (Conjoined twins: Medical Treatment)* The Times Law Report, 10 October 2000; [2001] Fam 147 CA

17 R. Jenkins (2000) Coroner records rare verdict on Siamese twin *The Times* 16 December

18 *Re T(a Minor) (Wardship: medical treatment)* [1997] 1 All ER 906; *Re C (a minor-refusal of parental consent)* [1997] 8 Med LR 166

19 HC (89)29 paragraph 4

20 R. Taylor (1998) *Guidelines for Services for Children and Young People with Brain and Spinal Tumours* RCoR, Issue No 53 (Winter 1998) p. 15

21 J.V. Cook, A. Pettett and others (1999) *Guidelines on Best Practice in the X-Ray Imaging of Children* St George's Healthcare Radiological Protection Centre, St George's Hospital, London

22 M. Drummond & C. York (2001) Evaluating paediatric practice and care *Synergy* (February 2001) pages 20–21

23 M. Hardy 2000 Paediatric radiography: is there a need for postgraduate education? *Radiography* (February 2000), **6**, 27–34

24 *Jolley* v. *Sutton London Borough Council* The Times Law Report, 24 May 2000; [2000] 3 All ER 409

25 *J (a Minor)* v. *Staffordshire County Council* CLR 1997 Vol 2, paragraph 3783

26 *Gough* v *Thorne* [1966] 3 All ER 398

27 *A* v. *The United Kingdom* (100/1997/884/1096) judgment on 23 September 1998

28 J. Hodgson (2000) Distraction techniques for use in Micturating Cysto-urethrograms *Synergy* (January 2000) pages 8–9

29 G. Cox (1999) Child's Play *Synergy* (October 1999) pages 14–15

30 Royal College of Anaesthetists and Royal College of Radiologists (1992) *Sedation and Anaesthesia in Radiology: Report of Joint Working Party* (July 1992)

31 *Re AB (Child Abuse: Expert Witnesses)* [1995] 1 FLR 181, [1995] 1 FCR 280

32 L.M. Howard (1994) Multidisciplinary Quality assessment: The case of the child development team Parts 1, 2 and 3 *British Journal of Occupational Therapy* **57**, 9, 10, and 11, 345–8, 393–6 and 437–440

Chapter 9
The Pregnant Patient

This chapter discusses the issues which arise when caring for pregnant patients Dental radiography and pregnant patients are considered in Chapter 25.

Standards of care

Reasonable standards of care require specific precautions for any woman of child bearing age who is or may be pregnant. Clearly in the context of diagnostic radiography every care must be taken to prevent the exposure of the fetus to X-rays. In the field of therapeutic radiography special procedures are required to minimise any potential harm to the child if the woman is pregnant, or to the child-bearing capacity of the woman. Therefore failure to make the appropriate inquiries and to take the necessary action which results in harm to the woman or baby could lead to claims for compensation. To succeed a woman would have to show that the health professional was in breach of the duty of care owed to her by failing to take account of her pregnancy or childbearing potential and as a consequence she has suffered harm. The health professional's employer would be vicariously liable (see Chapter 14).

The potential for damage

In a review article Osei and Faulkner[1] conclude that very early and later stages of fetal development are at lower risk exposure to diagnostic medical ionising radiation than the period in between. The authors also state that:

'In general, risks from medical X-ray examination(s) are so small, that a mother-to-be who realises that her developing child has been irradiated should have no cause for additional anxiety. In utero exposure to diagnostic X-rays represents a very low additional risk to the developing embryo or fetus when compared to the other effects.'

In spite of this conclusion, inadvertent irradiation of a pregnant woman could lead to litigation if the child is found to be suffering from disabilities, though it may be difficult for the parents to prove causation.

So far as child-bearing capacity is concerned, in certain circumstances retrieval of eggs prior to radiotherapy may be clinically indicated.

Protection of the fetus from irradiation – the '28 day and 10 day rules'

The NRPB issued a statement in 1993 on diagnostic medical exposures to ionising radiation during pregnancy[2]. A small group was set up with representatives of the NRPB, the College of Radiographers and the Royal College of Radiologists to develop a practical guide for practitioners and a booklet published[3]. The booklet introduces the terms used, gives practical guidance on the implementation of the advice and provides the scientific background to the advice. Following the obtaining of information about the patient, the women can be assigned to one of the following groups:

- No possibility of pregnancy
- Patient definitely, or probably pregnant

Subsequent care will depend upon whether a low dose or high dose procedure is required. In a woman of child-bearing potential, low dose X-rays should be done within 28 days of the last menstrual period, 'the 28 day rule'. High dose radiation procedures and all nuclear medicine procedures should be done within 10 days of the last menstrual period, 'the 10 day rule'.

In practice there may be situations where these rules may not be adhered to or where there may be uncertainties about dates. The radiologist would advise the referring clinician of the dangers and the clinician would have to balance the risks of harm to the woman and foetus against the benefits to be achieved by carrying out the investigation. In certain cases a pregnancy test would be carried out. If inadvertent radiation does occur, then there is a clear procedure to follow in notification to the Radiation Protection Officer who will undertake an investigation.

The guidance emphasises that:

'Subsequently, if it becomes obvious that a fetus has been inadvertently exposed, despite the above guidance, the small risk to the fetus of the exposure does not justify the greater risks of invasive fetal diagnostic procedures to the fetus and mother (particularly as they are unlikely to pick up any induced effect), nor does the risk justify those of a termination of the pregnancy to the mother'.

Mis-information from the patient

What if the woman fails to answer the questions correctly? What reliance can be placed upon her response? Since untruthful answers can be anticipated for a variety of reasons, it is preferable that every precaution is taken against the possibility of harm to a fetus or to her child-bearing potential even though the woman may have denied that pregnancy is a likely possibility.

What if a woman signs a form that she is not pregnant, would that be a valid defence if in fact it turns out that she is pregnant? A distinction would have to be made between the situation where a woman knew that she was pregnant but signed a form denying it and where a woman did not know that she was pregnant, though in fact she was. If the former can be established, then any claim by the woman could be defeated on the grounds that she gave false information and thereby contributed to the harm that she or the baby has suffered. (For details on contributory negligence see Chapter 14.) The baby could not sue the mother for causing any prenatal injuries by this false information (see below on the Congenital Disabilities Act). In the other situation, where the woman signed the form, not knowing that she was actually pregnant, its existence would be of little relevance since the radiographers should in any event have treated her as though she might be pregnant, in spite of the form being signed. It would appear that the form is only of value if there has been deliberate fraud by the woman which would be very hard to prove.

Alternatives to X-rays

If it is not possible to take an X-ray because the patient was pregnant then the results of other investigations must be looked at very carefully as the following case shows.

Case: *No X-ray because of pregnancy*[4]

Mrs Hutton was admitted to hospital on 1 January 1991 suffering from severe retrosternal pain, with a cough, general lethargy, nausea and vomiting, and heart-burn. ECGs were carried out, but a chest X-ray was not taken because a pregnancy test was positive. She was discharged four days later. The next day she suffered a pulmonary embolus and died. If she had been treated with heparin she would probably have survived to live a normal life. Her husband brought a medical negligence action and succeeded on the following grounds;

- The severe pain she suffered on admission was probably due to an intermediate sized pulmonary embolus.
- The ECGs showed a number of abnormalities.
- Factors existed which should have been interpreted as an indication of the possibility at least of a respiratory problem or a haemodynamic disturbance in the pulmonary circuit.
- The local consultant physician was negligent in that he not only put pulmonary embolism relatively low on his list of possibilities but discarded it altogether.

The claimant was awarded the agreed sum of £95 000.

Giving information and the patient's responsibilities

In securing consent to therapeutic or diagnostic investigations, risks relating to a fetus or to child-bearing abilities should be disclosed to the patient as part of the duty of care to inform (see Chapter 4). The standard to be followed in the giving of information is that set down in the Bolam test, i.e. it should be according to the reasonable standard of accepted practice which would be supported by a competent body of professional opinion.

In what circumstances can it be assumed that the patient will accept responsibility for certain side effects and therefore cannot hold the health professional liable if harm occurs?

Situation: voluntary assumption of risk

A young girl of 20 requires radiotherapy which could render her sterile. She agrees that she will accept that risk. However ten years later, when she is in remission from her illness, she wishes to start a family and is holding the health professionals liable for her sterility.

Liability would depend upon

- her level of mental capacity at the time she agreed to assuming the risk
- whether she was given the necessary information (and understood it) and
- whether there was any other reasonable action which could have been taken (and which any reasonable health professional would have taken) to avoid that particular side effect of the treatment.

There could be a failure to give her the correct information and/or also a failure to give her the clinically indicated treatment taking into account her situation. If failure to give her the correct information is alleged, to succeed in obtaining compensation, the patient would have to prove that, had she been given the correct information, she would not have gone ahead with the treatment she had or she would have taken other action of which she was not advised (see Chapter 4 on consent and giving information to patients).

Abortion laws

A termination of pregnancy is lawful provided that it is undertaken under the statutory provisions. The Abortion Act 1967 was amended by the Human Fertilisation and Embryology Act 1990 and section 1(1) is set out in Figure 9.1. The time limit of 24 weeks only applies to the first ground for termination of pregnancy. The other three grounds, including that of the child suffering from serious disabilities, do not have a time limit. Therefore where it is discovered that there is substantial risk that if the child were born it would suffer from such physical or

---

Figure 9.1 **Abortion Act 1967, section 1(1).**

Subject to the provisions of this section, a person shall not be guilty of an offence under the law relating to abortion, when a pregnancy is terminated by a registered medical practitioner if two registered medical practitioners are of the opinion, formed in good faith—

(a)   that the pregnancy has not exceeded its twenty-fourth week and that the continuance of the pregnancy would involve risk, greater than if the pregnancy were terminated, of injury to the physical or mental health of the pregnant woman or any existing children of her family; or

(b)   that the termination is necessary to prevent grave permanent injury to the physical or mental health of the pregnant woman; or

(c)   that the continuance of the pregnancy would involve risk to the life of the pregnant woman, greater that if the pregnancy were terminated; or

(d)   that there is substantial risk that if the child were born it would suffer from such physical or mental abnormalities as to be seriously handicapped.

mental abnormalities as to be seriously handicapped, a termination may be carried out at a very late stage in the pregnancy.

Section 1(2) states that in determining whether the continuance of a pregnancy would involve such risk of injury to health as is mentioned in paragraph (a) or (b) of subsection (1), account may be taken of the pregnant woman's actual or reasonably foreseeable environment.

Multiple pregnancies

The Human Fertilisation and Embryology Act 1990 added a further amendment to the Abortion Act 1967 to cover the situation where one or more fetus(es) in a multiple pregnancy is terminated. The termination may be justified either to protect the health or life of the mother or if there is a substantial risk that if the child were born it would suffer from such physical or mental abnormalities as to be seriously handicapped (i.e. section 1(1)(d)) of the Abortion Act 1967).

Emergency situations

In an emergency situation the requirements of section 1 are dispensed with and section 1(4) applies (see Figure 9.2).

Figure 9.2   Termination in an emergency, section 1(4).

Subsection (3) of this section, and so much of subsection (1) as relates to the opinion of two registered medical practitioners, shall not apply to the termination of a pregnancy by a registered medical practitioner in a case where he is of the opinion, formed in good faith, that the termination is immediately necessary to save the life or to prevent grave permanent injury to the physical or mental health of the pregnant woman.

Conscientious objection

The Abortion Act also gives a right to a person not to participate in a termination of pregnancy if they have a conscientious objection to it. See Figure 9.3.

Figure 9.3   Conscientious objection, section 4.

(1)   Subject to subsection (2) of this section, no person shall be under any duty, whether by contract or by any statutory or other legal requirement, to participate in any treatment authorised by this Act to which he has a conscientious objection: ...

(2)   Nothing in subsection (1) of this section shall affect any duty to participate in treatment which is necessary to save the life or to prevent grave permanent injury to the physical or mental health of a pregnant woman.

In the case of *Janaway* v. *Salford*[5] the House of Lords held that this protection did not apply to a secretary who wrote the referral letters for a termination of pregnancy. It held that the word participate should be given its natural meaning, i.e. actually taking part in treatment and the work of a secretary was too ancillary to the abortion procedure.

There is no decided case on whether a radiographer or radiologist assisting in radiography of a women who wanted a termination could exercise a right of conscientious objection. It depends upon whether the taking and interpreting of the X-ray would constitute taking part in the termination.

Ultrasound and the legal issues arising

Ultrasound is the emission of high frequency sound waves by an ultrasound probe to travel through the body and bounce off various layers of tissues. The probe then hears these echoes which are relayed onto a screen and the resulting pictures are interpreted.

The role that ultrasound can play in diagnosing conditions such as:

- placenta praevia
- abruptions
- incompetent cervix
- fetal distress
- congenital abnormalities
- infection
- multiple births and
- ruptured membranes

all of which can lead to premature labour, is described in an article by Gail Ashington[6].

Ultrasound and fertility treatment

Where a patient is receiving fertility treatment it would be possible for a practitioner to rely on the conscientious objection clause contained in section 38 of the Human Fertilisation and Embryology Act 1990.

'(1) No person who has a conscientious objection to participating in any activity governed by this Act shall be under any duty, however arising, to do so.
(2) In any legal proceedings the burden of proof of conscientious objection shall rest on the person claiming to rely on it.'

Reasonable standard of care

Unrealistic expectations may accompany the carrying out of a ultrasound scan. For example if an abnormality is not discovered, then the woman may wish to sue because this defect has not been detected. Does the reasonable standard of care require all abnormalities to be detected? Is a margin of error accepted by the courts? How is the reasonable standard of care defined?

These are similar to the issues which arose in the case brought against Kent

NHS trust in respect of standards of cervical screening[7] (considered in detail in Chapter 14). The Court of Appeal dismissed the appeal by the health authority and upheld the finding that the Health Authority was liable. It held that the Bolam test (the requisite standard being that of an ordinarily competent professional) was only appropriate where the exercise of skill and judgment of the screener was being questioned. In this case the Bolam test did not apply since the screeners were not expected to exercise judgment. The decision has been criticised on the grounds that cervical screeners are expected to exercise some professional judgment in deciding which slides should be subjected to further scrutiny. Clearly the role of the ultrasound practitioner and the task of inter-preting the pictures does require the exercise of professional judgment and it is hoped, in fairness to the practitioner, that the courts would hold that the Bolam test does apply to such activity.

Fetal sex determination

There appears to be an increasing interest in parents discovering the sex of the fetus as indicated in an article by Gail Ashington[8]. Motives will differ as will the views of the parents over whether they wish to know in advance. A termination of pregnancy on the grounds of the sex of the child would not come within the provisions of the Abortion Act 1967 (see above) unless genetic analysis of the parents indicates potential for a sex-linked congenital abnormality that creates a substantial risk of the child being born seriously handicapped. However many parents, after discovering the sex of the baby following the ultrasound scan, may seek a termination for reasons not connected with serious handicap. For example there may be cultural considerations where a boy is the preferred choice or, if parents have already several children of one sex, they may consider a termination if the fetus is not of the other sex.

The article by Gail Ashington promoted debate and information sharing – the Superintendent Sonographer in the ultrasound department at Milton Keynes, where they had a policy document on sexing the fetus, pointed out[9] the sheer number of ultrasounds carried out each year and the fact that the 15–20 minutes allocated time per ultrasound was to carry out the main investigations required. She added that there was a danger that increased pressure resulting from requests for sex determination might lead to the risk of overlooking some more subtle structural abnormalities. In another response[10], the Senior Ultra-sonographer at Norfolk and Norwich Healthcare Trust stated that guidelines were used in the department, on legal advice, and the policy now was:

● not to extend the examination time in order to sex the baby,
● to admit if there is any difficulty,
● to obtain verbal consent and document this in the mother's maternity notes, but
● not to record the sex in the notes.

In another response[11] a Superintendent Sonographer stated that it was their policy to sex the baby, but that a disclaimer as to the accuracy of sexing by ultrasound was displayed. The lack of availability of a follow-up scan was also explained if the sex could not be determined. There was no protocol to deal with the problem of the parents being divided over sex determination, but there was 'an unwritten directive to deny the ability to see the gender of this baby'.

From the correspondence there appeared to be dissatisfaction with the absence of general rules relating to giving such information to parents and it is clear that some departments work on an ad hoc basis with respect to individual parents.

Certain legal questions arise however.

Do parents have a legal right to know the sex of their baby?

The answer to this is probably not, unless it could be justified on the basis of concern over a particular congenital abnormality which is sex-linked.

Clearly the parents do have the right to access health records (see Chapter 6), but since the prime purpose of the ultrasound is not sex determination, but the identification of fetal abnormalities, the sex might not be identified and therefore not be recorded. Accordingly a statutory right to access records is of little value in this context.

Where, however, the parents would be justified in seeking a termination under the provisions of the Abortion Act 1967 (as amended) because of a serious sex-linked congenital disease which would lead to a seriously handicapped baby, a request for sex identification would be justified, and negligence in carrying out this identification could lead to litigation. Where identification is not certain this needs to be stated in the records and unequivocally to the parents so they know they are making their decision on imperfect information. In practice, parents concerned about a sex-linked congenital condition would be advised to seek an amniocentesis examination before going ahead with a termination on the basis of the ultrasound findings alone.

Do parents have a legal right NOT to know?

Health information cannot be forced upon people and if they refuse to ask questions, or do not listen to information, that is their concern. Their failure to take note of information may in some circumstances constitute contributory negligence (see Chapter 14) but this is unlikely in the situation of sex determination. On the other hand, if a parent did not wish to know the sex and was inadvertently told it by a sonographer or midwife, there would be no legal action the parent could take against the health professional or their employer. In these circumstances no actionable harm has been suffered.

Should parents give written consent that they wanted to have the information?

There are always advantages in obtaining written evidence of a particular discussion since, in the event of a dispute, that document can be produced. However, as is seen from the Chapter 4 on consent, in most circumstances consent by word of mouth is as valid as written consent. The advantages of obtaining consent in writing is that it can also be recorded that the parent has been notified that there can be no guarantee that the identification of the sex is 100% correct.

What action can parents take if the information proves to be incorrect?

If the parents were notified that the sex identification could not be guaranteed as absolutely accurate, then there would be no basis for a legal action. However there may be possible legal action if, on the basis of the sex identification made, a termination of pregnancy was carried out because of a serious risk of a sex-linked congenital abnormality. If the termination was then found to be unnecessary because the fetus was not of the identified sex, then the parents may have an action in negligence. It would have to be established:

(1)   that there was a duty of care owed in the sexing of the fetus (this may include the requirement that the sonographer knew that reliance would be placed upon the identification and that the parents would take action in seeking a termination);

(2)   that there was failure by the sonographer to follow acceptable professional practice in making the identification (since there are many difficulties in making a correct identification, including the position of the fetus, this breach of duty may be difficult to establish); and

(3)   that as a reasonably foreseeable consequence of this failure by the sonographer, an unnecessary termination was carried out.

Should the information be put in writing?
There are considerable advantages in having a printed form which warns parents of the difficulties of an accurate identification and the dangers of relying upon one scan to decide upon a termination of pregnancy.

Is a disclaimer effective?
Where there has been negligence in carrying out an examination, then a disclaimer is not effective in removing liability for that negligence should personal injury or death occur. This is because of the effects of the Unfair Contract Terms Act 1977 which is discussed in Chapter 14. If the notice is not a disclaimer, but a warning that 100% accuracy cannot be guaranteed, then it would be valid in law in making it clear that the patient was aware of the unreliability of any determination.

Should there be a national policy covering these issues?
Certainty of practice and consistent high standards throughout the country are desirable. It may be that the Royal College of Obstetricians and Gynaecologists and College of Radiographers could, in conjunction with other organisations such as the Patients' Association and the Confederation of Health Authorities and Trusts, draw up a recommended protocol.

Congenital abnormalities

The existence of congenital abnormalities is a justification for the termination of a pregnancy, without any limit of time. The Abortion Act requires that 'there is substantial risk that if the child were born it would suffer from such physical or mental abnormalities as to be seriously handicapped'. Negligent failure to identify correctly the existence of serious abnormalities could therefore be grounds for litigation by the parents. The baby itself does not however have any right to claim that it should never have been born as is shown in the case below.

Minor abnormalities may be revealed by the ultrasound such as a missing arm or leg which would not come within the definition of 'seriously handicapped' in section 1(1)(d) of the Abortion Act 1967. Professional judgment must determine the appropriate time to notify the woman of this defect. Where such an abnormality has not been identified from the ultrasound, it does not necessarily mean that the person carrying out the ultrasound has been negligent.

Case: *Rubella*[12]

Mrs McKay was pregnant and suspected that she had contracted German measles in the early weeks of her pregnancy. Blood tests were arranged to see if she had been infected. Unfortunately, she was wrongly informed that she had not been infected. When the baby was born it was found to be disabled as a result of the effect of German measles.

The Court of Appeal held that the child's claim for wrongful life (i.e. if there had been no negligence the child would have been aborted) could not be sustained. Although this child was born before the Congenital Disabilities (Civil Liability) Act 1976 was passed, the Court still held that an action for wrongful life could not stand, even under the provisions of the Act. This decision does not of course affect the rights of the mother to sue for damages resulting from the negligence in informing her of the results of the tests and Mrs McKay brought her own action on that point. The former decision was concerned solely with the rights of the child.

The Congenital Disabilities (Civil Liability) Act 1976

The Congenital Disabilities (Civil Liability) Act 1976 referred to in the McKay case was passed, as a result of the thalidomide tragedy, when children born to mothers who had taken that medication were disabled. There was uncertainty at the time as to whether the law enabled a child who was harmed whilst a fetus to obtain compensation for any injuries which occurred as the result of negligence since a fetus is not recognised in the UK law as having a legal personality. The Act gives a statutory right of compensation to a child who is born disabled as the result of an act of negligence which took place pre-birth. However as a matter of public policy the child cannot sue the mother for any pre-natal negligence by her which caused the harm (e.g. continuing to smoke or drink alcohol). An exception to this is if the mother was at the time driving a car; in this case, of course, the child is effectively suing the mother's third party risks insurers.

Situation: Pre-natal injury

A woman tells a radiographer that she is pregnant, but the radiographer fails to record this information and investigations were carried out on the woman in ignorance of that fact.

When the baby is born he is found to be suffering from severe disabilities which expert opinion suggests is due to the treatment that the mother received whilst pregnant. What rights does the child have?

In this situation there would be a *prima facie* case of negligence by the radiographer. Both the mother and child may have a right of action because of the radiographer's failure to follow accepted approved practice. Action could also be brought against the employing health authority or NHS trust because of its vicarious accountability for the actions of the radiographer (see Chapter 14). The action of the child would be under the Congenital Disabilities (Civil Liability) Act 1976. The representatives of the child would have to prove

- that there was a duty of care owed to the parent;
- that there was a failure to follow the reasonable standard of care (according to the Bolam test); and
- that this failure caused the harm which the child is suffering.

On the facts of the case it may be difficult to establish that negligence by the radiographer caused the harm suffered by the baby if there is conflicting expert evidence on this point. It is a defence under the Act if the reasonable standard of professional care at the relevant time was followed. Section 1(5) of the Congenital Disabilities (Civil Liability) Act 1976 states that:

'The defendant is not answerable to the child, for anything he did or omitted to do when responsible in a professional capacity for treating or advising the parent, if he took reasonable care having due regard to then received professional opinion applicable to the particular class of case; but this does not mean that he is answerable only because he departed from received opinion.'

Time limits for bringing action

If parents or others fail to take action on behalf of the child, the child has a right to sue in respect of the harm in his own right from the age of 18 years and it is only at that time that the three year limitation for bringing a civil action in respect of personal injuries starts to run. If the child is suffering from mental disabilities then the time limit does not start until the disabilities end, which would usually not be until death. Time limits are further discussed in Chapter 14.

Congenital Anomaly Register and the West Midlands Perinatal Institute

The Congenital Anomaly Register (CAR) was set up following the establishment of the National Confidential Enquiry into Stillbirths and Deaths in Infancy in 1983. The West Midlands Perinatal Institute started to investigate high rates of perinatal death in 1986 and subsequently expanded its role to include a standard region-wide antenatal care record and the establishment of a multi-disciplinary regional ultrasound group[13]. The Institute co-ordinates the registration of congenital anomalies, which is also provided pre-natally with the introduction of antenatal ultrasound screening. Departments have notification forms for congenital anomalies from the Institute and radiographers provide a good source of information. The Institute also provides training for midwives and doctors in ultrasound scanning. The training does not cover transvaginal scanning, since that is considered a separate skill for which specialist training must be given. Guidelines have been issued by the Royal College of Obstetricians and Gynaecologists on ultrasound scanning[14].

Conclusions

Special precautions must be taken by all diagnostic and therapeutic radiography and radiotherapy departments in relation to pregnant women. Whilst the scientific evidence of harm to the fetus from diagnostic X-rays is minimal, there is a public perception that pregnant women should not be X-rayed. Litigation is likely to follow inadvertent X-raying of a pregnant women, even though the causal links between the X-raying and any disabilities suffered by the child may be difficult to establish.

Regular monitoring is required of the standards of care in relation to pregnant women, and of the information which is given to them both by word of mouth and in writing. The provisions of the Human Rights Act must also be borne in mind in planning and providing services.

Consanguinity relationships can lead to congenital defects and the advantages of ultrasound in early diagnosis are discussed by Gail Ashington[15]. It is crucial, however, that patients are made aware of the limitations of ultrasound in pre-natal diagnosis and that an apparently normal scan may overlook an underlying abnormality.

 ## Questions and exercises

1   Prepare a protocol for the care of a pregnant woman undergoing investigations or treatment in your department.
2   If a pregnant woman consents to treatment which could harm her fetus, does the fetus have any right of action against health professionals who allowed the treatment to proceed?
3   What comments would you make on the law relating to the identification of gender in the fetus?

References

1   E.K. Osei & K. Faulkner (2000) Radiation risks from exposure to diagnostic X-rays during pregnancy *Radiography* **6**, 2, 131–44
2   NRPB Board (1993) *Statement on diagnostic medical exposures to ionising radiation during pregnancy* Documents of the NRPB Vol 4 No 4
3   C. Sharp, J.A. Shrimpton & R.F. Bury (1998) *Diagnostic Medical Exposures: Advice on Exposure to Ionising Radiation During Pregnancy* NRPB, the College of Radiographers and the Royal College of Radiologists, London
4   *Hutton* v. *East Dyfed Health Authority* [1998] Lloyds Law Reports (Medical) 335
5   *Janaway* v. *Salford HA* [1989] AC 537
6   G. Ashington (2000) The role of ultrasound in diagnosing respiratory distress syndrome *Synergy* (September 2000) pages 14–16
7   *Penny, Palmer and Cannon* v. *East Kent Health Authority* [2000] Lloyds Rep. Med. 41
8   G. Ashington (1999) Fetal sex determination *Synergy* (September 1999) pages 8–11
9   A. Ryder (1999) Letter *Synergy News* (December 1999) page 15
10 L. Samuels (1999) Letter *Synergy News* (November 1999) page 12
11 G. Fletcher (1999) Letter *Synergy News* (November 1999) page 12

12   *McKay* v. *Essex Area Health Authority* [1982] 2 All ER 771
13   G. Ashington (2000) Recording Congenital Anomalies *Synergy* (May 2000) pages 14–15
14   RCOG *Routine ultrasound screening in pregnancy: protocol, standards and training.* (see website www.rcog.org.uk/medical/ultrasound
15   G. Ashington (2000) The problems of consanguinity *Synergy* (January 2000) pages 12–13

Chapter 10
Death and Dying

The oncologist and therapeutic radiographer in particular find that they are caring for patients who are terminally ill. They therefore need to have a clear understanding of the law which applies in this field. In addition many radiographers and radiologists may become involved in forensic issues, where evidence is required for criminal proceedings including manslaughter or murder cases.

The extent of the duty to maintain life

The law draws a distinction between taking positive action to end life and withholding care. The former will always be illegal but the latter may or may not be legally permissible depending upon the prognosis of the patient. It is not, therefore, the duty of the health professional to continue to provide high technology care when the patient's prognosis is considered hopeless and the patient can be allowed to die.

Murder

The definition of murder derives from a 17th century case:

> 'Murder is when a man of sound memory, and of the age of discretion, unlawfully killeth within any country of the realm any reasonable creature in rerum natura under the King's peace, with malice aforethought, either expressed by the party or implied by law, so as the party wounded, or hurt, etc. die of the wound or hurt etc.' (Coke)

The original definition set a time limit of a year and a day in which the person must die of the wound or hurt. This limitation was removed in 1996.

Manslaughter

In certain circumstances what would have been a crime of murder may be reduced to manslaughter.

Manslaughter is divided into two categories: voluntary and involuntary. Voluntary covers the situation where there is the intention to kill or complete disregard as to the possibility that death could arise from one's deliberate actions (i.e. there is the mental requirement) but there are extenuating factors, such as provocation, death in pursuance of a suicide pact or diminished responsibility.

These can mean that a murder verdict might not be obtained but the defendant could be guilty of voluntary manslaughter.

Involuntary manslaughter exists when the mental intention (*mens rea*) for murder is absent but death results from a person's actions (*actus reus*) (see glossary). Such circumstances would include gross negligence or recklessness, for example by a health professional, and can give rise to a conviction for manslaughter in certain circumstances[1] (see Chapter 2).

Where the accused is convicted of manslaughter the judge has complete discretion over sentencing. In contrast where there is a murder conviction, at present the sentence is a mandatory one of life imprisonment.

Voluntary euthanasia

This means killing a person with that person's consent. This is unlawful. It could amount to murder which is punishable on conviction by life imprisonment, or it could be seen as manslaughter, where the judge has complete discretion over sentencing. Alternatively if the act amounts to assistance in a suicide bid (e.g. procuring poison which the patient administers himself) then it is illegal under section 2(1) of the Suicide Act 1961:

> 'A person who aids, abets, counsels or procures the suicide of another or an attempt by another to commit suicide, shall be liable on conviction on indictment to imprisonment [up to 14 years].'

Situation: Asking for help

> The wife of a patient who is in the terminal stages of lung cancer is concerned that he finds breathing difficult in spite of constant oxygen and is convinced he no longer wishes to carry on living. She asks the radiographer if she would help her husband out of his misery. What right of action does the radiographer have?

There is no grey area of law here. Any action on the part of the radiographer to assist the wife in ending her husband's misery would constitute a criminal wrong and they could both face murder proceedings, although the wife might plead diminished responsibility to reduce the charge to manslaughter.

The law on this issue has recently been reaffirmed in a case which attracted considerable publicity as it went through the appeal stages. Diane Pretty, who suffered from the terminal stages of motor neurone disease, finally lost her application for her husband to be given by the Director of Public Prosecution a promise of immunity from prosecution under the Suicide Act 1961 if he should assist her to die.

The House of Lords[2] held that the refusal to grant immunity was not an infringement of Articles 2, 3, 8, 9 or 14 of the Articles of the European Convention on Human Rights as set out in Schedule 1 of the Human Rights Act 1998. Any change in the law relating to euthanasia must be enacted through Parliament. Assistance by the husband to help her die would be an offence under section 2(1) of the Suicide Act 1961.

Even where the parents wish a grossly handicapped baby to die, any professional who intentionally speeded up the process of death could be guilty of causing the death of the child. In the case of *R* v. *Arthur*[3] a paediatrician was prosecuted for attempting to cause the death of a grossly handicapped baby who was suffering from Down's Syndrome and who had other disabilities when he prescribed dihydrocodeine and nursing care only. The judge stated unequivocally that:

> 'There is no special law in this country that places doctors in a separate category and gives them extra protection over the rest of us ... Neither in law is there any special power, facility or licence to kill children who are handicapped or seriously disadvantaged in an irreversible way.'

Dr Arthur was nevertheless acquitted by the jury who ignored the judge's exposition of the law, presumably because of the extremely distressing circumstances of the case.

In contrast to the Dr Arthur case, at the other end of life, Dr Nigel Cox[4] was convicted when he prescribed potassium chloride to a terminally ill patient and was sentenced to a year's imprisonment, although this was suspended for a year so he did not actually go to prison. He also had to appear before disciplinary proceedings of the Regional Health Authority, his employers and before the General Medical Council.

The Select Committee of the House of Lords[5] has reported that there should be no change in the law to permit euthanasia. This is also the view put forward by the Law Commission in its recent report[6].

Letting die

Do these cases mean that it is never lawful to permit a patient to die whatever the circumstances of his condition? The answer is that the law does not expect constant medical intervention whatever the prognosis and that in certain circumstances it is legally permissible to let die. The law draws a distinction between letting die and killing, between withdrawing life-sustaining treatment and taking positive steps to hasten death.

Adults

Where an adult wishes to die and refuses treatment, then crucial to the decision making and withholding of treatment is that person's mental capacity to make a decision or the existence of a living will (see below). A mentally competent person has the right to refuse treatment. However in this situation the practitioner should be careful not to undertake any action which could be interpreted as aiding or abetting a suicide attempt. She should also obtain independent advice on the mental competence of the patient to refuse treatment (see Chapter 4 and the law relating to consent).

Situation: Coming off a ventilator.

A tetraplegic patient attended by the therapeutic radiographer told her that he wished to be allowed to die and come off the ventilator. What is the legal situation?

This is the situation which arose in the Karen Quinlan case[7] in the USA where an extremely long court action resulted in a decision being made that she could come off the ventilator. In the case of *Re B* (2002)[8] the court held that a mentally competent adult could refuse to be on a ventilator.

Children

An example of the court permitting a child to be allowed to die is the case of *Re C*[9], where the Court of Appeal ordered that:

> 'The hospital do continue to treat the minor within the parameters of the opinion expressed by [the specialist paediatrician called to give expert evidence] in his report ... which report is not to be disclosed to any person other than the health authority.'

In a more recent case (*A National Health Trust* v. *D*)[10] Article 2 of the Human Rights Convention (disussed in Chapter 3) was invoked to justify further proactive treatment for a severely disabled child but the judge held that the overriding criterion may to act in the best interests of the child which could include allowing him to die (see below).

The Royal College of Paediatrics and Child Health (RCPCH)[11] has published a framework for practice in determining whether life saving treatment should be withheld or withdrawn.

Decision making in advance

Living wills

A living will, also known as an advance refusal of treatment or an advance directive is a statement made when a person is mentally competent over what treatments and care they would wish to refuse at a later time, when they no longer have the mental capacity to make decisions. There is at the time of writing no statutory provision (i.e. by Act of Parliament) for the recognition of a living will. However the House of Lords in the Tony Bland (see below) case stated that had Tony Bland when competent expressed any refusal of treatment then that would have been binding upon the health professionals caring for him (i.e. at common law living wills should be recognised). The Law Commission[6] had put forward recommendations relating to advance refusals of treatment but the government decided that it was not yet the time to give these statutory force[12]. The present law which relies on the recognition of the validity of living wills at common law provides more flexibility. The BMA has prepared guidelines[13] for the preparation of a living will. It suggests that as a minimum, the following information is included:

- Full name
- Address
- Name and address of general practitioner
- Whether advice was sought from health professionals
- Signature
- Date drafted and reviewed

- Witness signature
- A clear statement of your wishes, either general or specific
- The name, address and telephone number of your 'nominated person', if you have one.

Forms and guidance are also available from the Terence Higgins Trust.

If a health professional withholds treatment on the basis of a refusal of a patient contained in an advance directive and there is no reason to believe that it is invalid, then the health professional should not be held liable for a breach of the duty of care.

Situation: Refusing treatment.

> A patient, on hearing that he was suffering from carcinoma of the oesophagus, wrote an advance refusal of treatment that he would not wish to receive any artificial feeding. He is now finding it more and more difficult to swallow and artificial feeding is seen as the only option. The Consultant has stated that this should be commenced and refuses to accept that the living will has any significance to his clinical judgment. What is the law?

If there is no reason to doubt the validity of the living will and if there is no reason to believe that the patient changed his mind, then it is valid in law. There is therefore an obligation upon all health professionals to respect the wishes of the patient. If the consultant treats the patient contrary to the wishes expressed in a valid living will, then he is guilty of trespass to the person (see Chapter 4).

Insisting on treatment

Conversely there is no absolute right to insist upon treatment (see Chapter 3). A health professional would be failing in her obligations if treatment were provided, on the patient's insistence, that she knew was professionally contraindicated. If a patient in a living will, rather than just refusing treatment, attempts to direct that treatment should be given, this direction is likely to be of little effect if it is not supported by professional judgment as to its appropriateness.

Not for resuscitation orders

What is the legal significance of such orders?

The mentally competent patient

If a patient has the mental competence to understand the situation he is entitled to refuse to give consent to any treatment, even though it is life saving (see Chapter 4).

Children of 16 and 17

Whilst a child of 16 or 17 has a statutory right to give consent, a recent case has decided that such children cannot refuse treatment which is in their best interests (see Chapter 8). In the case of *Re W*[14] a girl of 16 years refused to be treated for anorexia nervosa, but her refusal was overruled by the court. If, however, a decision made by a minor is considered to be in his best interests, then it would be valid for all professional carers of that patient to accept that refusal of care and the instructions that the patient is not to be resuscitated.

The impact of the Convention of Human Rights (see Chapter 3) on the law relating to the right of a 16 or 17 year old to refuse life saving treatment has, at the time of writing, yet to be considered by the courts. This issue is, however, considered in the BMA book on consent and the rights of the child[15].

The mentally incapacitated

Where the patient is mentally incapacitated and the decision has been made by the consultant in charge of the care of the patient that he should not be resuscitated, then the legality of such a decision depends upon the prognosis of the patient and in dubious cases there are advantages in a declaration from the court being obtained (see below and Chapter 7).

Relatives do not have any right to make decisions on behalf of a mentally incapacitated adult. It is clear that, whilst the relatives should be fully consulted in the decision making, they do not have the right to refuse treatment that the health-care team consider to be in the patient's best interests.

Guidance

A joint statement from the British Medical Association, Resuscitation Council (UK) and the Royal College of Nursing[16] provides revised guidance on *Decisions Relating to Cardiopulmonary Resuscitation*. This guidance was commended to NHS trusts in a Circular by the NHS Executive[17]. Chief Executives of NHS trusts are required to ensure that appropriate resuscitation policies which respect patients' rights are in place, understood by all relevant staff, and accessible to those who need them and that such policies are subject to appropriate audit and monitoring arrangements.

The Commission for Health Improvement (CHI) has been asked by the Secretary of State to pay particular attention to resuscitation decision-making processes as part of its rolling programme of reviews of clinical governance arrangements put in place by NHS organisations. Guidance emphasises that there must be no blanket policies, each individual patient must be assessed personally and policy cannot depend solely on the age of the patient.

According to the Guidelines cardiopulmonary resuscitation (CPR) should only be withheld in the following 4 situations:

- The mentally competent patient has refused treatment
- A valid living will covering such circumstances has been made by the patient
- Effective cardiopulmonary resuscitation (CPR) is unlikely to be successful
- Where successful CPR is likely to be followed by a length and quality of life which it would not be in the best interests of the patient to sustain.

The Resuscitation Council, the BMA and the RCN issued a joint statement with further revised guidelines in 2001[18] amended in the light the Human Rights Act 1998. It emphasises that there is a presumption in favour of resuscitation and decisions should be made for each patient on an individual basis. An advance decision of 'Do Not Attempt Resuscitation' (DNAR) should only apply when there has been consideration of all relevant aspects of the patient's condition including but not limited to:

- the likely clinical outcome;
- the patient's known or ascertainable wishes; and
- the patient's human rights including the right to life and, conversely, the right to be free from degrading treatment.

The refusal by parents to consent to treatment for their children and other issues relating to the child are considered in Chapter 8.

Involvement of the court

When should the guidance of the court be obtained on a decision?

Where the patient is a mentally incompetent adult and there is no living will, then the withholding of for example, artificial feeding is a matter for court intervention as the Tony Bland case shows.

Case: Airedale NHS Trust v. Bland[19]

The patient was a victim of the football stadium crush at Hillsborough and it was established that, although he could breathe and digest food independently, he could not see, hear, taste, smell or communicate in any way and it appeared that there was no hope of recovery or improvement. The House of Lords had to decide if it was lawful to permit artificial feeding to be discontinued in the case of a patient in a persistent vegetative state. The House of Lords decided that it would be in the best interests of the patient to discontinue the nasal gastric feed and he was later reported as having died.

The House of Lords recommended that if any similar decisions were required to be made in the future there should be application before the courts. A court in Bristol gave consent in a similar case a few months after the House of Lords decision in Tony Bland's case[20].

A practice note has been issued by the Official Solicitor[21] for such situations.

There are, however, probably many occasions in practice when a patient is allowed to die without court approval being obtained. If a patient refuses treatment and it is clear that he has the capacity to refuse his consent, then this cannot be overruled. (See Chapter 4 and the case of *Re C*, the Broadmoor patient whose refusal of a life-saving amputation was held to be valid.)

Where the patient lacks mental competence, if the doctors, the relatives and the rest of the multi-disciplinary team are agreed that his prognosis is extremely poor and that aggressive treatment is inappropriate, there is unlikely to be a court hearing. The patient will be allowed to die and 'nature to take its course'.

The referral of a case of a dying patient to court is not necessarily the most appropriate means for such decisions to be made. Legislation is to follow the Lord Chancellor's paper *Making Decisions*[22] which followed closely the Law Commission's recommendations[6] on decision making and the mentally incapacitated adult. There needs to be clarification on when the court's intervention should be sought in the care of a terminally ill child or adult.

BMA guidelines

In the meantime in 1999 the BMA issued, following a consultation document[23] on withholding and withdrawing treatment, new guidelines for decision making[24]. This guidance distinguishes between situations where patients have the mental capacity and to make their own decisions and situations where such mental capacity is lacking. It covers babies, children and young people, and also covers decisions about the withholding or withdrawing of artificial nutrition and hydration. The guidance further suggests that where a member of the health-care team has a conscientious objection to the withdrawal or withholding of life-prolonging treatment, she should, wherever possible, be allowed to hand over the care of the patient to a colleague.

Can the court order doctors to treat?

Case: *Re J*[25]

J was born in January 1991 and suffered an accidental fall when he was a month old with the result that he was profoundly handicapped both mentally and physically. He was severely microcephalic, his brain not having grown sufficiently following the injury. He also had severe cerebral palsy, cortical blindness and severe epilepsy. He was in general fed by a nasal gastric tube. Medical opinion was unanimous that J was unlikely to develop much beyond his present functioning, that that level might deteriorate and that his expectation of life, although uncertain, would be short. The paediatrician's report stated that given J's condition it would not be medically appropriate to intervene with intensive procedures such as artificial ventilation if he were to suffer a life-threatening event.

In the Court of Appeal, Lord Donaldson, Master of the Rolls, said that the order of the judge, ordering specific treatment to take place, was wholly inconsistent with the law as stated in *Re J* (a different case)[26] and in *Re R*[27] and could not be justified on the basis of any known authority. Generally the court should be reluctant to order a course of treatment not supported by medical opinion as being in the best interests of the patient.

The reluctance of the court to interfere with the decision making of the doctors in the interests of the patient was seen in a later case in very different circumstances. In the case of *Re B* where the father of a girl of 10 suffering from leukaemia brought an action against the health authority for its refusal to fund a course of chemotherapy followed by a second bone marrow transplant operation[28] (see Chapter 3 for a fuller discussion of the case) the Court of Appeal took the view that the court should not intervene in such a decision but that the health authority should follow medical advice as to what was in the best interests of the child.

The situation has not significantly changed even with the advent of the Human Rights Act 1998. Such judicial decisions are confronting for parents who wish their handicapped child to survive at any cost.

Case: *A National Health Service Trust v. D July 2000*[10]

The child was born prematurely and found to be suffering from severe and irreversible lung disease and had a very short life expectancy. He also had heart failure, renal and liver dysfunction with a background of severe developmental delay. Following his admission to hospital the parents and doctors disagreed over whether he should be resuscitated. The hospital applied to the High Court for a declaration that it was not in the best interests of the child for his life to be prolonged, in view of his extremely poor state of health and the poor prognosis. The parents opposed the application.

The judge ruled that:

- In such cases the paramount consideration is the welfare of the child, which of course involves careful consideration of the parents' views, but those views cannot be allowed to override the court's view of the child's best interests.
- The court's high respect for the sanctity of human life imposes a strong presumption in favour of taking all steps capable of preserving it, save in exceptional circumstances.
- There was no question of the court directing treatment which a doctor was not prepared to give, or which was contrary to the doctor's clinical judgment.
- The doctors had made it plain that, when any decision was required the child's condition would be fully reassessed, including the possibility of artificial ventilation.
- A declaration would be made that full *palliative* care was in the best interests of the child and would allow him to die with dignity.
- There was no breach of either Article 2 (the right to life) or Article 3 (the right not to be subjected to inhuman or degrading treatment – including the right to die with dignity) of the European Convention for the Protection of Human Rights and Fundamental Freedoms.

Care of the dying patient

Children

The Association for children with life-threatening or terminal conditions and their families has been active in developing a Charter[29] for their care.

A report was also prepared by a working party on the care of dying children and their families by the British Paediatric Association, King Edward's Hospital Fund for London and the National Association of Health Authorities in 1988[30]. The aim of the report is to guide health authority members, managers and practitioners.

These matters are discussed in more detail in the author's work on the legal aspects of childhealth care[31].

Adults

Many of the books covering specific illnesses provide valuable advice on caring for the dying patient, which can be useful for health practitioners. Thus *Motor Neurone Disease* by Sue Beresford[32] provides helpful advice on terminal care. She emphasises the importance of honesty – 'honesty is vital but should never be brutal'. The many books by Kubler Ross are also to be recommended.

Situation Am I dying?

> A health practitioner was asked by a patient suffering in the terminal stages of MND – 'How much longer do I have?' The practitioner knew that he was dying but found it difficult to answer since the patient's wife refused to acknowledge to the patient the true position.

The answer to the question may require all the practitioner's skills and sensitivity. On the one hand she cannot lie to the patient (although in fact she would probably not know the exact answer to the question); nor should she collude with the spouse in keeping information from the patient. On the other hand she does need to attempt to create some understanding between patient and spouse and should be aware of organisations which could assist in this dilemma.

The role of the coroner

The doctor who attended the patient during the last illness must certify the death and state the cause unless the circumstances are such that the death should be reported to the coroner. These would include the following[33]:

(1)   Where the deceased was not attended in his last illness by a doctor.
(2)   Where the deceased was not seen by a doctor either after death or within the 14 days prior to death.
(3)   Where the cause of death is unknown.
(4)   Where death appears to be due to industrial disease or poisoning.
(5)   Where death may have been unnatural, or caused by violence or neglect or abortion, or attended by suspicious circumstances.
(6)   Where death has occurred during operation or before recovery from an anaesthetic.

Usually the individual coroner will make known his requirements in respect of the notification of deaths occurring in hospital. Some, for example, may require reporting of all deaths occurring within 24 hours of emergency admission[33].

Until the coroner has formally notified the doctor of his decision in relation to the deceased, the body remains under the control of the coroner, i.e. under his jurisdiction. He has the right to request a post mortem and there can be no action taken in respect of the body without his consent. His consent must be obtained even before the body can be viewed by the relatives[34].

Post mortem

If the coroner orders a post mortem, the relatives have no right to refuse this. This is so even when the religious views of the deceased would be against a post mortem[35]. On the other hand if the doctor requests a post mortem where the body is not under the jurisdiction of the coroner the person in charge of the body (usually the next of kin) could refuse to give consent. In any event the requirements of the Human Tissue Act 1961 and the Anatomy Act 1984 must be followed.

Inquest

Where a death has been reported to the coroner he will decide whether or not an inquest will be held. He is obliged by law to hold an inquest where there are reasons to suspect a criminal offence has caused the death, for industrial accidents and diseases and in the case of deaths in prison or police custody. The purpose of the inquest is to ascertain[36]:

- who the deceased was; and
- how, when and where the deceased came by his death.

Possible verdicts are:

- natural causes
- unlawful killing
- killed lawfully
- suicide
- accidental death
- misadventure
- an open verdict

- dependence upon a drug
- non-dependent abuse of drugs
- industrial disease
- neglect
- want of attention at birth
- attempted/self-induced abortion

An open verdict indicates that there is insufficient evidence to determine the cause of death, i.e. the evidence did not further or fully disclose the means whereby death arose. Once completed the inquest cannot be resumed but the High Court has the power under section 13 of the Coroners Act 1988 to order another inquest to be held.

The coroner's court

A practitioner might be required to give evidence at an inquest on the events which preceded death. It is essential that she obtains assistance from a senior manager or lawyer on the preparation of the statement which the coroner's office will require from her. If she is subsequently asked to attend the inquest she should have assistance in preparation for giving evidence (see Chapter 18 on giving evidence). It should be noted that the coroner's court is what is known as an inquisitorial one. This means that the the coroner is much more interventionist than a judge in other proceedings. He determines the witnesses who will give evidence, the course of the proceedings and he will disallow any question which in his opinion is not relevant or otherwise not a proper one. He can himself examine the witnesses often asking leading questions where information is not disputed to speed up the hearing. Hence the words 'inquisitorial' and 'inquest' (see glossary).

Where the death has been reported to the coroner, no certificate can be issued or registration take place until he has made his decision.

Other legal issues concerning bodies

Organ transplants

The donation of organs from a deceased person and from a living person are both regulated by law. The Human Tissue Act 1961 and the Corneal Tissue Act 1986 cover the use of organs of a deceased person and the Human Organ Transplants Act 1989 covers the transplant of organs from a live donor. There are many legal and ethical issues surrounding the question of organ donation and establishing when someone has actually died. These are considered in detail in *Brain Death and Ethics*[37], a book written some time ago but still valid.

Disposal where radioactive substances have been administered

Care must be taken in carrying out post mortems, and burying or cremating a body which contains radioactive substances. Guidance is provided by the IPEM[38]. This sets out the good practice to be followed to ensure that there is no breach of IRR99 or RSA. It recommends that the Radiation Protection Adviser (RPA) should be contacted for advice on whether or not there is any requirement for whole body or extremity dose monitoring. The guidance covers the dosages over which special precautions should be taken and the different procedures which are to be followed when a patient dies within 48 hours of diagnostic quantities of radioactive substances or within 48 hours of therapeutic quantities of radioactive substances.

Conclusions

In their care of terminally ill patients, practitioners need to be confident in their knowledge about the laws which apply. They may, for example, feel great empathy for a tetraplegic patient who no longer has the desire to live but they must be aware that to assist in his death would be to commit a crime under the Suicide Act. Similarly, in the care of patients suffering from chronic illnesses, practitioners must keep a clear distinction between the right of the mentally capable patient to refuse to be treated (including the right of the patient to make a living will) and the criminal act of killing the patient.

 ## Questions and exercises _____

1 In what circumstances could a patient facing a terminal illness refuse treatment? (see also Chapter 4)
2 Draw up the requirements for a valid living will.
3 Parents of a child suffering from leukaemia have suggested to you that further treatment, investigations and therapy should be stopped. What are the legal considerations in respect of this request and what action would you take?
4 Following the death of a patient in hospital, you are asked to provide a statement for the coroner. What principles would you bear in mind in preparing the statement? (see also Chapter 18)

References

1 *R* v. *Adomako* The Times Law Report, 4 July 1994; [1994] 3 All ER 79
2 *R* v. *Director of Public Prosecutions, ex parte Pretty (Secretary of State for the Home Department intervening)* The Times Law Report, 5 December 2001
3 *R* v. *Arthur* (1981) *The Times* 6 November 1981
4 *R* v. *Cox* [1993] 2 All ER 19
5 House of Lords: (31 January 1994) Committee on Medical Ethics, Session 1993–4 HMSO, London
6 Law Commission (1995) Report No 231 *Mental Incapacity* HMSO, London
7 *Re Quinlan* (1976) 70 NJ 10
8 *Re B (Consent to treatment: capacity)* Times Law Report, 26th March 2002
9 *Re C (a minor) (Wardship; medical treatment)* 1989 2 All ER 782
10 O. Wright & L. Peek (2000) Judge rules boy must be left to die *The Times*, 13 July 2000, *A National Health Service Trust* v. *D* The Times Law Report, 19 July 2000.
11 Royal College of Paediatrics and Child Health (1997) *Withholding or Withdrawing Life Saving Treatment in Children. A Framework for Practice* (September 1997) RCPCH, London
12 Lord Chancellor's Office (1999) *Making Decisions on behalf of mentally incapacitated adults.* HMSO, London
13 British Medical Association (April 1995) *Advance Statements about medical treatment: Code of Practice* BMA, London
14 *Re W (a minor) (medical treatment)* [1992] 4 All ER 627
15 British Medical Association (2001) *Consent, Rights and Choices in Health Care for Children and Young People* BMJ Books, London.
16 British Medical Association, Resuscitation Council (UK) and the Royal College of Nursing (1999) *Decisions Relating to Cardiopulmonary Resuscitation* BMA, London
17 NHS Executive *Resuscitation Policy HSC 2000/028* (September 2000)
18 Resuscitation Council (UK) British Medical Association and Royal College of Nursing (2001) *Decisions Relating to Cardiopulmonary Resuscitation A Joint Statement* (28 February 2001) BMA, London
19 *Airedale NHS Trust* v. *Bland* [1993] 1 All ER 821
20 *Frenchay Healthcare NHS Trust* v. *S* [1994] 2 All ER 403
21 Practice note [1996] 4 All ER 766
22 Lord Chancellor's Office (1999) *Making Decisions* HMSO, London
23 BMA's Medical Ethics Committee (1998) *Withdrawing and Withholding Treatment*: BMA, London
24 British Medical Association (1999) *Withholding and withdrawing life prolonging medical treatment* BMA, London
25 *Re J* [1992] 4 All ER 614, Times Law Report 12 June 1992
26 *Re J (a minor) (wardship; medical treatment)* [1990] 3 All ER 930
27 *Re R* [1991] 4 All ER 177
28 *R* v. *Cambridge and Huntingdon Health Authority, ex parte* B Times Law Report, 15 March 1995, [1995] 2 All ER 129
29 See B.C. Dimond (1996) *Legal Aspects of Childhealth Care* Mosby
30 R. Thornes (1998) *The care of dying children and their families* (from guidelines prepared by the British Paediatric Association, King Edward's Hospital Fund for London and the National Association of Health Authorities in 1988) Birmingham National Association of Health Authorities, Birmingham
31 B. Dimond (1996) *The Legal Aspects of Childhealth Care* Mosby, pages 210–12
32 S. Beresford (1995) *Motor Neurone Disease* Chapman and Hall, London

33   List taken from *the Registration of Births and Deaths Regulations* SI No. 2088 of 1987 (regulation 41(1)); See further B. Knight (1992) *Legal Aspects of Medical Practice* 5th edn. Churchill Livingstone, Edinburgh (pages 95–102)

34   B.C. Dimond (1995) Death in the Accident and Emergency Department *Accident and Emergency Nursing* **3**, 1, 38–41 (further details of the coroner's jurisdiction)

35   *R* v. *Westminster City Coroner, ex parte Rainer* (1968) 112 Solicitors Journal 883.

36   Coroners Act 1988, section 11(5)(b)

37   D. Lamb (1985) *Brain Death and Ethics* Croom Helm, London

38   Institute of Physics and Engineering in Medicine (2001) *Medical and Dental Guidance notes: A good practice guide to implement ionising radiation protection legislation in the clinical environment* IPEM, London

Section C
Professional Issues

Chapter 11
Professional Registration and Statutory Controls

This chapter will consider both the registration provisions of the General Medical Council and also those of the Health Professions Council. In the next two chapters the law relating to professional conduct and education is considered.

Medical practitioners

Introduction

The Medical Act 1983 (as amended) sets out the main provisions for the registration of persons as medical practitioners through the General Medical Council. Any person who satisfies the necessary educational qualifications and pays the requisite fee is entitled to be registered under section 3 as a fully registered medical practitioner. The Act provides protection of title, so that it is a criminal offence falsely to claim to be a registered practitioner[1]. The privileges of registered practitioners are set out in Part VI of the Act:

- only a registered practitioner can recover fees for medical advice or attendance or an operation (section 46);
- only registered medical practitioners can hold appointments as a medical officer in the forces, any hospital, prison or other public institution for the care of the sick (section 47); and
- certificates required for medical purposes are not valid unless the person signing it is fully registered (section 48).

General Medical Council (GMC)

The GMC is a corporate body the functions of which are to set standards of professional competence and conduct, to keep up-to-date registers of doctors, to supervise the basic training of doctors and co-ordinate all stages of medical education and to deal with doctors whose fitness to practice is in doubt. Seven committees are established under the Medical Act 1983 Act (as amended) and the Medical (Professional Performance) Act 1995:

- The Professional Conduct Committee
- The Health Committee
- The Preliminary Proceedings Committee
- The Education Committee
- The Assessment Referral Committee

- The Committee on Professional Performance
- The Interim Orders Committee.

In addition there are the president's advisory committee, the finance and establishment committee, the overseas committee, the registration committee, the committee on standards of professional conduct and the committee on medical ethics.

As currently constituted, the GMC consists of 104 members:

- 54 doctors elected by doctors on the register
- 25 members of the public nominated by the Privy Council
- 25 doctors appointed by educational bodies – universities, medical royal colleges and faculties.

Schedule 1 makes provision for the constitution of the GMC, its committees and branches.

The role of the GMC in relation to the education of doctors, the visits and inspections of courses and examinations leading to registration, is considered in Chapter 13 and its statutory powers to take action in relation to fitness to practise are considered in Chapter 12.

Registration

Under section 2 of the Act the GMC is required to keep two registers:

(1)   The register of medical practitioners containing four lists:
- the principal list
- the overseas list
- the visiting overseas doctors list
- the visiting European Economic Area (EEA) list
(2)   The register of medical practitioners with limited registration.

The main register contains about 190 000 names and is available to the general public, health authorities and trusts to check on the registration of individual practitioners.

Requirements for registration include qualification from a UK medical school or (for EEA nationals) qualifications elsewhere in the European Economic Area (EEA).

Doctors who qualify elsewhere can apply for limited registration, allowing them to practise in the UK under supervision in approved training posts. In addition all doctors applying for limited registration must have obtained a satisfactory score in the academic modules of the International English Language Testing system administered by the British Council. There have been proposals recently to increase the standard of communication in English of overseas doctors[2].

The GMC also holds a specialist register showing those doctors who have completed specialist training. Doctors must be included on this specialist register to obtain consultant posts in the NHS. The Specialist Training Authority of the Medical Royal Colleges was established on 12 January 1996 for the purposes of specialist medical training and the issue of Certificates of Completion of Specialist Training (see Chapter 13).

NHS hospital doctors are subject to the nationally negotiated *Terms and Conditions of Service of Hospital Medical and Dental staff* (the red book) but have contracts of service or employment with individual NHS trusts, Primary Care Trusts or health authorities. The terms on which they can work in the NHS and in private practice are nationally set down and in its recent NHS Plan the Government has stated its intention to prevent junior hospital consultants from working both in the NHS and in private practice for the first six years. There is a statutory procedure laid down for the appointment of consultants.

Royal College of Radiology (RCR)

The Royal College of Radiology is a registered charity and was incorporated by Royal Charter in 1975[3]. The objectives set down in the Charter are:

- the advancement of the science and practice of radiology and oncology
- the furtherance of public education
- the promotion of study and research.

Amongst its considerable educational and training activities, the RCR sets professional standards, the curriculum, the assessment of schemes of training, the programme of education and training in clinical radiology and oncology and the syllabus and examinations to become a Fellow of the RCR. In addition it initiates research, provides guidance and advice, liaises with the government and other organisations on policy matters and publishes scientific journals and reports.

Health professionals other than doctors or nurses

Reform of the 1960 Act

From the outset in 1960 radiographers were one of the professions supplementary to medicine covered by the Professions Supplementary to Medicine Act 1960. The whole scheme has remained in force for over 40 years but was the subject of a consultation exercise undertaken by JM Consulting under the aegis of a steering group chaired by Professor Sheila McLean. Following a consultation document issued in October 1995, a report was published in July 1996[4].

The report identified the weaknesses in the the 1960 Act. It also explored the developments which had taken place since 1960 including:

- the development of primary care
- the internal market
- the use of multi-disciplinary teams and the possibility of non-state registered professionals being employed in the NHS by GPs and
- the growth of private sector provision.

It highlighted the changes which have taken place within the professions including:

- strong professional associations with regulations for discipline
- the new professions that have sought state registered status
- developments within higher education (degree status for many professions and education provision being made outside the NHS), and
- changing attitudes in society and public expectations.

The report commented on the inappropriateness of the term 'Professions Supplementary to Medicine' and recommended new machinery for the regulation of the professions once so described. The recommendations included the establishment of a 'Council for Health Professionals', statutory committees and a panel of professional advisers.

Implementing the proposals

The government accepted these recommendation and in the Health Act 1999 took the preliminary steps to implement the new system for registration and professional control. A consultation paper was published in August 2000[5], stating that modernising professional self-regulation should be seen as a component part of a wider strategy to modernise the whole of the NHS to help deliver better health and faster, fairer care. It was followed by a draft order, published in April 2001[6].

The new scheme

In April 2002 a new Health Professions Council replaced the Council for Professions Supplementary to Medicine and its twelve boards, which regulated 120 000 health professionals. The key objectives of the reorganisation were:

- To reform ways of working, by requiring the Council to:
  ○ treat the health and welfare of patients as paramount
  ○ collaborate and consult with key stakeholders
  ○ be open and pro-active in accounting to the public and the profession for its work.
- To reform structure and functions by:
  ○ giving wider powers to deal effectively with individuals who present unacceptable risks to patients
  ○ creating a smaller Council comprising directly elected practitioners and a strong lay input
  ○ linking registration with evidence of continuing professional development
  ○ providing stronger protection of professional titles
  ○ enabling the extension of regulation to new groups.

The Council is charged with strategic responsibility for setting and monitoring standards of professional training, performance and conduct.

The Consultation paper[5] quoted from the NHS Plan that the key tests for regulatory bodies are that they must be:

- smaller (but with much greater patient and public representation)
- have faster, more transparent procedures and
- develop meaningful accountability to the public and the health service.

It stated that the GMC had been asked to explore introducing a civil burden of proof and making other reforms. It recommended that the procedures adopted by the new HPC would need to be consistent with those agreed for doctors.

The Consultation paper also stated that there needed to be formal co-ordination between the health regulatory bodies and therefore a UK Council of Health Regulators was to be established. Its initial task would be to help co-ordinate and act as a forum in which common approaches across the professions could be developed for dealing with matters such as complaints against practitioners.

Composition of the Health Professions Council

The Government proposed that the HPC should initially consist of 23 members (12 practitioners ie one from each of the professions covered and 11 lay members (who may or may not be members of other professions not covered by the HPC). The emphasis is on a smaller more effective body.

Fundamental functions of the HPC

These are set out in Schedule 3 to the 1999 Health Act and are not transferable by Order to another body:

- keeping the Register of members admitted to practise
- determining standards of education and training for admission to practise
- giving advice about standards of conduct and performance and
- administering procedures (including making rules) relating to misconduct, unfitness to practise and similar matters[7].

Section 60 of the Health Act 1999 enables an Order in Council to make provision for:

- modifying the regulation of any profession 'so far as appears to be necessary or expedient for the purpose of securing or improving the regulation of the profession or the services which the profession provides or to which it contributes'.
- regulating any other profession which appears to be concerned (wholly or partly) with the physical or mental health of individuals and to require regulation in pursuance of the section.

There is also an overarching duty of the HPC to 'safeguard the health and well-being of persons using or needing the services, as well as to work in partnership with employers, educators and other regulatory bodies'[8].

The HPC committees

There are four committees, identified as the statutory committees, of the Council:

- Education and Training Committee
- Investigating Committee
- Conduct and Competence Committee } Practice Committees
- Health Committee.

Flexibility is built in so that the Council may establish other committees to discharge its functions and can establish professional advisory committees whose function is to advise the Council and its statutory committees on matters affecting any of the relevant professions.

Consultation with registrants

The Council shall inform and educate registrants and the public about its work. Before establishing any standards or giving guidance the Council shall consult representatives of any group of persons it considers appropriate including, as it sees fit:

- representatives of registrants or classes of registrants
- employers of registrants
- users of the services of registrants
- persons providing, assessing or funding education or training for registrants and potential registrants.

The Council shall publish any standards it establishes and any guidance it gives.

The registration machinery

One of the main functions of the Council is to establish and maintain a register of members of the relevant professions. This entails establishing from time to time the standards of proficiency necessary to be admitted to the different parts of the Register, being standards the Council considers necessary for safe and effective practice under that part of the Register. The Register will show, in relation to each registrant, such address and other details as the Council may prescribe.

To be effective and enable practitioners to progress in their profession, there shall be one or more designated titles for each part of the Register indicative of different qualifications and different kinds of training and a registered professional is entitled to use whichever of those titles is appropriate in his case in accordance with set criteria.

The Council, having consulted the Education and Training Committee, can make rules in connection with registration, the register and the payment of fees.

The Council shall make the register available for inspection by members of the public at all reasonable times and shall publish the register in such manner and at such times as it considers appropriate.

Application to be registered

A person seeking admission to any part of the register shall be registered if the application is made in the prescribed form and manner and she:

- satisfies the Education and Training Committee that she holds an approved qualification awarded:
  - less than five years ago,
  - more than five years but she has met specified requirements as to additional education, training, and experience
- satisfies the Education and Training Committee that she meets prescribed requirements as to safe and effective practice; and
- has paid the prescribed fee.

Provisions for renewal of registration and readmission require the applicant to meet any set requirements for continuing professional development within the specified time.

The Council can make rules over the procedure to be followed and circumstances in which a registered professional's name may be removed from the register on her own application or after the expiry of a prescribed period.

Provision is made for definition of approved qualifications and European Economics Area qualifications.

Appeals

Appeal can be made under Article 37 against the decisions of the Education and Training Committee where an application for registration, readmission or renewal or the inclusion of an additional entry has been refused or where specific conditions have been imposed on an applicant. There is also the right to appeal if the name of a registered professional has been removed on the grounds that she is in breach of a condition in respect of continuing education. The appeal lies to the Council.

Under Article 38 an appeal can be made from any decision of a Practice Committee or any decision of the Council under Article 37 to the appropriate court. Proposals for a Health Professions Independent Appeals Tribunal were not included in the final statutory instrument (Health Professions Order 2001 S.I. 2002/254).

Offences

It is an offence to:

- falsely claim registration with intent to deceive, or
- use a title to which one is not entitled, or
- falsely represent oneself to possess qualifications in a relevant profession.

It is an offence fraudulently to procure registration or, after registration, fail to comply with any requirement imposed by the Council or a Practice Committee.

Protected titles

The Consultation Paper recommended that a registrant should be entitled to use the designated title corresponding to the part or parts of the Register in which she is registered, whether alone or prefixed by the word 'registered' and that no other person should be so entitled. The Consultation Paper notes that this provision could be unfair to non state registered practitioners who practise lawfully and safely and suggests 'grandparenting' arrangements to enable the registration of those who can show that they have practised lawfully, safely and effectively for a number of years, and if appropriate pass a test of competence for that purpose. Alternatively such persons might be required to undertake some additional training or experience before admission to the Register. To pass oneself off as registered is an offence under Article 39 (see above). The offence is committed whether such representation is express or implied.

New professional groups

Legislation is to be introduced to provide a mechanism for Parliament to extend the scope of the HPC to new groups, including complementary or alternative therapies.

Non-registered support workers

The registered practitioner is increasingly expected to work with support from non-registered practitioners known variously as imaging assistants, technicians, health support workers, care assistants and other such titles. The legal aspects relating to the supervision of the activities of non-registered practitioners and delegation to them are considered in Chapter 14 on negligence and Chapter 27 on the scope of professional practice. The care workers in a wide range of specialisms are now receiving training through the National Vocational Qualifications scheme, which provides a basic training at specified levels.

The General Social Care Council established under the Care Standards Act 2000 has issued a draft Code of Practice to be followed by social workers and is intended to regulate the standards and training of support workers.

Conclusions

The General Medical Council has changed and is still changing to meet the modern requirements of openness about its performance and results, and has stronger powers to protect the public[9]. The new provisions for the revalidation of doctors (see Chapter 13), the concept of clinical governance (see Chapter 22) and the role of the National Clinical Assessment Authority (see Chapter 12) will all have a considerable impact on the role and function of the GMC. At the time of writing the shadow Health Professions Council is in being, with a massive agenda in terms of setting out the details, rules and procedures for its proper functioning. It is therefore too soon to determine whether the correct balance has been struck between self-regulation and state control so that the safety of the public is protected. There are likely to be continued changes to our system of registration for all health professionals over the next few years, including the admission to state registration of some of the complementary or alternative therapies.

The provisions relating to professional misconduct are discussed in the next chapter.

 Questions and exercises _____

1 Analyse the changes made to the functions and constitution of the General Medical Council and consider the extent to which they will ensure the accountability of the profession to the general public.
2 Draw up a table illustrating the relationship between the Health Professions Council, and the Society and College of Radiographers and the universities providing education for student radiographers.
3 Do you consider that the functions of the registered radiographer should be protected rather than just the title?

4 Do you consider that there is justification for the separation of diagnostic and therapeutic radiographers into two entirely separate professions with a change of title for the latter?

References

1 Medical Act 1983, section 49
2 Press reports, August 2000
3 RCR, 38 Portland Place, London WIN 4JQ (0207 636 4432), website www.rcr.ac.uk
4 *The Regulation of Health Professions: Report of a review of the Professions Supplementary to Medicine Act (1960) with recommendations for new legislation*, Conducted and Published by JM Consulting Ltd, July 1996
5 NHS Executive (2000) *Modernising Regulation: The New Health Professions Council*: (consultation document) (August 2000), Department of Health, London
6 Department of Health *Establishing the new Health Professions Council* (April 2001) Department of Health, London; Health Profession Order 2001 S.I. 2002/254
7 Health Act 1999, Schedule 3 paragraph 8(2)
8 Health Professions Order 2001; S.I. 2002/254 Article 3
9 General Medical Council (1999) *Changing Times Changing Culture* GMC, London

Chapter 12
Professional Standards and Misconduct

An overview and the sources of the law are dealt with here. For details of the actual procedures for a misconduct enquiry or hearing readers should contact the relevant professional body or visit their website.

In this chapter the professional control proceedings of the registration bodies are considered; firstly the powers and functions of the GMC and secondly the arrangements for control by the new Health Professions Council.

Registered Professionals come under several different forms of accountability:

- The professional conduct machinery of their own registration body
- Disciplinary proceedings established by employers (see Chapter 22 on employment law and below)
- Civil action for negligence or breach of statutory duties (see Chapter 14)
- Criminal prosecution (see Chapter 2)
- Complaints machinery (see Chapter 19)

It is the first form of accountability that is considered in this chapter for both doctors and other health professionals (other than nurses, health visitors or midwives).

General Medical Council

The Medical Act 1983 lays down the powers and duties of the General Medical Council to ensure high standards of professional practice and conduct. A general framework for professional proceedings is set out in the Act, but it has been amended in recent years in order to widen the powers of the GMC in dealing with doctors who are considered unfit to practise[1]. More recently, in the light of the scandals of Shipman, Ledward, Neale and others (see Chapter 22) there have been strong calls for the powers of the GMC in the control of professional conduct to be further strengthened and for there to be greater lay (i.e. non-medical) representation on the Council.

Advising on professional standards

Under Section 35 of the Medical Act 1983, the General Medical Council has the power to provide advice to doctors on standards of professional conduct or on medical ethics. The GMC publications include:

- *Good Medical Practice*[2]
- *Confidentiality: Protecting and Providing Information*[3] and
- *Seeking Patients' Consent: The Ethical Considerations*[4]

Access to these publications is available via the GMC website[5]

The GMC and its committees have powers to assist in carrying out functions in respect of professional conduct, professional performance or fitness to practise and it can require any practitioner (apart from the person who is the subject of the investigation) or any other person to provide any relevant information or document[6].

Professional conduct and fitness to practise

Part V of the Medical Act 1983, as amended in particular by the Medical (Professional Performance) Act 1995, covers the provisions relating to professional conduct and fitness to practise. Schedule 4 to the 1983 Act (as amended) sets out the provisions for proceedings before the professional conduct, health and preliminary proceedings committees. The GMC now has five committees which can hear allegations against doctors:

- The Professional Conduct Committee
- The Preliminary Proceedings Committee
- The Health Committee
- The Assessment Referral Committee
- The Committee on Professional Performance.

Criminal convictions and serious professional misconduct

Under Section 36 of the Medical Act 1983, the General Medical Council can take action where the Professional Conduct Committee

- either finds that the registered medical practitioner is convicted of a criminal offence, or
- judges him to have been guilty of serious professional misconduct.

Serious professional misconduct is not defined in the Act but replaces the earlier term of 'infamous conduct in any professional respect'. Case law has determined that serious professional misconduct is not restricted to conduct which is morally blameworthy but could include seriously negligent conduct[7].

The action which can be taken by the Professional Conduct Committee is:

- Erasing the name from the register
- Suspending registration for a maximum of 12 months
- Making the registration conditional on compliance with specified requirements for a maximum period of 3 years
- Issuing a warning
- Postponing a decision to obtain more evidence

The conditions under the third point above, which the Committee can impose for the protection of members of the public or in the doctor's own interests include:

- limiting the specialities the doctor can work in
- requiring the doctor to be supervised
- preventing the doctor from prescribing controlled drugs
- requiring the doctor to correct something that is wrong with his conduct or practice.

Stages of a professional conduct complaint

These are as follows:

- Assessment by a medically qualified GMC member, a professional screener, who reviews the case for and against the doctor.
- Reference, if appropriate, to the Preliminary Proceedings Committee which can take into account character, previous history and mitigation.
- Consideration by the Professional Conduct Committee which makes a decision on 'serious misconduct' and, if appropriate, can remove a doctor from the register.

The functions of the Preliminary Proceedings Committee are set out in section 42 of the Act. It has to decide if an allegation under section 36 or 37 should be referred for inquiry by the Professional Conduct Committee or the Health Committee.

Section 40 enables a doctor to appeal to the Privy Council against a decision of the Professional Conduct Committee. The doctor can also appeal to the High Court to have an order for immediate suspension of registration to be lifted.

Professional performance

New provisions on professional performance came into force in July 1997 as a result of the Medical (Professional Performance) Act 1995. This Act established two new Committees: the Assessment Referral Committee and the Committee on Professional Performance. Under a new Section 36A of the Medical Act 1983 the Committee on Professional Performance is given power when the standard of professional performance of a fully registered person is found to have been seriously deficient to direct:

- that the registration is suspended for up to 12 months; or
- that the registration is conditional on compliance for up to three years with specified requirements.

If a registered practitioner fails to comply with the conditions, then he can be suspended for up to 12 months. The Committee has the power to extend the period of suspension for periods of 12 months at a time, and in certain circumstances can make a direction extending a period of suspension indefinitely[8]. Further information can be obtained from the GMC[9].

There are four stages for any review of professional performance:

- screening
- assessment of performance by the Assessment Referral Committee
- remedial training and reassessment
- consideration by the Committee on Professional Performance.

At any stage the process is halted if the requirements are met, i.e. if the initial screening is satisfactory things go no further.

Stage 4 only applies where doctors

- have particulaly serious deficiencies identified by an assessment,
- have failed to cooperate with the procedures, and
- have not made sufficient improvement in performance.

Fitness to practise

The Health Committee of the General Medical Council can determine whether a doctor is fit to practise. Its jurisdiction is set out under section 37 of the Medical Act 1983. The Health Committee has the power, if it judges a doctor's fitness to practise to be seriously impaired by reason of his physical or mental condition, to:

- suspend the registration for up to 12 months, or
- make the registration conditional on compliance with specified conditions for a period not exceeding three years.

Failure to comply with the conditions can lead to suspension of registration for up to 12 months. As with professional performance, there are powers to extend the suspension for further periods for up to 12 months at a time and, in certain circumstances, there can be an indefinite suspension.

Emergency action

Under section 38 the Professional Conduct Committee, the Committee on Professional Performance and the Health Committee have powers, on giving an order for erasure or suspension, to direct the immediate suspension if satisfied that to do so is necessary for the protection of members of the public or would be in the best interests of the doctor.

Appeals

Section 40 sets out the rights of appeal from the various orders of the Committees and of the GMC. Full details and the procedure for hearings generally can be found in the GMC booklet *Facing a complaint*[10].

Interim orders

Under Section 41A, where the interim orders committee is satisfied that

- it is necessary for the protection of members of the public or
- it is otherwise in the public interest or
- it is in the interests of a fully registered person

for a person's registration to be suspended or be made subject to conditions, the committee may make the appropriate order.

Examples of professional misconduct

A senior House Officer at Stafford General Hospital was suspended for six months for inadequate examinations of three A&E patients. He failed to arrange specialist investigation of a deep facial laceration, check a road accident victim with a serious head injury for possible fracture of the spine or properly examine the eyes and central nervous system of a patient known to have had a fit. The GMC Professional Conduct Committee recommended that the doctor took a refresher course training during his suspension and return to the committee for review after six months[11].

In January 2002 two consultant radiologists, who ran the East Devon sector of the national breast screening programme, were found guilty of serious professional misconduct[12]. They were allowed to stay on the register on the understanding that they would not carry out breast examinations again and would be recalled in two years for their progress to be assessed. They had failed to notice the signs of breast cancer in 82 patients. Eleven women died and others needed aggressive treatment which could have been avoided had their condition been diagnosed earlier. Compensation claims amounting to over £1.5 million are being brought.

Professional misconduct can include management functions. In *Roylance* v. *General Medical Council*[13] the Privy Council held that serious professional misconduct could include failures by a Chief Executive, who was also a registered medical practitioner, because he did not respond to concerns about the professional standards of paediatric heart surgeons.

Role of the Royal College of Radiologists

In 1995 the Royal College of Radiologists issued *The College and Its role in Performance Review*, detailing the circumstances in which the College could have a part to play in issues relating to standards of performance. Subsequently it announced that it was withdrawing that publication[14] and instead referred to the *Consultant's Handbook* of the British Medical Association[15] covering disciplinary procedures, personal health and performance matters and departmental organisation and management problems.

The RCR would not normally be involved in disciplinary matters but it could be asked to provide the names of external assessors under the intermediate procedure set up by a Trust to resolve cases of alleged professional misconduct or incompetence where the outcome will fall short of dismissal. In addition the RCR could provide the names of professional members for an enquiry panel under HC(90)9[16] or the name of a member to serve on the review panel established by the medical staff committee of a Trust to deal with concerns about a consultant's failure to fulfil contractual responsibilities. The RCR may also be asked to provide names for the National Counselling Service for Doctors or to nominate a GMC screener under the fitness to practice procedures.

The RCR will also assist the GMC in its performance review procedures by arranging for remedial training of a member or could provide Fellows to advise on departmental, organisation and management problems, provided that the Fellow acts in their own name and not on behalf of the College.

Other disciplinary proceedings against doctors

Doctors employed in NHS trusts

The Department of Health has provided guidance for terms for the disciplining of employed doctors to be included into the contract of employment which each doctor has with their employer[16]. These terms cover intermediate procedures, suspension from duty, the holding of an inquiry and appeals to the Secretary of State.

Reforms of the present procedure are being considered by the Secretary of State for Health[17].

General practitioners

As self-employed practitioners, GPs have a contract for services with the NHS. The details in the terms of service covering disciplinary proceedings were set out in 1992[18] and enabled a GP to be brought before a Medical Services Committee of the FHSA. After 1996 a new complaints procedure was introduced into the NHS and complaints against GPs would follow the procedure which applied in hospitals (see Chapter 19). Medical Service Committees were abolished and Disciplinary Committees established under the health authority to investigate any alleged breach of the practitioner's terms of service. In the past a health authority could apply to the NHS Tribunal that the GP should be removed from its list on the grounds that continued inclusion would be prejudicial to the efficiency of the services[19] or where there has been fraud[20]. The Health and Social Care Act 2001, section 16, abolishes the NHS Tribunal.

Increasing control on professional practice

In 2000 a spate of scandals of criminal and professional misconduct by doctors hit the press. Dr Shipman was convicted of 15 murders; the Richie Report[21] was published on the malpractice by Dr Ledward, the gynaecologist; there was an announcement that another gynaecologist, Dr Neale (who had been struck off from the Canadian register 15 years ago) was facing professional conduct proceedings from the General Medical Council in relation to allegations of mistreatment of over 50 women[22]; and an announcement in 2000 that over 200 patients had to have their histology reports revised following failures by Dr Elwood, a Consultant pathologist, (seven patients were wrongly diagnosed and suffered serious consequences as a result)[23].

The Chief Medical Officer, the top medically qualified adviser to the Secretary of State for Health, issued a consultation document *Supporting Doctors; Protecting patients*[24]. This document put forward proposals for preventing, recognising and dealing with poor clinical performance of doctors in the NHS in England. Its most significant proposal is routine annual appraisal of consultant staff. It also recommends the setting up of Assessment and Support Centres to be run jointly by the NHS and the medical profession which would give impartial advice and support to the local employer regarding doctors referred to it and also provide support to the doctors.

The GMC proposed appraisal and assessment for revalidation of its registered practitioners every five years[25]. The summary document for the GMC proposals invited feedback by 25 September 2000 (see Chapter 13).

National Clinical Assessment Authority

The National Clinical Assessment Authority (NCAA) was established in April 2001[26], (following the Chief Medical Officer's report[24]), as a special health authority and as one of the central elements of the NHS's work on quality. Its aim is to provide a support service to health authorities and hospital and community trusts who are faced with concerns about the performance of an individual doctor. The Authority deals with concerns about doctors by providing advice, taking referrals and carrying out targeted assessments where necessary. The NCAA does not seek to take over the role of the employer or act as a regulator.

On 4 December 2001 the GMC, CHI and the NCAA signed up to a memorandum of understanding setting out their respective roles[27].

Health Professions Council

Duties in respect of conduct and fitness to practise

Part V of the order for the new Health Professions Council[28], sets out the provisions for fitness to practise procedures for health professionals who are not doctors, dentists, midwives or nurses (see Chapter 11). The Health Professions Council is required to establish three practice Committees, an Investigating Committee, the Conduct and Competence Committee and the Health Committee. In relation to Fitness to Practice, the order requires the Health Professions Council to:

- establish and keep under review the standards of conduct, performance and ethics expected of registrants and prospective registrants and give them such guidance on these matters as it sees fit; and
- establish and keep under review effective arrangements to protect the public from persons whose fitness to practise is impaired.

Allegations

A procedure is laid down for dealing with allegations made against a registered person to the effect that her fitness to practice is impaired by reason of:

- misconduct
- lack of competence
- a conviction or caution in the UK for a criminal offence (or a conviction elsewhere for what would also be a crime in England and Wales)
- her physical or mental health, or
- a determination by a UK statutory body responsible for a health or social care

profession that she is unfit to practise that profession (or a determination by a licensing body elsewhere to the same effect).

Allegations can be referred to a panel of screeners and at least two of them (with one lay person and one registrant from the professional field of the person under scrutiny) shall consider whether the allegation is well founded. The Council has power to make rules relating to the appointment and functions of the Screeners.

The Investigating Committee (Article 26) investigates any allegation referred to it following a set procedure. If the committee considers that there is a case to answer it must notify in writing with reasons the registered professional concerned and the person making the allegation. It has powers, where it concludes that there is a case to answer, to undertake mediation, refer the case to screeners for them to undertake mediation, to the Health Committee or the Conduct and Competence Committee.

The Conduct and Competence Committee (Article 27), after consultation with the other Practice Committees, shall consider:

- any allegation referred to it by the Council, Screeners, the Investigating Committee or the Health Committee and
- any application for restoration referred to it by the Registrar.

The Health Committee (Article 28) shall consider any allegation referred to it by the Council, Screeners, the Investigating Committee or the Conduct and Competence Committee and also any application for restoration referred to it by the Registrar, and Article 29 sets out the procedure to be followed. Articles 30 to 35 cover further procedural details, including the appointment of legal assessors who have the general function of giving advice to screeners, the statutory committees or the Registrar on questions of law. Medical assessors can also be appointed to give relevant advice.

Appeals

An appeal from any decision of a Practice Committee lies to an appropriate court. Earlier proposals for the establishment of a Health Professions Independent Appeals Tribunal were not contained in the final order.

Conclusions

Standards of professional practice are constantly being raised and the onus is on the professional personally to ensure that her competence is maintained and that she upholds the reasonable standards of professional practice. She therefore has the responsibility of ensuring that she obtains the necessary training and instruction to remain competent and to develop safely in new areas of practice. Re-registration will require evidence of ongoing professional development. High standards of professional practice are central to the Government's plan for the NHS[29].

At present, in spite of the considerable changes to professional regulation in recent years and the enhanced powers of the GMC, there are still considerable differences between the professional registration bodies both in the definition of professional misconduct and the procedure for dealing with it. It is highly likely that the next few years will see stronger powers given to the registration bodies for the protection of the public and there will be a move towards a uniformity across all health professionals (including doctors, nurses and those formerly described as the professions supplementary to medicine) in the definition of professional misconduct and the procedures laid down to both prevent it and deal with it. Proposals contained in the NHS Reform and Healthcare Professions Bill 2002 for the establishment of a Council for the Regulation of the Healthcare Professions will, if enacted, speed the process of uniformity of professional regulation.

 Questions and exercises _____

1   A colleague tells you that she has been reported to the HPC for alleged professional misconduct. Advise her on the procedure which will be followed and how she could defend herself.

2   Do you consider that the following conduct by a registered practitioner should be the subject of professional conduct proceedings:
   ● A parking fine
   ● An offence of shop-lifting
   ● Being cited in a divorce as an adulterer
   ● Being found guilty of a breach of the peace following a New Year's Eve party?

3   A radiologist and a radiographer are found guilty of professional misconduct in stealing drugs from the X-ray department. Explain the differences in how they would be dealt with by their respective professional registration bodies. (Research suggested sources)

References

1   *The Medical Act 1983 (Amendment) Order* SI No 1803 of 2000
2   GMC (1998) *Good Medical Practice* (July 1998) GMC, London
3   GMC (2000) *Confidentiality: Protecting and Providing Information* GMC, London
4   GMC (1998) *Seeking Patients' Consent: The Ethical Considerations* (November 1998) GMC, London
5   www.gmc-uk.org
6   The Medical Act 1983, Section 35A and The Medical Act 1983 (Amendment) Order SI No 1803 of 2000
7   *McCandless* v. *General Medical Council* [1996] 1 WLR 167
8   Medical Act 1983, s 36A(4) as inserted by the Medical (Professional Performance) Act 1995
9   GMC (1999) *Performance Procedures: A Guide to the Arrangements* (June 1999) GMC, London
10 GMC (1997) *Facing a complaint* (November 1997) GMC, London
11 GMC (2000) *News Issue*, (1 July 2000)
12 J Bale (2002) Cancer scandal doctors allowed to keep working *The Times* 18 January 2002

13 *Roylance* v. *General Medical Council* [1999] Lloyd's Rep Med 139 (PC)
14 Royal College of Radiologists (1995) *The College and its role in Performance Review* (AJC/cmj/4481) RCR, London
15 British Medical Association *The Consultant's Handbook* BMA, London
16 Department of Health (1990) *Disciplinary Procedures for Hospital and Community Medical and Dental Staff* HC(90)9 DoH, London
17 Department of Health (1999) *Supporting Doctors, Protecting Patients* DoH, London
18 National Health Service (Service Committees and Tribunal) Regulations 1992 SI No 664 of 1992
19 NHS Act 1977, section 46(6)
20 Health Act 1999, section 40 (amending Section 46 of the NHS Act 1977)
21 Department of Health (2000) *Inquiry into the practice of Dr Ledward* (chaired by Jean Richie) Stationery Office, London
22 M. Horsnell (2000) Patient tells GMC of pain and suffering after two operations *The Times*, 14 June
23 Department of Health *NHS Standards watchdog to investigate locum doctor's employment at 4 trusts* Press release 2000/348 (13 June 2000)
24 Chief Medical Officer (2000) *Supporting Doctors; Protecting patients* DoH, London; available on the internet http://www.doh.gov.uk/cmoconsult1.htm
25 General Medical Council (2000) *Revalidating Doctors Ensuring Standards, securing the future: A Summary GMC, London*
26 National Clinical Assessment Authority (Establishment and Constitution) Order 2000 SI No 2961 of 2000
27 *Accessible on the NCAA website: www.ncaa.nhs.uk*
28 Health Professions Order 2001; S.I. 2002/254
29 Department of Health (2000) *NHS Plan* DoH, London

Chapter 13
Education and Training

This chapter considers the legal framework for defining the content and establishing high standards of pre-registration and post-registration education and training of both the doctors and radiographers. (Reference should also be made to Chapter 28 on the legal aspects of research.)

Radiologists

General Medical Council

Under section 5(1) of the Medical Act, the Education Committee of General Medical Council[1] has the general function of promoting high standards and co-ordinating all stages of medical education. For the purpose of discharging this function the Education Committee must:

- Determine the extent of the knowledge and skill which is to be required for the granting of primary UK qualifications ('the prescribed knowledge and skill') and secure that instruction given in universities in the UK to persons studying for such qualifications is sufficient to equip them with knowledge and skill to that extent.
- Determine the standard of proficiency which is to be required from candidates at qualifying examinations ('the prescribed standard of proficiency') and secure maintenance of that standard.
- Determine patterns of experience which may be recognised as suitable for giving general clinical training for the purpose of the practice of their profession to those engaging in employment in a resident medical capacity in approved hospitals or institutions for the purpose of obtaining the necessary experience to qualify for registration ('the prescribed pattern of experience').

It must secure that the requirements of article 23 of Directive 93/16/EEC are satisfied. (This is designed to facilitate the free movement of doctors and the mutual recognition of their diplomas, certificates and other evidence of formal qualifications.)

Under section 6 universities granting any primary UK qualification are obliged to provide the Education Committee with information on the courses, etc. and the Education Committee can appoint inspectors to attend any of the qualifying examinations. The role of the inspectors is to secure the maintenance of the prescribed standard of proficiency required from candidates. The inspectors report to the Committee their opinion on the sufficiency of every examination that they attend and on other matters directed by the Education Committee. Reports from the inspectors which go to the Committee must be forwarded to the institution which held the examinations.

Visitors are appointed by the Education Committee of the GMC under section 7 of the 1983 Act to visit institutions where instruction is given to medical students. Visitors are subject to directions from the Privy Council and they report to the Education Committee on the sufficiency of instruction given and on any other matters relevant to the education. Any report from the Visitors must be sent to the institution, which is permitted to respond to that report.

The ultimate sanction is that if the Education Committee is concerned about the course of study, then it can make representations to the Privy Council, which can make an order that a qualification obtained at that institution is not one which can lead to registration.

The experience required for full registration by virtue of primary UK qualification is set out in section 10 of the Act and requires a person, after passing the primary qualification to have been engaged for the prescribed period in employment in a resident medical capacity in one or more approved hospitals, institutions or medical practices. Visitors can also be appointed by the Education Committee to visit any approved hospital or approved institution to report to the committee on the extent to which general clinical training given by employment in a resident medical capacity is such as to provide the experience required[2]. (Alternative requirements for the experience are provided for in section 14.)

Specialist training and register

The GMC also holds a specialist register listing those doctors who have completed specialist training. Doctors must be included on this specialist register to obtain consultant posts in the NHS. The Specialist Training Authority of the Medical Royal Colleges was established on 12 January 1996 for the purposes of specialist medical training and the issue of Certificates of Completion of Specialist Training.

Overseas and European Economic Area qualifications

Changes have been made to the criteria for recognition of overseas doctors and those qualified in the EEA. These are considered in detail by Diana Kloss[3], in the Butterworths standard textbook on medical law.

Revalidation

Proposals have been put forward for consultation by the GMC for a three stage process of revalidation:[4]

- a folder of information describing the work of the doctor which will be regularly reviewed in an annual appraisal;
- periodic revalidation, being a recommendation by a group of medical and lay people that the doctor remains fit to practise, or that the GMC should review the doctor's registration; and

- action by the GMC, usually revalidation of the doctor's registration, or occasionally detailed investigation under the fitness to practice procedures.

The RCR has provided a practical guide[5] on clinical governance and revalidation for its members. This gives step by step advice on how to carry out an audit of different activities for use both in the implementation of clinical governance and also for the purposes of securing revalidation.

Role of the Royal College of Radiologists

The RCR has a major role to play in the education and training for those specialising in radiology and oncology. To become a Fellow of the RCR doctors must have trained for a minimum of five years and study the syllabus and complete the examinations set by the RCR. An information pack is available from the training administrator of the RCR[6]. The Education Board of the Faculty of Clinical Radiology of the Royal College of Radiologists has also published a guide on structured training in radiology[7]. Its aim is to define the present curriculum in each year of training and to set down the overall structure of trainee assessment during the period of Higher Specialist Training. A second edition was published in 1999[8] and an appendix covering the curricula for sub-specialty training in 2000[9].

Radionuclide imaging – the way training develops
The Joint Committee of Higher Medical Training of the Royal Colleges of Physicians of the UK (JCHMT) has issued curricula for higher specialist training[10]. Martin Wastie, Regional Adviser for nuclear medicine, has suggested that the Royal College of Radiologists should formulate a policy making radionuclide imaging a sub-specialty of diagnostic imaging and setting out a curriculum. He states that 'with their knowledge of other diagnostic imaging techniques radiologists are the ideal people to interpret radionuclide scans and are in a unique position to advance this vital aspect of nuclear medicine'. He also comments that 'most radiologists report between 10–15 000 investigations a year and would look with envy at someone who is only expected to report 2400'.

Radiographers

Health Professions Council

Under the Health Act 1999 one of the statutory duties of the HPC which are not transferable by Order to another body is the determining of standards of education and training for admission to practice (see Chapter 11).

Education and Training Committee
One of the statutory committees which must be set up by the Health Professions Council is an Education and Training Committee. This will advise the Council on the performance of the Council's functions in relation to:

- the establishing of standards of proficiency
- the establishing of standards and requirements in respect of education and training

- the giving of guidance on education and training standards to registrants, employers and others.

The Council is required to establish from time to time:

- the standards of education and training necessary to achieve the standards of proficiency it has established, and
- the requirements to be satisfied for admission to such education and training which may include requirements as to good health and good character.

The Education and Training Committee shall ensure that universities and other institutions are notified of the standards and requirements and shall take appropriate steps to satisfy itself that those standards and requirements are met. The Education and Training Committee can approve courses of education or training, qualifications, institutions, such tests of professional competence, education, training and experience which would lead to the award of additional qualifications which would be recorded in the register. The Council is required to publish a statement of the criteria which will be taken into account in deciding whether to give approval. The Council is also required to maintain and publish a list of the courses of education or training, qualifications and institutions which are or were approved under the Order.

Visitors

The Council may appoint persons, known as Visitors to visit any place or institution which gives or proposes to give a relevant course of education, examination or test of competence. A Visitor cannot exercise these functions at any institution with which he has a significant connection. A Visitor can be a member of the Council or its committees, but not an employee of the Council. Visitors are to be selected with due regard to the profession with which the education and training they are to report on is concerned and at least one of the Visitors shall be registered in that part of the register which relates to that profession.

Any institution must give to the Education and Training Committee or the Council 'such information and assistance as the Committee may reasonably require in connection with the exercise of its functions under this Order'.

Withdrawing approval

The Committee can refuse or withdraw of approval of courses, qualifications and institutions. Where approval is withdrawn the Committee has to use its best endeavours to secure that any person who is undertaking the education or training concerned or studying for the qualification concerned is given the opportunity to follow approved education or training or to study for an approved qualification or at an approved institution. The procedures are designed to maintain standards but not disadvantage individuals who have the misfortune to be studying on a course or at an institution where approval is withdrawn.

Post registration training

The Health Professions Council may make rules requiring registered professionals to undertake such continuing professional development as it shall specify.

Wales

The National Assembly for Wales is empowered to create or designate a body with whom the Council may enter into any arrangements for the approval of pre-registration courses etc and the standards for continuing professional development under articles 16(5) and 20(4) respectively.

College and Society of Radiographers

The Society of Radiographers was inaugurated in 1920 and is a professional body and trade union, affiliated to the Trades Union Congress. The College of Radiographers is the charitable subsidiary of the Society. Its objective is to support education, research and other activities in support of the science and practice of radiography and its allied sciences. The Society commissions the College to deliver professional and educational services for its members. Guidance was provided to the CPSM (in future to the HPC) on the content of the educational qualifications leading to the securing of the necessary educational qualifications for state registration of therapeutic and diagnostic radiographers.

Special statutory requirements

Under Regulation 11 of the Ionising Radiation (Medical Exposure) Regulations 2000[11] certain requirements are set out in relation to training. Regulation 11(1) states that no practitioner or operator is permitted to carry out a medical exposure or any practical aspect without having been adequately trained. A certificate issued by an institute or person competent to award degrees or diplomas or to provide other evidence of training shall, if such certificate so attests, be sufficient proof that the person to whom it has been issued has been adequately trained. However allowance is made for practical training providing this is done under the supervision of people who are themselves adequately trained.

Under Regulation 11(4) any employer shall keep and have available for inspection by the appropriate authority up-to-date records of all practitioners and operators engaged to carry out medical exposures or any practical aspect of such exposures showing the date or dates on which training qualifying as adequate training was completed and also the nature of the training.

By Regulation 11(5), with agency staff the agency is responsible for keeping the records and supplying them to the employing Trust on request.

Content of training

Training which satisfies the requirements of Schedule 2 of the Ionising Radiation (Medical Exposure) Regulations 2000 must be provided by employers and (the expression 'adequately trained' is construed in this light.). The requirements set out in Schedule 2 are comprehensive and a useful check list for educational programmes. Practitioners and operators must successfully complete training (both theoretical knowledge and practical experience) in two aspects of their work.

- Firstly they must receive training in such of:
  ○ fundamental physics of radiation
  ○ management and radiation protection of the patient
  ○ statutory requirements and advisory aspects

as are relevant to their functions as practitioner or operator.

- Secondly they need to study whichever of:
  ○ diagnostic radiology
  ○ radiotherapy
  ○ nuclear medicine

are relevant to their specific area of practice.

Education issues

Wastage

One of the concerns raised in the 1997/8 annual report of the Radiographer's Board was the wastage from training courses for therapeutic radiographers. It was estimated that there was a loss of over 25% from students taking these courses, in contrast with a government estimate of 10% in placing contracts for such courses. The result would be that there was likely to be a significant shortfall in those entering the workforce. The Joint Validation Committee for radiographers had therefore made a strong recommendation that the Board and the College of Radiographers should draw the attention of the NHS Executive to the situation.

Feedback from students

Developments in the effectiveness of pre- and post-registration training and professional practice depend heavily upon the research undertaken by staff working in both academic and clinical environments[12].

In order to prevent serious wastage taking place it was essential to obtain more feedback from students. A survey was conducted by Georgina Gerrard of the views of clinical oncology trainees in each region of the UK[13]. The problems which were identified included:

- excessive service commitment
- disparity of teaching between centres, and a feeling of isolation in some small centres
- poor supervision of trainees in some clinics and radiotherapy planning sessions
- lack of exposure to specialist areas, e.g. head and neck oncology
- lack of protected study time for research
- frequent examinations on some masters courses.

Suggestions for improving training included

- creating new consultant, specialist registrar staff grade and clinical assistant posts

- reducing the clinic size if a doctor is absent rather than using another doctor to cross-cover
- consultant participation in more organised teaching
- inclusion of trainees in smaller centres (perhaps via video conferences and learning on the internet)
- rotation to other centres and to other oncological specialties, especially closer integration with medical oncology
- protected study time.

Post-registration training

Duty of employer to provide facilities

It could be argued that, since the health-care employer has a duty of care at common law to its patients, it must, as part of this duty, ensure that its staff are competent. In addition as part of the contractual duty that it owes to its employees, it must provide competent fellow staff. Should the employer fail to fulfil this duty, and harm befall a patient or employee as a result, then the employer could be directly liable in negligence. Thus one can assume that the employer's duty includes the duty to ensure that staff are kept competent and that therefore paid study leave should be made available as an implied condition of the contract of employment.

This logic has not, however, so far been categorically established in the courts. The uncertainty has meant that there is wide variation across the country as to the rights of employees in obtaining paid study leave and funded professional development. Registered nurses and midwives now have to prove that they have undertaken at least five study days (or comparable training) every three years in order to be reregistered. Similar provisions are being introduced for professionals registered under the Health Professions Council. Doctors are also required to undergo continuing professional development. In order to remain on the register they will have to show that they have completed a specified number of post-registration professional development days. However there is no agreement that NHS trusts will automatically fund this activity and practice varies from Trust to Trust.

Responsibility of the practitioner

It therefore remains the responsibility of individual practitioners to maintain their post-registration competence, experience and knowledge. In an article for *Synergy*[14], Suzanne Henwood suggests that practitioners should have a more strategic approach to CPD, should identify the particular style most suitable to them and then consider the various CPD opportunities listed. Finally she emphasises the importance of evaluation to ensure that CPD carried out is effective in terms of outcomes and the costs invested. She comments:

> 'Individuals must take some of the responsibility for assessing the effectiveness of their own CPD activity, but we could offer a greater degree of peer support to encourage this to occur on a more formal basis.'

If the Trust or private hospital employer is unwilling to fund post-registration courses or study leave, the individual practitioner may have to be prepared to be responsible for the cost herself. A practitioner could not defend a failure to maintain her competence on the grounds that the employer has not funded study leave or further training. Registered nurses and midwives also have a responsibility to complete a personal profile of their professional development to be reregistered and such a record might also be extremely useful for radiographers[15].

Training role of the registered practitioner

Educating and supervising students
It cannot be assumed that only full time clinical teachers have responsibilities in education and training. Increasingly, the colleges are looking for practitioners to provide not only clinical supervision for pre-registration students, but also to provide a mentoring role for students and newly qualified registered staff. The responsibilities of the senior practitioner in relation to supervision and delegation cannot be underestimated.

Training of assistants
It must not be forgotten that as the dependence on assistants increases so resources must be allocated to ensure that they are appropriately trained. There appears little doubt that the skill-mix ratio in radiography will change as there are more assistants employed in ratio to the registered practitioner. In Chapter 27 the legal issues relating to delegation and supervision are discussed.

The Workforce Development Confederations

From April 2001 the role of the Education and Training Consortia has been subsumed in the remit of the new Workforce Development Confederations. Their function is to ensure the supply of appropriately trained health and social care staff in England, including medical and dental staff. In relation to radiography the Confederations will commission pre- and post-registration courses in radiography and will also be responsible for the supply of clinical placements. Funded by the government, the Confederations have a Chief Executive and each Trust and health authority are members of the appropriate area Confederation.

Individual placements for students are funded on an individual basis, in England and Wales from a Department of Health bursary; in Scotland and Northern Ireland from its Higher Education Funding Council.

Administrative failures

Lecturers and other educationalists should be aware that administrative weaknesses or inefficiencies could give rise to court hearings and complaints. Thus in one case a would-be physiotherapy student was wrongly informed through the admissions system by the University of Salford that he was being offered a place. He wrote accepting the offer, and then learnt later that a mistake had been made, and there had never been a place for him. His application for specific performance of the contract and a mandatory injunction compelling the University to give a place failed because the Court of Appeal[16] held that, while there probably was a binding agreement that the University would accept him for the degree course in physiotherapy, it was not just to compel the University to provide a place for a student whose academic record was not good enough. Even though the prospective student failed on the facts in this case, it is clear that a contract is created between the student and the institution when an offer for a place is accepted with obligations on both sides.

Conclusions

The effects of the recent statutory changes to the composition and functions of professional registration bodies may have significant implications for the delivery and standards of education for both doctors and for other health professions. The maintenance of high standards for admission to the respective professional registers is likely to be accompanied by greater flexibility and role expansion of the different health professionals which is considered in Chapter 27. The effectiveness of the new Workforce Development Confederations in securing the appropriate number of qualified staff is still to be evaluated.

Questions and exercises

1 A student reports to you, her tutor, that she was aware unsafe equipment is being used in an X-ray department of a Trust. What action would you take and what action would you advise her to take?

2 Obtain a copy of the memorandum of agreement between your college and the NHS trust (or Workforce Confederation) which takes your students on placements. To what extent does it determine responsibility for the negligence of the student or for responsibility for harm to the student whilst on clinical placement? (see also Chapters 14, 15 and 27)

3 There are strong advantages in every health professional having a profile by which they can identify both on-going professional development and also potential areas of further development. Consider the extent to which this could be used in personal negotiation with senior management to obtain trust support for an individual's professional development and define a development plan to ensure your continued professional competence.

4 What improvements do you consider could be made in ensuring the integration of theoretical and clinical training for the pre-registration student?

5 Design a protocol which could be used for those practitioners who act as mentors for junior colleagues.

References

1 *Halsbury's Laws of England* 4th ed. Vol. 30 2000 reissue, paras. 78–84
2 Medical Act 1983, section 13

3   D. Kloss (1998) 'The Health Care Professions' in I. Kennedy and A. Grubb (eds) *Principles of Medical Law* Butterworths, London

4   General Medical Council (2000) *Revalidating Doctors* GMC, London

5   G. de Lacey, R. Godwin & A. Manhire (2000) (eds) *Clinical Governance and Revalidation* Royal College of Radiologists, London

6   RCR, 38 Portland Place, London W1N 4JQ (0207 636 4432)

7   The Education Board of the Faculty of Clinical Radiology of the Royal College of Radiologists (1995) *A guide on structured Training in Radiology* (EBCR(95)1) RCR, London

8   The Education Board of the Faculty of Clinical Radiology of the Royal College of Radiologists (1999) *A Guide on structured Training in Radiology* 2nd edn., (EBFCR(99)1) RCR, London

9   The Education Board of the Faculty of Clinical Radiology of the Royal College of Radiologists (2000) *Appendix covering the curricula for subspecialty training in 2000.* (EBCR(00)1) RCR, London

10 M. Wastie (1998) *Radionuclide* Royal College of Radiologists Issue No 53 Winter 1998, page 14

11 The Ionising Radiation (Medical Exposure) Regulations 2000 SI No. 1059 of 2000

12 G. Marshall & P. Harris (2000) A study of the role of an objective structured clinical examination (OSCE) in assessing clinical competence in third year student radiographers *Radiography* (May 2000) Vol 6, pages 117–122; D. Manning, J. Leach & S. Bunting (2000) A comparison of expert and novice performance in the detection of simulated pulmonary nodules *Radiography* (May 2000) Vol 6 pages 111–116; D. J. Manning, S. Bunting & J. Leach (1999) An ROC evaluation of six systems for chest radiography *Radiography* November (1999) Vol 5, pages 201–209

13 G. Gerrard (1997) Clinical Oncology Training: Views of clinical oncology trainees in each region of the UK Royal College of Radiographers Issue No 51 (Summer 1997) page 7

14 S. Henwood (2000) What is effective CPD and how do I evaluate it? *Synergy* (August 2000) pages 6–9

15 A. Alsop (1991) The Professional Portfolio – Purpose, process and Practice *British Journal of Occupational Therapy* **58**, 7, 299–302

16 *Moran* v. *University of Salford* Lexis, 12 November 1993; *The Times* 23 November 1993

Section D
Accountability in the Civil and Criminal Courts

Chapter 14
Negligence

Introduction

Litigation is increasing as the expectations of patients in relation to health care grow and publicity about compensation awards raises hopes of vast settlements.

The employed practitioner is unlikely to be sued personally. This is because the employer is indirectly responsible in law for the wrongful acts of its employee whilst the employee is acting in course of employment. This is known as vicarious liability and is explained further below. The employed practitioner might however be held personally liable for 'Samaritan' acts, if harm is caused, in a situation where the employer could argue that it is not vicariously liable because the employee was not acting in the course of employment.

Even if the practitioner is an employee, she still needs to have an understanding of the law relating to negligence, so that she is appropriately prepared to defend any allegations against her.

Civil actions

These include those actions which are brought in the civil courts by an individual or organisation, usually with the aim of obtaining compensation or other remedy which the court is able to order. The main group of civil actions affecting health professionals are called torts, i.e. civil wrongs excluding breach of contract. Within this group are included negligence, trespass, breach of statutory duty, defamation, nuisance and others. In each case the burden will usually be upon the person bringing the action (known as the claimant, but prior to April 1999 referred to as the plaintiff) to establish, on a balance of probabilities, the existence of each of the elements which make up a cause of action. Thus in an action for trespass to the person (see Chapter 4) the claimant must show that there was a direct interference or touching of his person and that it was without his consent or other lawful justification.

Principles of negligence

Negligence is the most common tort brought in situations where the claimant alleges that there has been personal injury or death, or damage or loss of property caused by another. Compensation is sought for the loss which has occurred. To succeed in the action, the claimant has to show the following elements:

- that the defendant owed to the person harmed a duty of care;
- that the defendant was in breach of that duty;
- that the breach of duty caused reasonably foreseeable harm to the claimant.

These four elements – duty, breach, causation and harm are discussed below.

Duty of care

The law recognises that a duty of care will exist where one person can reasonably foresee that his or her actions or omissions could cause reasonably foreseeable harm to another person. A duty of care will always exist between the health professional and the patient, but it might not always be easy to identify what it includes. Where there is no pre-existing duty to a person, the usual legal principle is that there is no duty to volunteer services. There may however be a professional duty to volunteer help in certain circumstances.

In the case of *Donoghue* v. *Stevenson*[1] the House of Lords defined the duty of care owed at common law (i.e. judge-made law) as being:

> 'You must take reasonable care to avoid acts or omissions which you can reasonably foresee would be likely to injure your neighbour. Who then in law is my neighbour? The answer seems to be persons who are so closely and directly affected by my act that I ought reasonably to have them in contemplation as being so affected when I am directing my mind to the acts or omissions which are called in question.'

Despite there being such a straightforward definition laid down by the House of Lords there is often difficulty in deciding how far and to whom, precisely, the duty of care extends. Cases are decided on their particular facts. For example, in a case involving the escape of Borstal boys who caused serious damage to a yacht[2], the House of Lords held that a duty of care was owed by the Home Office to any persons who were injured or whose property was damaged as a result of the failure to keep the boys under proper control.

Breach of duty

Determining the standard of care
In order to determine whether there has been a breach of the duty of care, it will first be necessary to establish the required standard. The courts have used what has become known as the 'Bolam test' to determine the standard of care required by a professional. In the case from which the test took its name[3] the court laid down the following principle to determine the standard of care which should be followed:

> 'The test is the standard of the ordinary skilled man exercising and professing to have that special skill.' (Judge McNair, page 121)

The Bolam test was applied by the House of Lord in a case[4] where negligence by an obstetrician in delivering a child by forceps was alleged:

'Where you get a situation which involves the use of some special skill or competence, then the test as to whether there has been negligence or not ... is the standard of the ordinary skilled man exercising and professing to have that special skill. If a surgeon fails to measure up to that in any respect (clinical judgment or otherwise) he has been negligent and should be so adjudged.'

The House of Lords found that the surgeon was not liable in negligence and held that an error of judgment may or may not be negligence. It depends upon the circumstances.

This standard of the reasonable professional man following the accepted approved standard of care can be used to apply to any professional person – architect, lawyer, accountant as well as any health professional. The standard of care which a practitioner should have provided would be judged in this way. Expert witnesses would give evidence to the court on the standard of care they would expect to have found in the circumstances giving rise to the claim. These experts would be respected members of the profession of radiographers or radiologists, possibly a head of a department or training college, and lawyers would look to the leading organisations of individual professional groups to obtain recommended names. The experts would be expected to place themselves in the situation of the practitioners at the time the alleged negligent act took place and give their opinion on the standard of care that they would have expected to have been followed at that time not the standards at the time of the court hearing. This is significant, since many cases take several years to come to court in which time standards may have changed.

In a civil action, the judge would decide, in the light of the evidence which has been given to the court, what standard should have been followed (see Chapter 18 on the expert witness).

Experts can, of course, differ and a case may arise where the expert giving evidence for the claimant states that the accepted approved standard of care was not followed by the defendant or its employees but in contrast the expert evidence for the defendant states that a reasonable standard of care was followed. Where such a conflict arises the House of Lords in the *Maynard* case[5] has laid down the following principle:

'It is not enough [to establish negligence by the defendant] to show that there is a body of competent professional opinion which considers that theirs was the wrong decision, if there also exists a body of professional opinion, equally competent, which supports the decision as reasonable in the circumstances.'

The determination of the reasonable standard of care has been more recently considered by the House of Lords in the case of *Bolitho* v. *City Hospital Hackney*[6]. In this case the House of Lords stated that:

'The court has to be satisfied that the exponents of the body of opinion relied on can demonstrate that such opinion has a logical basis. In particular in cases involving, as they often do, the weighing of risks against benefits, the judge, before accepting a body of opinion as being responsible, reasonable or respectable, will need to be satisfied that, in forming their views, the experts had directed their minds to the question of comparative risks and benefits and had reached a defensible conclusion on the matter.'

The Lords commented that the adjectives 'responsible, reasonable and respectable' (in the Bolam case) all showed that experts relied on had to demonstrate that their opinion had a logical basis, and referred to cases where this was not so. However it was stated that

'It will very seldom be right for a judge to reach the conclusion that views held by a competent medical expert are unreasonable'.

Following the Woolf Reforms (see Chapter 2) parties to personal injury litigation are encouraged to agree upon an expert witness.

It follows from the *Bolitho* judgment that there will be exceptional cases where a judge decides that expert opinion given by a defendant is not reasonable. This occurred in the following case[7].

Case: *Marriott* v. *West Midlands Health Authority*

The claimant fell downstairs at his home, suffered a head injury and was unconscious for about 20–30 minutes. He was admitted to hospital and, following X-rays and neurological observations, he was discharged the next day. He remained lethargic with no appetite and had headaches. He called the GP who was informed of the history, gave him neurological tests but found no abnormality. He told the claimant's wife to call him if the condition deteriorated and advised him to take pain killers for his headache. Four days later his condition suddenly deteriorated and he became unconscious and was returned to hospital. A massive left extradural haematoma was operated upon. A linear fracture of the skull was discovered. The claimant was left with hemiplegia, dysarthria and was severely disabled.

The claimant sued the health authorities and the general practitioner. There was disputed expert evidence over the correct course which should have been followed by the GP. The trial judge found against the GP and the GP appealed against this decision. The Court of Appeal dismissed the appeal and held that the judge was entitled to subject a body of opinion to analysis to see whether it could properly be regarded as reasonable. Despite expert evidence to the contrary, the judge was entitled to find it could not be a reasonable exercise of a GP's discretion to leave such a patient at home.

National standards
The White Paper[8] issues on the NHS and the Health Act 1999 which are discussed in Chapter 21 are likely to lead to increasing emphasis on standard setting. The National Institute of Clinical Excellence (NICE), the Commission for Health Improvement (CHI) and the National Standards Frameworks also give more guidance on standards to be achieved in all departments of a hospital and community care. It is anticipated that these standards will be incorporated into the Bolam test of reasonable professional practice. Practitioners will be expected to follow the results of clinical effectiveness research in their treatment and care of the patients and patients will be able to use these national guidelines to argue that inadequate care has been provided. For example in January 2001 the

Government published its national standards for cancer services[9] (see Chapter 21). If a hospital fails to meet these standards and a claimant can show that he has suffered consequential harm, then this failure could be used as evidence in a claim for compensation for negligence. In addition to showing that there has been vicarious liability on the part of the Trust, a claimant may also be able to establish the Trust's direct liability for the inadequate services.

Other organisations will be involved with NICE in determining the appropriate standards for different clinical areas. For example the NHS Executive is working in conjunction with the Society of Radiographers, the Royal College of Radiologists, the Health Service Breast Screening Programme and the National Training Organisation to prepare occupational standards in mammography[10]. Once the standards are finalised, it is likely that they will have considerable weight in determining the Bolam test of approved accepted practice.

However a recent decision of the Court of Appeal has emphasised that the highest standards are not those which have to be implemented in the law of negligence. The Court of Appeal suggested that where there was more than one acceptable standard, competence should be gauged by the lowest of them[11]. The Bolam test applied where there was a conscious choice of available courses made by a trained professional. It was inappropriate where the alleged neglect lay in an oversight.

Legal significance of guidelines

It should be emphasised that the publication of national guidelines will never remove the need for individual professional discretion to be exercised to ensure that the specific circumstances of the patient are taken into account in determining what would be the reasonable standard of care. As J.R. Hampton put it in a Guest editorial in *Radiography*[12], guidelines are only as good as the evidence upon which they are based and to cover all the variables in any guideline could result in a textbook which will be rapidly out of date. He wrote:

> 'Guidelines are seldom going to be truly evidence-based. They can only be for the obedience of fools and the guidance of wise men.'

Has there been a breach of the duty of care?

Once it has been established in court what the reasonable standard of care should have been, the next stage is to decide whether what took place was in accordance with that standard, i.e. has there been a breach of the duty of care. Gross negligence which results in death could be followed by criminal proceedings (see Chapter 2). In the civil courts evidence will be given by witnesses of fact as to what actually took place. The role of witnesses is considered in Chapter 18.

Causation

The claimant must show that not only was there a breach of the duty of care, but that this breach of duty caused actual and reasonably foreseeable harm to the claimant. This requires both factual causation to be established, and also evidence that the type of harm which occurred was reasonably foreseeable. A third factor which can cause problems for a claimant is that there must be no other intervening cause which breaks the chain of events from the negligent act to the harm suffered.

Factual causation

There may be a breach of the duty of care and harm but there may be no link between them. In the classic case of *Barnett* v. *Chelsea HMC*[13] a casualty doctor failed to examine patients who came in vomiting severely. The widow of one failed to obtain compensation, since the patient would have died anyway. There was no factual causation between the failure to examine and the death of the patient.

The onus is on the claimant to establish that there is this causation link between the breach of the duty of care and the harm which occurred. In the following case, the claimants failed initially to establish causation, and ultimately the House of Lords ordered a new hearing on the issue. At the end of the day, faced with more protracted litigation, the parties then agreed to a settlement.

Case: *Wilsher* v. *Essex Area Health Authority*[14]

A premature baby was being treated with oxygen therapy. A junior doctor mistakenly inserted the catheter to monitor the oxygen intake into the vein rather than an artery. A senior registrar when being asked to check what had been done failed to notice the error. The baby was given excess oxygen. The parents claimed compensation for the retrolentalfibroplasia that the baby suffered, but failed to prove that it was the excess oxygen which had caused the harm. They therefore failed in their claim.

It was agreed that there were several different factors which could have caused the child to become blind and the negligence was only one of them. It could not been presumed that it was the defendant's negligence which had caused the harm.

An example of a case involving a radiologist where there was a breach of the duty of care, but there was no liability because of the absence of causation is the Canadian case of *Meyer* v. *Rogers*[15].

Case: (*Meyer* v. *Rogers*)

Liability for using a dye which caused an allergic reaction was alleged in this case. Meyer suffered from a urinary tract problem and attended for an intravenous pyelogram (IVP), a diagnostic procedure recommended by an urologist. She signed a form titled 'Authorisation of medical and/or surgical treatment'. A radiologist administered the dye, hypaque. Meyer died from an allergic reaction. Her estate argued that the urologist was negligent in:

● failing to communicate Meyer's allergies to the radiologist,
● failing to suggest alternative procedures, and
● failing to warn her of the risks inherent in the dye.

Evidence showed that the death occurred in 1 in 100,000 cases. The radiologist had acted in accordance with the advice of the Canadian Association of Radiologists in not warning Meyer of the risk.

It was held that:

- There was no evidence to support any of the claims against the urologist.
- It was the responsibility of the radiologist to warn of the risk and he should have done so.

However the non-disclosure of material information was not causative of Meyer's death, because, on the balance of probabilities, a reasonable person in M's position would have consented to the IVP.

Negligence not affecting outcome

In some cases there may be negligence in overlooking signs of disease but the circumstances are such that even had the cancer been diagnosed when the patient first presented no cure would be possible. In such cases any award is limited to additional pain and suffering that might have arisen through lack of ameliorative care. In *Eaton* v. *Dale*[16] expert evidence from a clinical oncologist stated that the tumour from which the patient had died was highly aggressive and it was unlikely to have been curable even if treated when she first reported the symptoms. The claim was settled for £4000 for pain and suffering and loss of amenity for a four and a half month period. The case below is similar.

Case: *SH* v. *Salford Health Authority Date of Settlement 1991*[17]

The claimant attended Hope Hospital in April 1990 where a chest X-ray indicated that neoplastic disease seemed likely with either metastatic disease or two separate primaries. However, no steps were taken to confirm the possible diagnosis. She was treated for stress-related back pain at the pain clinic. A second X-ray was carried out in July 1990. The report suggested that the appearances were strongly suspicious of carcinoma and recommended that an isotope scan be carried out which was not done.

In August 1990 she was seen privately, where the consultant suspected a pulmonary primary lesion with metastatic disease. This diagnosis was confirmed in September by a bone scan and X-rays. She was admitted to hospital and received a single dose of palliative radiotherapy. In November she died suffering from lung cancer with extensive bone metastases. The cancer could not have been cured even if diagnosed earlier. However had they investigated the possibility of lung cancer with metastatic disease, she could have received palliative radiotherapy and appropriate pain relief earlier.

The claim was settled with an award of £3500 for the four to five months of pre-death avoidable pain and suffering.

Reasonably foreseeable harm

The harm which might arise may not be within the reasonable contemplation of the defendant so that even though there is a breach of duty and there is harm, the defendant is not liable. For example a practitioner may have delivered the wrong dose and therefore be in breach of the duty of care, but the client may have become more ill because of her underlying medical condition not because of the wrong dose. In the case of *Jolley* v. *Sutton London Borough Council*[18] (where a boy of 14 was paralysed when a boat that he and his friends had jacked up fell upon him) the House of Lords held that, even though the exact type of mischief carried out by children could not be foreseen, the Council were liable, subject to a reduction of 25% contributory negligence. The risk which should have been contemplated was that if children meddle with a rotten boat, then injuries are likely to occur (see Chapter 8 for further discussion of occupier's liability).

An intervening cause breaking the chain

It may happen that any causal link between the plaintiffs breach of duty and the harm suffered by the client is interrupted by an intervening event.

Situation: intervening act

A radiographer fails to set the dials of the X-ray machine correctly, but as the X-ray is progressing the patient suffers a cardiac arrest and dies. The dosage is such that it would have caused serious harm to the patient, but there is no suggestion that the wrong dose caused the arrest.

In this situation the negligence of the practitioner has not caused the death of the patient so her employer would not be vicariously liable. There may however be subsequent disciplinary and even professional misconduct proceedings taken against the practitioner because of her professional misconduct.

Harm

To succeed in an action for negligence the claimant or his representative must establish that he has suffered harm which the court recognises as being subject to compensation. Thus personal injury, death, loss or damage to property are the main areas of recognisable harm. In addition the courts have ruled that nervous shock (now known as post traumatic stress syndrome) can be the subject of compensation where an identifiable medical condition exists within strict limits of liability. A test of proximity to the defendant's negligent action or omission has been set by the House of Lords[19].

Some of the types of harm covered by the effect of personal injury are illustrated below in the section showing how compensation is calculated.

Loss of a chance

Case: *Hotson* v. *East Berhshire Health Authority*[20]

A 13 year old boy fell out of a tree and suffered a slipped femoral epiphysis. He attended the A&E department, but the doctor failed to carry out an X-ray of the hip. The boy suffered considerable pain and returned to hospital five days later when the fracture was diagnosed. He developed avascular necrosis of the femoral head which medical evidence suggested occurred in 75% of patients. Expert evidence for the claimant was that as a result of the delay in diagnosis he lost a 25% chance of avoiding this complication. The judge awarded the boy £150 damages for the pain suffered by him for the five days, which he would have been spared by prompt diagnosis and treatment. In addition the boy was awarded 25% of the damages which would have been awarded if the entire injury had been attributable to negligence (i.e. 25% of £45 000) for the loss of the chance of recovery.

The House of Lords allowed the health authority's appeal, holding that the claimant had not established that the defendant's negligence had caused the avascular necrosis. The question of causation was to be determined on the balance of probabilities with the onus on the claimant.

This issue of the 'loss of a chance' is particularly important in litigation concerning radiology since, where there has been a failure to detect a malignancy, then the claimant has to argue that this failure has prevented the possibility of a cure. Statistical evidence of how many people die even when the malignancy is detected earlier is not always helpful to the claimant who would have to prove that he is in the group which would have benefited from the earlier diagnosis.

In order to obtain compensation when there has been negligence in diagnosis, the claimant may have to rely upon the specific consequences of delayed diagnosis such as further protracted treatment, additional pain and suffering, or other harm, rather than being able to claim that he would or could have been cured.

Vicarious and personal liability distinguished

As stated above it is unlikely that an employee will be sued personally, since the employer would be vicariously liable for her actions. To establish the vicarious liability of the employer the claimant must show:

- the employee;
- was negligent or was guilty of another wrong;
- whilst acting in the course of employment.

An independent practitioner would have to accept personal and professional liability for her actions but she may also be vicariously liable for the harm, caused during the course of employment, by anyone she employs. A practitioner who is an employee but who also works as an independent practitioner would have to have indemnity cover in respect of the private practice.

An employer is not liable for the acts of independent contractors, i.e. self-employed persons who are working on a contract for services, unless there is fault in selecting or instructing them.

The employer may challenge whether the actions were performed in the course of employment. For example, a practitioner may have undertaken training in a complementary medicine such as acupuncture. If she decided to use these new skills whilst at work without the agreement, express or implied, of the employer and through her use of the remedies caused harm to the patient, the employer might refuse to accept vicarious liability on the grounds that the employee was not acting in the course of employment. (Complementary therapies are considered in Chapter 26.)

Vicarious liability in a health-care context

The development of this principle in a hospital contest is, interestingly, one of the earliest cases involving alleged negligence by a radiographer, *Gold* v. *Essex* in 1942. In earlier cases the court had held that the hospital was not liable for its qualified professionals in their professional work. This was the view taken by the High Court in this case but the Court of Appeal broke new ground.

Case: *Gold* v. *Esses County Council*[21]

A child of 5 years was treated by a radiographer employed by Essex County Council at one of the County Hospitals. Because the radiographer failed to provide adequate screening material in giving Grenz-ray treatment for the removal of warts the child suffered injury to her face. The first dose of 1000 units was administered but it did not remove the warts. A second dose was therefore administered. On this occasion the radiographer did not use rubber lead-lined material as a screen for the face as he had on the previous occasion, but only lint as a protection. The mother was given lead-lined gloves as a protection for her as she held the child's head in place. After the treatment, the child developed ulcers on her face. The face became very inflamed and painful and the result was that the lower part of one side of her face was permanently disfigured. The medical evidence was that the disfigurement would be permanent and might possibly worsen.

In the High Court the judge was clear that there had been negligence by the radiographer. He was negligent in not using the proper screening. However he felt bound by an earlier case of *Hillyer* v. *St Bartholomew's Hospital*[22] in which it was stated that nurses and other such persons are servants of the hospital for general purposes but within their professional work they cease to be under the orders of the defendants.

The judge therefore held that the County Council were not liable for the actions of the radiographer. The Court of Appeal however held that as the radiographer was under a contract of service with the respondents, they were liable for his negligence under the doctrine of *respondeat superior* (i.e. the principle of vicarious liability).

In a recent court decision the House of Lords has widened the scope of vicarious liability still further. It ruled that the owners of a boarding school were vicariously liable for sexual abuse carried out by a warden[23]. The owners had been responsible for the care of vulnerable children and employed the warden to carry out that duty on its behalf. The sexual abuse had taken place while the employee had been engaged in duties at the very time and place demanded by his employment. The court held that the warden's wrongs were so closely connected with his employment that it would be fair and just to hold the defendants vicariously liable.

The self-employed practitioner

Where a practitioner is self-employed then she must ensure that she takes out public indemnity cover for any alleged negligence, since she alone would be personally liable for any harm caused by her negligence and there would be no employer who would be vicariously liable. Those practitioners who work in the private sector should check to ascertain whether they are under a contract for services, in which case they are self-employed professionals and would have to have their own personal insurance cover, or whether they have a contract of service, in which case they are employees for whom the employer would be vicariously liable.

Defences to an action

The main defences to an action for negligence are listed below:

- Allegations of fact are disputed.
- It is denied that all the elements of negligence are established.
- The defendant alleges contributory negligence on the part of the claimant.

- The defendant claims exemption from liability.
- The time set for bringing the claim has expired.
- The defendant alleges the claimant voluntarily assumed of the risk.

Disputed allegations of fact

Many cases will be resolved entirely on what facts can be shown to exist. Thus the effectiveness of the witnesses for both parties in establishing the facts of what did or did not occur will be the determining factor in who wins the case. Reference should be made to Chapter 18 on record keeping and giving evidence for further discussion on the nature of evidence and the role of the witnesses. In theory, it might appear before the court hearing that one party has a particularly strong case but, unless the facts on which its case rests can be proved in court, the actual outcome of the case might be that the opponent wins.

Basically every case depends on the evidence available and whether the witnesses of fact (either about the event or about the extent of the injuries), including the parties themselves, can be believed.

Elements of negligence are not established

The claimant must establish, on a balance of probabilities, that all elements required to prove negligence are present, i.e. duty, breach, causation and harm. If one or more of these cannot be established then the defendant will win the case.

Contributory negligence

If the claimant is partly to blame for the harm which has occurred then there may still be liability on the part of the professional but the compensation payable might be reduced in proportion to the claimant's fault. In extreme cases, such a claim may be a complete defence if 100% contributory negligence is claimed. In determining the level of contributory negligence, the physical and mental health and the age of the claimant would be taken into account.

Situation: Contributory negligence

A patient is told by the therapeutic radiographer to return to the hospital if he suffers specified symptoms. The radiographer fails to ensure that the patient has the appropriate medication to take home. The patient suffers from some distressing symptoms at home, but fails to return. His sufferings are aggravated by the fact that he is not on the correct medication.

There is a clear breach of duty by the radiographer, but the patient is also at fault and this would be taken into account in assessing any compensation payable.

The Law Reform (Contributory Negligence) Act 1945 enables an apportionment of responsibility for the harm which has been caused which may result in a reduction of damages payable. The Court can reduce the damages 'to such extent as it thinks just and equitable having regard to the claimant's share in the responsibility for the damage' (section 1(1).

For contributory negligence by a child see Chapter 8.

Exemption from liability

It is possible for people to exempt themselves from liability for harm arising from negligence but the effects of the Unfair Contract Terms Act 1977 mean that this exemption only applies to loss or damage to property. A defendant cannot exclude liability for negligence which results in personal injury or death either by contract or by a notice.

Where exemption from liability for loss or damage to property is claimed by the defendant, it must be shown by the defendant that it is reasonable to rely upon the term or notice which purported to exclude liability. The provisions of the Unfair Contract Terms Act 1977 are shown in Figure 14.1.

Figure 14.1 **Unfair Contract Terms Act 1977 – sections 2 and 11 (extracts).**

2(1) A person cannot by reference to any contract term or to a notice given to persons generally or to particular persons exclude or restrict his liability for death or personal injury resulting from negligence.

2(2) In the case of other loss or damage, a person cannot so exclude or restrict his liability for negligence except in so far as the term or notice satisfies the requirement of reasonableness.

[The 'reasonableness' test is explained in section 11]

11(3) In relation to a notice (not being a notice having contractual effect) it should be fair and reasonable to allow reliance on it, having regard to all the circumstances obtaining when the liability arose or (but for the notice) would have arisen.

11(5) It is for those claiming that a contract term or notice satisfies the requirements of reasonableness to show that it does.

The effect of this legislation is that notices which purport to exempt a department for liability for negligence are invalid if that negligence leads to personal injury or death. However a notice which excludes liability for loss or damage to property may be valid if it is reasonable for the negligent person or organisation to rely upon it.

Limitation of time

Actions for personal injury or death should normally be commenced within three years of the date of the event which gave rise to the harm or three years from the date on which the person had the necessary knowledge of the harm and the fact that it arose from the defendant's actions or omissions.

Exceptions

There are however some major qualifications to this general principle and these are shown in Figure 14.2.

Figure 14.2 **Situations where the limitation of time can be extended.**

- Those suffering from a disability:
  - Children under 18 – the time does not start to run until the child reaches 18 years.
  - Those suffering from a mental disability – time does not start to run until the disability ends. In the case of those who are suffering from severe learning disabilities or brain damage this may not be until death.
- Discretion of the judge. The judge has a statutory power to extend the time within which a claimant can bring an action for personal injuries or death, if it is just and equitable to do so.

The implications of the rules relating to limitation of time, are that in those cases which might come under one of the exceptions to the three year time limit, records should be kept and not destroyed. This is particularly important in the case of children and those with learning disabilities. For example in the case of *Bull* v. *Wakeham*[24] the case was brought 18 years after the claimant's birth. In a news report in 1995[25] a man then 33 obtained compensation of £1.25 million because of a failure to diagnose severe dehydration a few weeks after birth.

Knowledge

Claimants are assumed to have the necessary knowledge (and so the 'clock' starts running) when they know or it is reasonable to expect them to know the following facts:

- that the injury in question was significant;
- that the injury was attributable in whole or in part to the act or omission which is alleged to constitute the negligence, nuisance or breach of duty;
- the identity of the defendant;
- if it is alleged that the act or omission was that of a person other than the defendant, the identity of that person and the additional facts supporting the bringing of an action against the defendant.

Knowledge that any acts or omissions did or did not, as a matter of law, involve negligence, nuisance or breach of duty is irrelevant. The claimant cannot bring an action out of time if he knew all the facts more than three years ago but has only just found out that they could give rise to a claim.

A person is not fixed with knowledge of a fact ascertainable only with the help of expert advice so long as he has taken all reasonable steps to obtain and, where appropriate, to act on that advice.

Clearly if a person is exposed to radiation, a considerable time may take place before evidence of harm occurs. It is when this harm becomes known to the claimant, or the claimant should have reasonably known that fact from the evidence available, that the three year time limit starts to run.

An example of a case involving a claim being made out of time and the destruction of X-rays is *Hammond* v. *West Lancashire Health Authority*[26] (further considered in Chapter 6). The difficulties that would be encountered by the Health Authority if the case could proceed even though it was brought out of time were of their own makeing, arising from the premature destruction of X-rays and records.

In contrast, in the following case[27] the Court of Appeal refused an appeal against the judge's decision not to exercise his discretion to extend the limitation period set by the Act.

Case: *Fenech v. East London and City Health Authority*

On 5 July 1960 the claimant gave birth to her first child. Afterwards the doctor suturing her episiotomy informed her that the needle which he had been using had broken. In fact a two inch piece of the needle had been left inside the wound. The claimant experienced pain in the area of the episiotomy, but was too embarrassed to discuss her symptoms with her general practitioner. She gave birth to five more children. In 1983 she came under the care of a female gynaecologist and underwent a number of negative investigations and operations over a period of 11 years. The fragment of the needle was identified on a hip X-ray when she was being reviewed by orthopaedic surgeons in 1991 but it was not till a repeat X-ray in 1994 that she was informed of the needle's presence. She issued proceedings in January 1997 and the issue of limitation was tried as a pre-liminary point. At the County Court her claim was held to be statute barred: although she had not attained actual knowledge until 1994, she had had constructive knowledge 'long before 1994'. She appealed to the Court of Appeal on the grounds that the judge had erred in refusing to take into account her embarrassment when considering when she ought reasonably to have sought medical advice and the defendant could not prove that such earlier advice would have led to an earlier detection of the needle fragment.

The Court of Appeal dismissed the appeal on the grounds that she should have sought medical advice earlier, she failed to give the gynaecologist sufficient information about her symptoms and, whilst the 1991 X-ray had revealed the fragment of the needle, its significance and relationship to her gynaecological problems were not realised by the orthopaedic specialists who were reviewing her for a hip replacement.

Voluntary assumption of risk

Volenti non fit injuria is the Latin tag for the defence that a person willingly undertook the risk of being harmed. It is unlikely to succeed as a defence in an action for professional negligence since the professional cannot contract out of liability where harm occurs as a result of her negligence (see the Unfair Contract Terms Act considered above). The defence of *volenti non fit injuria* would not be available to an employer as a defence against a radiographer who argued that she had been exposed to radiation as a result of the work. The employers have a duty of care to ensure that exposure levels are kept under control (see Chapters 15 and 16) and it cannot be argued successfully that a radiographer accepts a risk of being radiated as an occupational hazard. This can be contrasted with a 1969 case[28] involving injury to an adult rugby player who was held to have willingly accepted the risk[28].

Calculation of compensation

In some cases of negligence, liability might be accepted by the defendant, but there might be disagreement between the parties over the amount of compensation. In other cases, there might be agreement over the amount of compensation and liability alone might be disputed. In others, both liability and quantum might be in dispute.

The compensation awarded to anyone suffering personal injuries through another's negligence is made up of different parts.

- There are the 'special damages' which are the out of pocket expenses incurred as a result of the injury – prescriptions, travel, cost of care etc. to the date of the agreement or trial.
- There is loss of earnings – past and projected into the future.
- There is the cost of future care and anticipated future expenses.

The above are all subject either to direct proof or arithmetic calculation.

- There are also what is known as 'general damages', compensation (insofar as money can compensate) for pain, suffering and loss of amenity.

The award of general damages is in the discretion of the judge, based on previous decisions and case law, but to bring about some measure of uniformity the Judicial Studies Board publishes guidelines on what type of injury or disability warrants what level of award.

Once a figure is arrived at there are still adjustments to be made:

- Social security receipts have to be paid out of the compensation awarded.
- The court takes into account the fact that the award for future loss or costs is being made at once and therefore the claimant is benefiting from the ability to obtain interest on the lump sum.

Calculations are made as to what interest can be expected. It is difficult to balance matters fairly but the House of Lords has ruled that, in the award of compensation, victims should not be expected to speculate on the stock market and therefore lower levels of return based on index-linked government securities should be used as the basis of calculation[29]. The effect of this ruling is to increase the capital amount awarded to victims. In the case itself James Thomas, a cerebral palsy victim as a result of negligence at birth was awarded £1 285 000 by the High Court judge, but in a very controversial decision this was reduced by the Court of Appeal by £300 000 on the basis that the capital could be invested in the higher returns (but more risky) equities. The House of Lords restored the original amount.

A report by the Law Commission[30] in 1999 recommended that compensation for non-pecuniary loss (i.e. pain suffering and loss of amenity) should be increased and this could be implemented through the decisions of the courts on damages. The Court of Appeal in a judgment in March 2000[31] decided that a modest increase was required to bring some awards up to a figure which was fair, reasonable and just. It recommended that damages for claims above £10 000 should be raised by a maximum of about 35% with increases tapering downwards. The Court of Appeal acknowledged that the life expectancy has increased for many seriously injured claimants who can now survive for many years. The Judicial Studies Board has been asked to provide new guidelines. There is likely to be a significant impact upon the NHS as a result of this judgment, though not perhaps as much as if the Law Commission recommendations had been supported in full.

The Kent cervical screening case

The Court of Appeal has held that the Bolam test is not always the appropriate test to use for negligence as the following case shows.

Case: *Penney, Palmer and Cannon* v. East Kent Health Authority[32]

The claimants brought an action on the grounds that their cervical smears were negligently examined and reported as negative between 1989 and 1992. As a consequence they were deprived of the opportunity of obtaining early treatment which would have prevented the development of endocervical carcinoma. Screening was carried out by qualified biomedical scientists or by qualified cytology screeners. They were not qualified to diagnose; their only function was to report what, using their expertise, they were able to see. If the screener detected an abnormality in the smear or was in doubt whether what he saw was abnormal he should pass the smear on to a senior screener known as a checker. The checker would re-examine the slide and, if he endorsed the screener's classification, pass the slide on to the pathologist for a final decision. The pathologist would then either re-classify the smear or, if he confirmed the abnormality, would refer the patient to a gynaecologist for colposcopy or biopsy. The five experts who gave evidence agreed that if the screener was in doubt about what he saw on the slide he should not have classified the smear as negative. The defendants argued that expert evidence by three independent pathologists constituted a reasonable body of opinion such as to provide them with the so called Bolam defence.

The trial judge held the claimants should win:

- He preferred the views of the claimant's experts as to whether, in the light of what the cytoscreeners saw, it was negligent to fail either to classify the smears as borderline or to refer the smears to the checker/and or to the pathologist.
- The Bolam principle did not apply because Bolam concerned acceptable and unacceptable practice; whereas no question of acceptability arose in the instant case because the cytoscreeners were wrong in their classification of the smears.

Even if the Bolam principle was relevant, the defendant's experts' views did not stand up to logical analysis because the cytoscreeners did not have the ability to draw a distinction between benign and pre-cancerous cells and so should have classified the smears as borderline.

The Court of Appeal dismissed the Health Authority's appeal and upheld the finding that it was liable. It held that the Bolam test was appropriate where the exercise of skill and judgment of the screener was being questioned. In this case however the Bolam test did not apply since the screeners were not expected to exercise judgment.

Comment on the Kent case

Firstly it must be emphasised that the Court of Appeal has not abandoned the Bolam test, but has held that it is not the appropriate test where professional judgment is not used.

Secondly there could be criticism of the view held by the trial judge that cytoscreeners only observe and record, rather than exercise judgment. It does not follow that in the observations which they are making, there is not a requirement of professional judgment and practice. This was the point urged by the health authority.

Thirdly there was recognition in the Court of Appeal that there is about a 5% false negative reading in the Cervical Screening Programme, yet this was not used to defend the reasonable standard of practice of the screeners.

Fourthly it is interesting to note that the screeners were not called to give evidence nor was there evidence by any one involved in the training and management of the screeners. The only evidence before the court was that of the experts, the Wells Report (an independent report conducted on cervical screening services at the hospital between 1990 and 1994), a generic report provided by the defendant's experts and various journals.

There may be a danger that hindsight influenced the decision and it would be dangerous to use the judgment out of its immediate context.

Following this decision, it is clear that the principles could apply to radiological screening.[33]

Situations involving radiographers and radiologists

Of specific interest to radiographers and radiologists is liability in the following areas.

Failures in assessment

An example of compensation being paid when cancer was wrongly diagnosed is the case of *Pawson* v. *St. Helens*[34] where an unnecessary mastectomy was carried out.

In another case[35] alleged failure to interpret X-rays led to a misdiagnosis and the claimant (aged 67 at the time) was told that she was terminally ill and advised to move to a nursing home. When the error in diagnosis was discovered she was discharged from the home but was no longer self-dependent.

There can also be failure to diagnose cancer. In *Judge* v. *Huntingdon*[36] the claimant's chance of survival went allegedly from 80% to nil because the lump in her breast was not investigated properly on her first visit but only excised on a second consultation.

Case: *Crawford* v. *North Manchester Health Authority (1996)*[37]

In March 1991, the deceased then aged 43 saw her GP complaining of pain in her right hypochondrium. A week later she attended hospital for X-rays and an ultrasound scan. No abnormality of the pancreas, spleen or right kidney was found, but the report stated that a small cyst was present in the left kidney in its upper pole. The GP reassured her but in fact she was suffering from a hypernephroma (malignant kidney tumour) which remained undiagnosed under November 1992. By the time of the diagnosis, her illness was terminal and she died on July 1993.

Proceedings were issued in March 1994 alleging negligence in relation to taking insufficient views of the left kidney. The claimant's case was that, had the condition been diagnosed at the time of the first ultrasound scan in March 1991, she would have undergone a nephrectomy and on the balance of probabilities she would not have developed metastasis. This is because 80% of patients with this condition survive if the diagnosis is achieved early.

A £10,000 payment into court was rejected. The defendants admitted negligence and causation and the case was settled at £57,500.

Failures in communication

Crucial to the reasonable standard of care of the patient is the communication between different departments within the Trust and with the patient. Communication between health and social services professionals is essential in ensuring that the client receives the appropriate standard of care. This is particularly important where one person is designated as the key worker on behalf of the multi-disciplinary team. However the Court of Appeal[38] has stated that the courts do not recognise a concept of team liability and it is therefore for each individual professional to ensure that her practice is according to the approved standard of care. Nor should a professional take instructions from another professional which she knows would be contrary to the standard of care which her profession would require.

Failures in communication between the health professionals

Case: Failure to follow up cytology report[39]

The claimant noticed a lump on her breast. The cytology report suggested a biopsy to confirm the diagnosis of fibroadenoma or fibrosystic disease. However no biopsy was performed. Two subsequent six-month reviews were carried out where she was assured that everything was normal. A year after the report her GP referred her to a consultant surgeon. His report noted 'probably carcinoma'. She was referred for radiotherapy and died after less than two years.

It was held that there was negligence. The registrar's interpretation and report failed to achieve the requisite standard of care. The claimant should not have merely received six-monthly reviews, especially as the cytology report suggested that the clinicians carry out further investigations.

Whose responsibility?

An American case where a radiologist was held responsible for not following up a case caused consternation amongst UK radiologists[40]. As described in the Newsletter of the RCR:

'A US radiologist reported a pre-operative chest X-ray as showing a 1.5 cm nodular density in the upper right lobe. The report was forwarded to the referring clinician but the clinician denied receiving it. Because the radiologist did not contact the referring clinician directly concerning the findings, the radiologist was found to be culpable.'

Following the report of this case several radiologists contacted the College. The current advice of the College is as follows:

'Provided the radiograph is interpreted appropriately and a timely report is produced and the report dispatched by an agreed and robust method of communication, it is the responsibility of the referring clinician to read the report and act upon it. In the view of the College, the radiologist cannot be held responsible for the failure of a referring clinician to follow up the results of their own clinical referrals.'

The MDU, in commenting on this case, stated that the Bolam principle is still essential to the defence of medical negligence claims. This principle allows for variations in clinical management providing that, if called into account, the management is supported by a responsible body of medical opinion. Admittedly the House of Lords in *Bolitho*[6] accepts that there can be exceptional situations where a judge decides that a body of expert opinion called in evidence cannot be logically supported as not being responsible or respectable. Nevertheless, the College Newsletter article concludes:

'The College will continue to issue advice to its members and Fellows across a wide range of issues. Provided such advice is based on good practice, it appears reasonable to assume that the Judiciary will regard the College as a "responsible body of men" and that its opinions constitute a "respectable body of professional opinion".'

Communicating 'bad news'

Policies are necessary to ensure that 'bad news' is communicated in an appropriate way, but there may be many logistic and other considerations.

Case: An HIV positive health worker[41]

It was alleged by 114 of the patients who had been notified that the two defendant health authorities were negligent in choosing to inform patients by letter as opposed to face to face and that the facilities offered by the letter were not properly provided. The High Court judge found in favour of the plaintiffs on the grounds that the health authorities did not exercise due care in that they should have realised that the best method of communicating the news was face to face and that there was a foreseeable risk that some vulnerable individuals might suffer psychiatric injury going beyond shock and distress. The health authorities appealed.

    Court of Appeal found for the defendants. The Exeter model (giving information face to face via the GP) should not have been adopted by the judge, without consideration of the different circumstances in this case (the numbers involved, Easter and the risk of the story breaking prematurely to the papers). There was a duty on the defendants to take only such steps as were reasonable to inform the patients, having regard to the possibility of psychiatric injury. However there was no evidence of negligence in fulfilling this duty.

Radiographers and communication with patients

Patients are anxious to have any information as soon as possible and therefore may question the radiographer on what is seen in the X-ray. Many diagnostic radiographers work under specific instructions that they must not give any hint to the patient about the significance of the X-ray investigations until the doctor has had a chance to see the X-ray and meet the patient. In practice however, as radiographers develop their reporting role, they may also have the responsibility, in less complex cases, of informing the patient of preliminary results. It is important that whatever practice is followed, this is supported by clear guidelines and protocols and radiographers have the necessary training (see Chapter 27).

Therapeutic radiographers may also find that they are asked questions by the patient about their condition: How long do I have? and similar questions. They must be very careful in responding to such questions and should discuss with the multi-disciplinary team what role they play in communication with the patient. This also applies to the information about the side effects of the treatment. If it is clear to a therapeutic radiographer that a patient has consented to treatment, yet has not been provided with basic information about the risks and side effects of the treatment, then the radiographer should ensure that a meeting between clinician and patient is facilitated.

Where the radiographer takes on the responsibility of obtaining the consent of the patient to treatment, then this should be seen as an expanded role, and the radiographer needs to have the necessary training (see Chapter 27). The consent and the giving of information and instructions to the patient is considered in Chapter 4.

Advice for radiologists to avoid litigation

Paul Butt describes the increase in litigation involving radiologists and provides some advice to radiologists based on his experience in cases involving radiological negligence in orthopaedic cases[42]. He considers that radiologists need to be ready for a large increase in the number of negligence actions.

Some of the specific lessons which he draws are:

- Do not do hand X-rays to assess finger abnormalities.
- Scaphoid fractures are *never* excluded on one examination. It is a moot point whether this is well enough known that a radiologist need not mention it in his report.
- Monteggias are still common, are still missed and it is indefensible not to see the elbow on a forearm fracture.
- It is not clear who should suggest a hip X-ray in a child with a knee pain but someone has to do it and it is not a bad idea for it to be the radiologist. A significant number of children with slipped upper femoral epiphyses will

present nothing but knee pain; the damages for a missed SUFE can be enormous.

- If a clinician has clinical doubts about his patient do not reassure him because the X-ray was negative. All radiological examinations have false negatives and you are almost certainly dealing with one. It is quite all right to reassure a clinician about his radiological doubts in a patient with no clinical suspicion (after all, that is a regular function of the specialist).

He describes several case studies which illustrate these points. He emphasises the danger of excluding conditions with inappropriate investigations (e.g. cervical spine examination failed to show a cervical rib).

'Spinal cord injury without radiological abnormality (SCIWORA) is a well known entity in older people and it is the brave radiologist who rules it out with standard X-rays'.

Paul Butt also states:

'It is quite sensible to write a detailed report at the time that something goes wrong because one knows well that six years down the line memories will be blurred. It is important to be sure that critical points are entered into that report.'

The experience from the USA

Even though the American laws and experience differ from ours, some benefit is derived from the actions for negligence which are being heard in the USA. Leonard Berlin[43] describes some recent cases brought against radiologists in the USA where breast cancer has been missed. He states:

'Radiologists have become the specialists most frequently sued in malpractice law-suits involving breast cancer; likewise mammography has become the most prevalent procedure involved in medical malpractice lawsuits filed against radiologists. Indeed, the allegation that an error in the diagnosis of breast cancer has occurred is now the most prevalent condition precipitating medical malpractice lawsuits against all physicians.'

He analyses the background against which this increase has occurred, showing the popular perceptions:

- that there is a high risk of developing and dying from breast cancer
- that radiologists can achieve 100% perfection and accuracy in the interpretation of mammography, and
- that early detection will cure breast cancer are

not based upon undisputed scientific findings.

In the USA, of course, juries are used in civil cases to determine liability (including causation) and also to fix quantum. Emotional concerns can therefore affect the outcome, both in terms of liability and in the amount awarded. In the UK juries are not used in civil cases (apart from defamation) and both liability (with all the complex issues of causation) and the amount of compensation awarded are determined by the judge. However undoubtedly the high and unrealistic expectations of patients can influence the number of complaints and cases, even though many may founder along the way.

Leonard Berlin makes the following suggestions to stem the rising tide of breast cancer litigation in the USA:

- Radiologists who interpret mammograms should constantly strive to increase their expertise.
- Every effort should be made to optimise mammographic examinations technically.
- Organisations which have made exaggerated claims about cancer risks should modify their positions and advertising campaigns to present a more realistic portrayal of breast cancer risks.
- Radiological organisations and others should educate the public about the actual rates of sensitivity and accuracy of mammography and about the reality that early diagnosis of breast cancer does not necessarily guarantee a cure.
- Radiologists involved in litigation should ensure that defence lawyers have the scientific evidence relating to accuracy of mammography and the relationship between early detection on mammography and breast cancer prognosis.

Evidence that there are similar myths and false expectations in the UK is provided by Sainsbury[44]. The result is that litigation for delays or failures in diagnosing breast cancer is increasing in the UK.

Students and unregistered assistants

Supervision and delegation

Exactly the same principles apply to the delegation and supervision of tasks as to the carrying out of professional activities. The professional delegating a task should only do so if she is reasonably sure that the person to whom the task is delegated is reasonably competent and experienced to undertake that activity safely for the care of the patient. At the same time, she must ensure that the person undertaking the activity has sufficient supervision to ensure that the delegated activity can be carried out reasonably safely. Should harm befall a patient because an activity was carried out by a junior member of staff, a student or an assistant it is no defence to argue that the harm occurred because that person did not have the ability, competence or experience to carry out that task reasonably safely[38].

It is essential that delegation is on a personal basis and takes into account the individual assistant's personal knowledge, experience, skill and training. (This topic is further considered in the context of the scope of professional practice in Chapter 27.)

The contribution of the non-registered junior staff

There is a danger that the real contribution which can be made to the care planning and multi-disciplinary decision making by persons such as assistants, technicians and support workers may not be recognised or may be treated dismissively. Many support workers may develop a close rapport with patients and it is essential that any relevant information which they posses should be made known to the team and listened to.

Chapter 4 of the inquiry report about the homicide committed by Jason Mitchell[45], a mentally disordered person, considers the assessments made of Jason by professional staff in disciplines other than psychiatry and nursing and points out:

> 'They contained observations and insights into Jason Mitchell's thoughts and feelings which were rarely recorded in the medical and nursing notes and which could present a different perspective on his case. They tended to be recorded in detail, but were marginalised.'

Attention is drawn in the report to the contribution of a technical instructor in the occupational therapy department at West Park Hospital whose report on Jason Mitchell is given in full as an addendum to the chapter. The Inquiry noted that her report was not included in the Mental Health Review Tribunal papers. In general her report had been ignored or discounted by the doctors central to the care and treatment of Jason Mitchell but in the Inquiry's view 'the material in her report ought to have prompted at least an assessment, if not a further therapeutic involvement, with a qualified and experienced clinician, possibly a psychologist'. The Inquiry concluded that

> 'Jason Mitchell's case illustrates how contributions from an unqualified member of staff were disregarded, and consequently how important data were put out of sight and mind. Nothing relevant to the assessment and treatment of a patient should be ignored, whatever its origins.'

Litigation and the NHS – general issues

Proof of the facts and documentation

It is clear from many of the cases considered above that the factual evidence was the main point in dispute. Absence of documentation or low standards in record-keeping may lead to cases being lost, (see Chapter 6, case of *Hammond* v. *West Lancashire*[26]). In every area of professional practice, it is essential to ensure that comprehensive clear records are kept, not only in the interests of patient care but also for the defence of the practitioner in the event of any dispute or complaint. Reference should be made to Chapter 18 on record-keeping.

Often the exact circumstances of a case are unknown to the claimant who has to obtain some information through the disclosure of his health records and other information during the stages leading up to a hearing, including the exchange of witness statements.

Sometimes a claimant might be assisted by the application of a legal doctrine, *'res ipsa loquitur'*. This literally means 'the thing speaks for itself'. It applies where the claimant is able to show that:

- what has occurred would not usually occur if reasonable care were taken
- the circumstances were entirely under the control of the defendants
- the defendants have not offered any explanation of what occurred.

If these elements can be shown, on a balance of probabilities, by the claimant then he has made out a *prima facie* case that there was negligence by the defendants[46]. The burden of proof however remains with the claimant to satisfy. An obvious example of where the doctrine might apply would be the amputation of the wrong limb, or leaving a swab in the patient after an operation, or using the incorrect dye in a diagnostic test.

No fault liability

Weaknesses in the pre- April 1999 system of obtaining compensation for personal injury had led to suggestions that a system of 'no fault' liability should be introduced. Countries such as Sweden, Finland and New Zealand have adopted no fault liability systems. In such a scheme, as the result of an arrangement between insurance companies, employers and the state, a compensation fund is set up from which payment is made to injured persons. It is not necessary to prove that the defendant (or its employees) had been at fault, but only that something which had not been anticipated occurred which caused harm to an individual. The Pearson Report which considered reforms in 1978[47] did not recommend no fault liability in the case of medical negligence, but there are strong calls for its introduction.

Alternative dispute resolution (ADR)

An alternative which is being considered by the Department of Health is the introduction of an alternative form of dispute resolution such as mediation or arbitration. This would have the advantage of a cheaper, speedier, resolution and there is much to recommend any system which ensures that any money paid out is to the benefit of the person who has suffered the harm, rather than to the benefit of the lawyers. The Woolf Reforms (see Chapter 2) have recommended that mediation should become an essential part of the litigation process.

Clinical Negligence Scheme for Trusts (CNST)

The Clinical Negligence Scheme for Trusts (CNST)[48] was established by the NHS Executive in 1994, to provide a means for Trusts to fund the cost of clinical negligence litigation and to encourage and support effective management of claims and risk. The scheme covers claims arising from incidents on or after 1 April 1995. The NHS Litigation Authority (NHSLA), a Special Health Authority, administers the scheme (see below). Membership is voluntary and open to all NHS trusts in England. Each Trust can choose its own level of self-retention and the scheme will contribute to the cost of claims in excess of this figure. Funding is on a 'pay as you go' non-profit basis. Actuaries appointed by the NHSLA analyse the available data and predict the total amount expected to be paid out to the member trusts in respect of damages, costs and other expenses which will be incurred in the ensuing financial year. This amount is then apportioned between the member trusts. Individual Trust contributions are based on a range of criteria, such as activities, budget, numbers of doctors by discipline, nurses and other professionals. These contributions can be reduced if a trust meets certain risk management criteria (the CNST Risk Management Standards). As the scheme matures it is possible that other criteria such as claims experience will influence individual trust contributions. It has not prepared standards specifically for radiography and radiotherapy departments but most of its standards would be expected to apply to these departments.

Standards set by the CNST

The assessment is based on nine 'core' standards. In addition, there are separate standards for maternity care, mental health and ambulance services which are applicable only to Trusts which provide such services. There are three levels of criteria: level one criteria represent the basic elements of a clinical risk management framework while levels two and three are more demanding. Many standards are concerned with the implementation and integration into practice of policies and procedures, monitoring them and acting on the results.

Advice on the standards and general aspects of risk management is given in the *NHSLA Review*, and at workshops and seminars. (See also Chapter 18.)

NHS Litigation Authority (NHSLA)

The NHS Litigation Authority (NHSLA)[49] exercises functions in connection with the establishment and the administration of the scheme for meeting liabilities of health service bodies to third parties for loss, damage or injury arising out of the exercise of their functions. Membership and claims issues of the CNST are dealt with by the NHSLA. Risk management matters are dealt with on behalf of the NHSLA by the CNST assessment team at Willis Ltd, working closely with and overseen by the NHSLA.

Guidance on NHS indemnity for clinical negligence claims has been issued by the NHS Executive[50].

The Law Commission recommended changes to the present system relating to the quantifying of damages for personal injury[51] in 1996 and has suggested, amongst other recommendations that the NHS should be able to recover the costs arising from the treatment of road traffic and other accident victims. It is estimated that this might bring in £120 million to the NHS. More radical measures will be necessary to make any serious reduction in the present costs of the NHS.

The future

The ever increasing cost of litigation to the NHS will continue to be a major item on the agenda for NHS reform. In April 2000 the National Audit Office (NAO) announced that it was to investigate how clinical negligence claims are handled by reviewing NHS trusts and health authorities, analysing the data-base of the NHS Litigation Authority, analysing information held by the Legal Services Commission and obtaining information from other sources[52]. The NAO reported in May 2001 that almost £4 billion would be required to meet the costs of known and anticipated claims in the NHS[53]. It made far reaching recommendations in relation to the number of claims, the costs of settling them and the time taken, suggesting action to be taken by the NHSLA and the Legal Services Commission to bring cases to a conclusion. It recommended that the DoH, the Lord Chancellor's Department and the Legal Services Commission should investigate alternative ways of satisfactorily resolving the small and medium sized claims. The Department of Health should also consider how to provide Trusts with financial and other incentives to reduce incidents that lead to claims.

In July 2001[54], the Secretary of State announced that the findings of the National Audit Office Report were so bleak that urgent action was essential. This had stated

- That the NHS must make provision of about £4 billion for claims already put forward and those anticipated from known incidents.
- That the number and value of claims continues to rise.
- That claims are taking on average about $5\frac{1}{2}$ years to settle.
- That nearly half the claims settled in 1999–2000 cost more in legal and other costs than the claims themselves.

Plans are therefore in hand for the biggest overhaul of the system of NHS clinical negligence compensation that has ever been seen. The Department of Health proposed that the Chief Medical Officer, Professor Liam Donaldson, should chair a committee to look at suggestions to make the system faster and fairer, not only for NHS patients but also for doctors, nurses and other health-care professionals. The Committee would include clinicians, and patient representatives. Its task would be to consult on various proposals for reforming the system with the aim of a White Paper being published by the Government in 2002. The possibilities which would be explored included:

- A no-fault liability system (see above)
- Structured settlements so that patients receive periodic payments (these are already legally possible but the NHSLA does not favour them)
- A scheme for fixed tariffs for specific injuries (comparable to the Criminal Injuries Compensation scheme or the Vaccine Damage Payments scheme)
- Greater use of mediation or other ways of resolving disputes.

A consultation paper was issued by the Department of Health[8] in August 2001.

Since it is unlikely that the present scheme for compensation through the civil courts could be abolished (such a step would probably be contrary to Article 6 of the Human Rights Convention), the success of any alternative scheme would probably be seen in the extent to which claimants are prepared to accept the swift certainty of a tariff award rather than sue through the civil courts.

Questions and exercises _____

1   Explain the difference between vicarious liability and personal liability.
2   Take any situation where harm nearly occurred to a patient, and work out what the patient would have had to prove to obtain compensation if he had suffered an injury.

3 How would you define the reasonable standard of care in relation to any chosen treatment or investigation provided by yourself?
4 Prepare a protocol to ensure safe delegation to and supervision of a health care assistant.
5 To what extent do you consider that a system of no-fault liability combined with mediation could replace the current system of liability for personal injury in health cases?

References

1 *Donoghue* v. *Stevenson* [1932] AC 562
2 *Home Office* v. *Dorset Yacht Co Ltd* [1970] 2 All ER 294
3 *Bolam* v. *Friern Hospital Management Committee* [1957] 1 WLR 582
4 *Whitehouse* v. *Jordan* [1981] 1 All ER 267
5 *Maynard* v. *West Midlands Regional Health Authority* [1985] 1 All ER 635
6 *Bolitho* v. *City and Hackney Health Authority* [1997] 3 WLR 1151
7 *Marriott* v. *West Midlands Health Authority* [1999] Lloyds Rep. Med. 23
8 Department of Health (1997) *The New NHS – Modern Dependable* HMSO, London
9 Department of Health (2001) *The Manual of Cancer Service Standards* (January 2001) DoH, London
10 L. Lee Occupational standards in mammography *Synergy* (October 2000) pages 4–7
11 *Michael Hyde and Associates Ltd* v. *JD Williams and Co Ltd* (2000) The Times Law Report, 4 August 2000
12 J. R. Hampton (2000) From Evidence to Guidelines *Radiography* (May 2000) Vol 6, pages 75–77
13 *Barnett* v. *Chelsea HMC* [1968] 1 All ER 1068
14 *Wilsher* v. *Essex Health Authority* [1986] 3 All ER 801
15 *Meyer* v. *Rogers* [1991] 2Med LR 370
16 *Eaton* v. *Dale* (1993) AVMA Medical and Legal Journal (1993) 4(4) 12
17 *SH* v. *Salford Health Authority* Date of Settlement 1991 (unreported) discussed in J. Waxman & D. Simons (1999) *Cancer and the Law Blackwell Science*, Oxford (in association with AVMA)
18 *Jolley* v. *Sutton London Borough Council* (1998) The Times Law Report, June 23 1998 CA
19 *Alcock* v. *Chief Constable of South Yorkshire* [1992] 1 AC 310
20 *Hotson* v. *East Berkshire HA* [1987] AC 750
21 *Gold* v. *Essex County Council* [1942] 2 All ER 237 CA
22 *Hillyer* v. *St Bartholomew's Hospital* (Governors) [1909] 2 KB 820
23 *Lister and Others* v. *Hesley Hall Ltd* (2001) Times Law Reports, 10 May 2001
24 *Bull* v. *Wakeham*, Transcript 2 February 1989
25 J. Laurance (1990) Man handicapped as a baby 33 years ago wins £1.25m. *The Times* page 5, 15 November 1995
26 *Hammond* v. *West Lancashire HA* [1998] Lloyd's Rep. Med 146
27 *Fenech* v. *East London and City Health Authority* [2000] Lloyds' Rep. Med 35
28 *Simms* v. *Leigh Rugby Football Club Ltd* [1969] 2 All ER 923
29 *Wells* v. *Wells* [1998] AC 345
30 Law Commission Report No 257 *Personal Injury Compensation for non-pecuniary loss* 19 April 1999
31 *Heil* v. *Rankin* [2000] 2 WLR 1173
32 *Penney, Palmer and Cannon* v. *East Kent Health Authority* [2000] Lloyds Rep. Med.

41

33 P. Butt (2000) The Bolam Principle: a precious but fragile resource *RCoR* Issue No 60 Winter 2000 page 12–3

34 *Pawson* v. *St Helens and Knowsley Hospitals NHS Trust* (1996) Clinical Risk – *AVMA Medical and Legal Journal* (1996) 2(4) 133 (date of settlement 1 February 1996) reported in J. Waxman & D. Simons (1999) *Cancer and the Law* Blackwell Science, Oxford (in association with AVMA)

35 *MW* v. *Bolton Health Authority and Another* (1995) AVMA (1995) Medical and Legal Journal (1993) 4(2) 12

36 *Judge* v. *Huntingdon Health Authority* [1995] 6 Med LR 223; Kemp and Kemp L8-160; Times Law Reports 9 March 1995; Clinical Risk – AVMA Medical and Legal Journal (1995) 1(3) 127

37 *Crawford* v. *North Manchester Health Authority* (1996) Clinical Risk – AVMA Medical and Legal Journal (1997) 3(4) 123; Health Care Risk Report (1997) 3(8) 2

38 *Wilsher* v. *Essex Area Health Authority* [1986] 3 All ER 801 CA

39 *Taylor* v. *West Kent Health Authority* [1997] 8 Med LR 251

40 AJ Cowles (1998) Bolam Redefined *Newsletter of the RCoR* Issue No 53 (Winter 1998) page 12

41 *AB and Others* v. *Tameside & Glossop HA* [1997] 8 Med LR 91

42 P. Butt (1998) Radiological Negligence *Newsletter of the RCR* Issue No 52 (Summer 1998) page 14

43 L. Berlin (1999) Malpractice Issues in Radiology. The missed breast cancer: perceptions and realities *American Journal of Radiology* Vol 173, 1161–1167

44 R. Sainsbury *et al* (1999) Effect on survival of delays in referral of patients with breast cancer symptoms: a retrospective analysis *Lancet* 353, 1132–5

45 L. Blom-Cooper *et al* (1996) *The Case of Jason Mitchell: Report of the Independent Panel of Inquiry* Duckworth, London

46 *Ratcliffe* v. *Plymouth and Torbay HA, Exeter and Devon HA* [1998] Lloyd's Rep. Med 162

47 Pearson Report (1978) *Royal Commission on Civil Liability and Compensation for Personal Injury* HMSO, London

48 A disc setting out standards information is available from the CNST: helpline 0845 300 12230

49 National Health Service Litigation Authority (Establishment and Constitution) Order 1995 SI No 2800 of 1995

50 HSG(96)48 *NHS Indemnity: Arrangements for Clinical Negligence Claims in the NHS*

51 Law Commission (1996) *Damages for Personal Injury: medical, nursing and other expenses* Stationery Office, London

52 www.nao.gov.uk/publications/workinprogress/negligence1.htm

53 National Audit Office (2001) *Handling Clinical negligence claims in England; Report by the Comptroller and Auditor General* (HC 403) Session 2000–2001 3 May 2001 Stationery Office, London

54 Department of Health Press release 2001/0313 *New Clinical Compensation Scheme for the NHS* 20 July 2001

Chapter 15
Health and Safety

This chapter covers the basic principles of law relating to the health and safety at work, taking examples from radiography and radiology practice. The theme is continued in Chapter 16, looking at the legislation relating to radiation and ionising regulations etc. and Chapter 17 which considers the law relating to equipment and consumer protection.

Many of the areas considered in this chapter are covered in the Health and Safety information prepared by the Society and College of Radiographers and Royal College of Radiologists.

Statutory provision

Health and Safety at Work Act 1974

The Health and Safety at Work Act 1974 (HASAW) is enforced through the criminal courts by the Health and Safety Executive (HSE) which has the power to prosecute for offences under the Act and under the Regulations. The HSE also has powers of inspection and can issue enforcement or prohibition notices. Health and Safety Inspectors are not liable for any economic loss suffered by an organisation as a result of their issuing such a notice[1]. Since the abolition of the Crown's immunity in relation to the health and safety laws (by the National Health Service Amendment Act 1986) prosecutions and notices can be brought against the health authorities. Trusts also do not enjoy any immunity from health and safety legislation.

The basic duty on the employer is set out in Figure 15.1.

Figure 15.1 **Duty under the Health and Safety at Work etc. Act 1974, section 2(1).**

It shall be the duty of every employer to ensure, so far as is reasonably practicable, the health, safety and welfare at work of all his employees.

Section 2(2) of the 1974 Act gives examples of the various duties which must be carried out but these do not detract from the width and comprehensiveness of the general duty.

An example of a prosecution brought by the Health and Safety Executive (HSE) is shown below.

Case: Health and safety prosecution[2]

Norfolk and Norwich Health Care Trust was prosecuted for breaches of health and safety legislation following the death of a patient. A routine cardiac angiography in May 1996 resulted in a fatal air embolism as air was injected into a patient's heart. A radiographer began a procedure, fitting an uncharged automated syringe, which was then cancelled. The empty syringe was left in the machine at the morning session. At the start of the afternoon session, a different radiographer returned and assumed that the syringe had been charged. A doctor then connected it to the patient's heart. The NHS trust admitted that it failed to take the necessary steps to ensure safe control of all stages of the procedure. The judge commented on the failure to ensure a safe system of work to protect patients and employees. The Trust was fined £38 000 plus £17 000 costs. The Trust has now established a protocol for the procedure which has been approved by the HSE.

Where a criminal prosecution is brought, this does not preclude other proceedings. Thus, on the facts of this case, there would also have been civil liability for the harm to the patient as well as disciplinary action for those at fault and also the facts may have been referred to professional registration bodies.

The Act also places a specific responsibility upon all employees. This is shown in Figure 15.2.

Figure 15.2   Statutory duty of the employee, HASAW, section 7.

It shall be the duty of every employee while at work —

(a)   to take reasonable care for the health and safety of himself and of other persons who may be affected by his acts or omissions at work; and

(b)   as regards any duty or requirements imposed on his employer or any other person ... to co-operate with him so far as is necessary to enable that duty or requirement to be performed or complied with.

It is also a criminal offence for any person to interfere with health and safety measures (see Figure 15.3).

Figure 15.3   Health and Safety at Work Act 1974, section 8.

No person shall intentionally or recklessly interfere with or misuse anything provided in the interests of health, safety or welfare in pursuance of any relevant statutory provisions.

General health and safety duty of employer to non-employees

Under section 3 of the 1974 Act the employer has a general duty of care to persons not in his employment (see Figure 15.4).

Figure 15.4   **Health and Safety at Work Act, section 3(1).**

It shall be the duty of every employer to conduct his undertaking in such a way as to ensure, so far as is reasonably practicable, that persons not in his employment who may be affected thereby are not thereby exposed to risks to their health and safety.

This duty would therefore cover patients, visitors and the general public. Nevertheless, the Court of Appeal has held[3] that, provided the employer has

- taken all reasonable care in laying down safe systems of work
- ensured that the employees had the necessary skill and instruction and were subject to proper supervision
- provided safe premises, plant and equipment

it was not guilty of an offence under section 3 of the 1974 Act if an employee was negligent and caused harm to others.

Safety Representatives and Safety Committees Regulations 1977

These regulations brought into force the requirement in the HASAW that employers should permit the safety representative appointed by the recognised trade union to inspect the workplace, get information held by the employer relating to health, safety or welfare and have paid time off for training and carrying out their functions. Each employer is required to set up a health and safety committee to consider matters relating to health and safety.

For those workplaces which are not covered by SRSC, the Health and Safety (Consultation with Employees) Regulations 1996 apply and require employers to consult with workers or their representatives on all matters relating to employees' health and safety.

Regulations under the Act

The detail of the legislation has been provided by Regulations (statutory instruments – see Chapter 2) since the outset. These are subject to regular updating and amendment. The key Regulations are shown in Figure 15.5.

Many of these have been revised by subsequent regulations and the date of revisions up to the time of writing is shown in the Figure.

Management of Health and Safety at Work Regulations

These basic regulations cover such topics as

- risk assessment
- health and safety arrangements
- health surveillance
- health and safety assistance

Figure 15.5   **Health and Safety Regulations.**

- Management of Health and Safety at Work Regulations 1992 (SI No. 2051) (re-enacted 1999, SI No 3242 of 1999)
- Provision and Use of Work Equipment Regulations (SI No. 2932 of 1992) (re-enacted 1998, SI No 2306 of 1998)
- Manual Handling Operations Regulations 1992 (SI No. 2793 of 1992) (considered in detail below)
- Workplace (Health, Safety and Welfare) Regulations 1992 (SI No. 3004) (amended by S.I. 1999/2024)
- Personal Protective Equipment at Work Regulations 1992 (SI No 2966) (amended in relation to ionising indications by the Ionising Radiations Regulations 1999, SI No 3232 of 1999 – see Chapter 16)
- Health and Safety (Display Screen Equipment) Regulations 1992 (SI No. 2792)

- serious and imminent danger and danger areas
- information for employees
- co-operation and co-ordination
- capabilities and training
- employee's duties to temporary workers and other specialist categories.

The revised regulations incorporate a number of changes required as a result of European Council Directives:

- to introduce measures to improve safety and health of workers[6]
- to encourage health and safety of temporary or fixed term employees[7]
- to provide for the protection of young people[8] and pregnant and breast feeding women[9].

The Code of Practice

A Code of Practice was approved in conjunction with these regulations[4] and like the regulations has subsequently been revised[5].

The Code now sets out:

- The general principles and purpose of risk assessment
- Health and safety arrangements
- Health surveillance
- Procedures for serious and imminent danger and for danger areas
- Contacts with external services
- Information for employees
- Co-operation and co-ordination
- Capabilities and training
- Employee's duties
- Risk assessment, certificate and notification, in respect of new or expectant mothers
- Protection of young persons.

This Code does not have legal force but, as the preface states:

'Although failure to comply with any provision of this Code is not in itself an offence, that failure may be taken by a Court in criminal proceedings as proof that a person has contravened the regulation or sections of the 1974 Act to which the provision relates. In such a case, however, it will be open to that person to satisfy a Court that he or she has complied with the regulation or section in some other way.'

Risk assessment

The law
Regulation 3(1) requires:

'Every employer shall make a suitable and sufficient assessment of —
(a)   the risks to the health and safety of his employees to which they are exposed whilst they are at work; and
(b)   the risks to the health and safety of persons not in his employment arising out of or in connection with the conduct by him of his undertaking,
for the purpose of identifying the measures he needs to take to comply with the requirements and prohibitions imposed upon him by or under the relevant statutory provisions'

There is a duty under regulation 3(3) to review the assessment when there is reason to suspect that it is no longer valid or there has been significant change in the matters to which it relates.

Where more than five people are employed there must be a record of the significant findings of the risk assessment and any group of employees identified as being especially at risk.

The guidance
The guidance in the Code of Practice emphasises that risk assessment must be a systematic general examination of work activity, with a recording of significant findings, rather than a reactive procedure.

The definition of risk includes both the likelihood that harm will occur and its severity. The aim of risk assessment is to guide the judgment of the employer or self-employed person as to the measures they ought to take to fulfil their statutory obligations laid down under HASAW and its regulations.

The key words 'suitable' and 'sufficient' are not defined in the Regulations but the guidance defines such a risk assessment as one that—

'(a)   should identify the significant risks arising out of work...
(b)   should enable the employer or the self-employed person to identify and prioritise the measures that need to be taken to comply with the relevant statutory provisions
(c)   should be appropriate to the nature of the work and should identify the period of time for which it is likely to remain valid.'

How is the risk assessment to be carried out?
Figure 15.6 sets out the requirements of a valid risk assessment set out in
paragraph 18 of the guidance.

***Figure 15.6*   Requirements of valid risk assessment.**

(a)   to ensure that all relevant risks or hazards are addressed:
(b)   ensure all aspects of the work activity are reviewed, including routine and non-
      routine activities ... Where workers visit members of the public in the home, e.g.
      nurses, employers should consider any risks arising from potential dangers;
(c)   take account of non-routine operations, e.g. maintenance, cleaning operations ...
(d)   take account of the management of incidents such as interruptions to the work
      activity, which frequently cause accidents, and consider what procedures should
      be followed to mitigate the effects of the incident;
(e)   be systematic in identifying hazards and looking at risks ...;
(f)   take account of the way in which work is organised, and the effects this can have
      on health;
(g)   take account of risks to the public;
(h)   take account of the need to cover fire risks.

Paragraphs 19–23 of the guidance suggests how hazards should be identified,
people at risk identified and the risks from these hazards evaluated.

Recording

The record should represent an effective statement of hazards and risks which
then leads management to take the relevant actions to protect health and safety.
It should be linked with other health and safety records or documents. It should
be in writing unless in computerised form and should be easily retrievable.

   The record should make note of:

• significant hazards
• existing control measures in place
• the persons who may be affected by the risk.

Preventive and protective measures

The following principles apply:

• If possible avoid the risk altogether.
• Evaluate risks that cannot be avoided by carrying out a risk assessment.
• Combat risks at source rather than by palliative measures.
• Adapt work to the requirements of the individual.
• Take advantage of technological and technical progress.
• Implement risk prevention measures to form part of a coherent policy and
  approach, progressively reducing those risks which cannot be prevented or
  avoided altogether.
• Give priority to those measures which protect the whole workplace and all
  those who work there, and so yield the greatest benefit.
• Ensure that workers, whether employees or self-employed, understand what
  they need to do

The existence of a positive health and safety culture should be central within an organisation. This means that the avoidance, prevention and reduction of risk at work must be accepted as part of the organisation's approach and attitudes to all its activities. It should be recognised at all levels of the organisation from junior to senior management.

Risk management and the radiographer/radiologist

Apart from dangers from radiation, the radiographer and radiologist would share common health and safety hazards with other hospital employees and thus models of risk assessment and management which are applied to other health professionals would also apply to radiography, radiology and oncology. Thus hazards relating to the safety of equipment, cross-infection risks, safe working practices or to violence at work would all apply to practitioners who should be involved in the system of the assessment of risk.

Each practitioner should therefore be able to carry out a risk assessment of health and safety hazards in relation to colleagues, clients, carers and the general public. Manual handling and risk assessment is considered below.

The Board of Faculty of Clinical Radiology of the RCR has issued guidelines on risk management in Clinical Radiology[10]. The Report follows the categories of risk identified in the NHS executive publication on risk management in the NHS[11]:

- Direct patient care
  - Injury to patient
  - Treatment factors
  - Complications of investigations
- Indirect patient care
  - Security of patient
  - Inadequate facilities
- Health and Safety
  - Hazardous substances
  - Patient handling
- Organisational risks
  - Failure of information technology systems
  - Failure of communication
  - Fabric and structure

The report makes 36 recommendations which should provide guidelines for risk management in Radiology Departments including recommendations on reporting, allocation of activities, communication with patients and many other areas.

The Society of Radiographers has a health and safety section which can provide expert advice on health and safety issues. For example following an inspection by the Society's health and safety representative at a hospital in Cumberland, it was reported that there were breaches of recommended space levels. This led to relocation of some radiographers and a new CT control room is to be built[12].

Reporting of Injuries, Diseases and Dangerous Occurrences Regulations 1995

The regulations (RIDDOR 95) which were introduced in 1985 governing the reporting of injuries, diseases and dangerous occurrences were replaced by new regulations which came into force on 1 April 1996. There is now one set of regulations in place of the four sets under the 1985 regulations. The list of reportable diseases has been updated as has the list of dangerous occurrences.

Following the successful HSE pilot scheme in Scotland[13], in February 2000 it was announced[14] that funding was to be made available to the HSE to set up a centralised national workplace accident and incident reporting system instead of the 500 different addresses which have to be used at present. It will be legally possible for reports to be made by telephone. The National Patient Safety Agency which will administer this scheme is considered in Chapter 21.

Protection of employees who report health and safety hazards

Additional protection has been given by the Trade Union Reform and Employment Rights Act 1993 against dismissal in health and safety cases and was consolidated in the Employment Rights Act 1996. The Public Interest Disclosure Act 1998 is intended to strengthen protection given to employees who report health and safety hazards. This is considered in Chapter 22 on employment.

Occupier's liability

The Occupier's Liability Acts 1957 and 1984 are enforceable in the civil courts if harm has occurred to a visitor (1957 Act) or trespasser (1984 Act)

The Occupier's Liability Act 1957

Under this Act the duty of care owed by the occupier (of whom there may be several) is what is reasonable in the circumstances to ensure that visitors will be safe for the purposes for which they are permitted to be on the premises.

The occupier would be the person in control of the premises. This would normally be the NHS trust in respect of hospital property and the ward sister would be acting as the agent of the occupier in respect of the safety of her ward. The Radiography Manager could be the occupier of the X-Ray Department. There can however be several occupiers. For example if painters employed by independent contractors come onto the premises they may also be in occupation of the premises and could be responsible for harm which occurs as a result of their lack of care.

A visitor is a person on the premises with the express or implied consent of the occupier. In the context of hospitals the term would therefore include patients, staff, visitors, tradesmen and any one else with a *bona fide* reason to be there and who is not excluded by the occupier. It could also include those accompanying patients (see below).

The nature of the duty owed to visitors

The duty is set out in section 2(2) of the Act and section 2(3) clarifies the duty further in relation to specific circumstances as shown in Figure 15.7.

Figure 15.7 **Occupier's Liability Act 1957 sections 2(2) and (3).**

2(2) The common duty of care is a duty to take such care as in all the circumstances of the case is reasonable to see that the visitor will be reasonably safe in using the premises for the purposes for which he is invited or permitted by the occupier to be there.

2(3) The circumstances relevant for the present purpose include the degree of care, and of want of care, which would ordinarily be looked for in such a visitor, so that (for example) in proper cases —
(a)   an occupier must be prepared for children to be less careful than adults; and
(b)   an occupier may expect that a person, in the exercise of his calling, will appreciate and guard against any special risks ordinarily incident to it, so far as the occupier leaves him free to do so.

The Occupier's Liability Act 1957 and children is considered in Chapter 8.

The Occupier's Liability Act 1984

The 1957 Act does not cover trespassers. Until the 1984 Act was passed the law relating to the nature of the duty owed to a trespasser was according to the common law (i.e. the decisions of judges).

Whether or not a duty is owed by the occupier to trespassers, in relation to risks on the premises, depends upon the following factors set out in section 1(3) and shown in Figure 15.8.

Figure 15.8 **The Occupier's Liability Act 1984 – section 1(3).**

(a)   [if the occupier] is aware of the danger or has reasonable grounds to believe that it exists;
(b)   [if the occupier] knows or has reasonable grounds to believe that the other is in the vicinity of the danger concerned or that he may come into the vicinity of the danger (in either case, whether the other has lawful authority for being in that vicinity or not); and
(c)   the risk is one against which, in all the circumstances of the case, [the occupier] may reasonably be expected to offer the other some protection.

In applying these factors to decide if a duty is owed to a trespasser, it would be rare for a duty to be owed to an adult. It is, however, more likely to be a duty owed to a child trespasser. Thus, for example, if a child on hospital premises is expressly told that he cannot go through a particular door or into another section of the hospital and he disobeys those instructions, then he becomes a trespasser for the purposes of the Occupiers' Liability Acts. Although he is not protected by the 1957 Act, it is likely that a duty would then arise under the 1984 Act depending on the child's age and understanding.

The nature of the duty owed to trespassers

Once it is held that a duty of care is owed to a trespasser, section 1(4) of the 1984 Act defines the duty as follows:

'The duty is to take such care as is reasonable in all the circumstances of the case to see that he does not suffer injury on the premises by reason of the danger concerned'.

The duty can be discharged by giving warnings, but in the case of children, this may have limited effect – it would depend upon the age of the child (see Chapter 8).

Control of Substances Hazardous to Health Regulations

All health workers have responsibilities under the COSHH Regulations[15]. The radiographer who uses different substances in her work should be specifically alert to the need to ensure that the regulations are implemented.

Assessment

The five stages of assessment set out in the guide issued by the Health and Safety Executive[16] are shown in Figure 15.9.

Figure 15.9   Stages in COSHH assessment.

(1)   Gather information about the substances, the work and the working practices
(2)   Evaluate the risks to health
(3)   Decide what needs to be done
(4)   Record the assessment
(5)   Review the assessment

There must be clarity over who has the responsibility of carrying out the assessment, but the guidance emphasises the importance of involving all employees in the process.

All potentially hazardous substances must be identified. These will include:

● domestic materials such as bleach, toilet cleaner, window cleaner, and polishes
● office materials such as toner and correction fluids
● the medicinal products in the treatment room
● materials and substances used in radiography and oncology.

An assessment has to be made as to whether each substance could be inhaled, swallowed, absorbed or introduced through the skin, or injected into the body (needles). The effects of each route of entry or contact and the potential harm must then be identified.

There must then be an identification of the persons who could be exposed and how.

Once this assessment is complete, decisions must be made on the necessary measures to be taken to comply with the regulations and who should undertake the different tasks. In certain cases health surveillance is required if there is a reasonable likelihood that the disease or ill-effect associated with exposure will occur in the workplace concerned. Radiographers should be particularly vigilant about any substances used in their activities such as developing and cleaning fluids and ensure that a suitable risk assessment is undertaken and its results implemented.

Managers need to ensure that the employees are given information, instruction and training.

Records should show:

- the results of the assessment
- what action has been taken and by whom and
- regular monitoring and review of the situation.

In 1999 the 1994 Regulations were replaced by new regulations. These were designed to provide further protection for workers by providing a mechanism to speed up the introduction of new Maximum Exposure Limits and for approving changes to the list.

Allergies and COSHH

Occupational asthma was recognised in 1991 to be of concern to radiographers[17] in a survey carried out by the Society of Radiographers.

'Occupational Asthma caused by processing chemicals is an acquired allergic reaction. Early symptoms include a metallic taste in the mouth, sore throat, headaches, sinus problems and catarrh. These worsen until the sufferer experiences shortness of breath, tight chest and chest pains. Sensitation (reaction) can happen after a single extreme exposure or the sufferer may have previously worked months or even years with the substances before the onset of symptoms.'

In September 2000 it was announced that a radiographer had won £150 000 compensation after becoming sensitised to a cocktail of processing chemicals.[18] She had worked at Pembury Hospital, Tunbridge Wells for 20 years. Complaints had been made about the ventilation system at the hospital.

Similar reactions can arise from latex and the dangers of latex are considered by Jackie Wall in an article in *Synergy*[19]. She points out the ignorance of staff over which products contain latex and emphasises the importance of each hospital having a latex sensitivity policy with the objective to clarify management and employee responsibilities. A Latex Allergy Support Group provides useful information[20]. Allergy response to latex can be against either the latex protein, a natural compound in the rubber, or the chemicals used in processing the rubber products.

Concerns also arise with gluteraldehyde and a motion was carried at the Radiographers Conference in 2000 asking the Health and Safety Executive to authorise laboratories to test for gluteraldehyde levels and to ensure that the tests are carried out. It was stated that 'radiographers are having to abandon their careers because of poor working conditions'[21].

On 3 May 2000 the Health and Safety Commission held a conference to prepare a draft strategy and consultation paper[22] on occupational asthma. It has published a strategy to reduce occupational asthma by 30% by 2010, an Asthma Project Board has been set up. The COSHH regulations are designed to ensure that any such exposure on the part of employees is prevented if at all possible.

The Society of Radiographers has published guidance[23] on occupational asthma and the COSHH regulations following a survey it carried out in 1991 and repeated in 1997.

Failure to provide adequate ventilation

Case: *Ogden v. Airedale Health Authority*[24]

A claim was brought by an employee against his health authority on the grounds that he was sensitised to X-ray chemicals resulting in occupational asthma and other airways obstruction. He alleged that the sensitation occurred in the course of his employment as a radiographer at Airedale Hospital and was caused by his employer's negligence and/or breach of statutory duty. The matters relied upon to support his allegations were:

- Failure to ensure that the environment in which he worked was so far as reasonably practicable free from fumes likely to be harmful to him
- Failure regularly to monitor his workplaces for such fumes
- Failure adequately to ventilate the workplaces
- Failure to provide him with protective equipment (in particular goggles, masks and an aspirator)
- Failure to warm him of the risk of exposure to fumes
- Failure to heed or act upon complaints made in 1987 concerning problems of temperature and chemical fumes in the A&E X-ray department of the hospital.

It was also alleged that there were breaches of the Control of Substances Hazardous to Health Regulations 1988.

The defendants denied all allegations, including causation and the alleged injuries suffered. They also raised a defence that the claim was out of time, but this was decided in favour of the claimant.

The result was that the claimant's case succeeded on the following grounds:

- During the time of the claimant's employment at Airedale Hospital there were in use in his place of work chemicals which were capable of having an irritant effect upon the health of the employees, and some of which were sensitisers capable of producing skin allergy and asthma and that during some of the activities which staff were required to carry out such as the mixing of chemicals there was a likelihood of the recommended exposure limits being exceeded.
- By the time a report was compiled in 1990 the defendants were well aware of the chemical constituents of most but not all of the chemicals in use in the X-ray department of the hospital and of the fact that such chemicals contained irritants and there was a risk of sensitation.
- The defendants were well aware that their radiographers were complaining that the chemicals used in the department were causing them health problems; during the whole of the claimant's employment at the hospital, the defendants knew that the chemicals in use contained irritants.

- If the defendants did not in fact know that the chemicals contained irritants they ought to have done so.
- The defendants ought to have taken steps to keep the level of chemical fumes in the X-ray department as low as possible. Their primary strategy should have been to seek to control the fumes at source.
- Until 1988 the defendants did little to safeguard radiography staff at the hospital against the irritant effects of chemicals they were working with.
- In failing to take the precautions as regards local exhaust ventilation, the provision of protective equipment, the laying down and enforcement of a proper warning system for dealing with spillages, the issuing of warnings to staff as to the hazards associated with X-ray chemicals and the precautions to be taken when handling them, the defendants were guilty of negligence.
- Failure to take such precautions, as they either knew or ought to have known, put the health of the radiographers at risk, and the risk went beyond mere irritation but included the risk of employees becoming sensitised which, if it occurred, might well lead to a radiographer being obliged to give up his employment and career as in fact had happened to the claimant.
- The claimant was suffering from occupational asthma induced by exposure to X-ray chemicals and that such exposure was caused by the negligence and breach of statutory duty of the employers.

Common law duties

Implied terms of the contract of employment

Some of the terms in the contract of employment are implied by the law. These include the obligation of the employer to safeguard the health and safety of the employee by

- employing competent staff
- setting up a safe system of work and
- maintaining safe premises, equipment and plant.

The employee must obey the reasonable instructions of the employer and take reasonable care in carrying out the work. Contracts of employment should ideally state clearly the duty upon the employer to take reasonable care of the employee's safety and also the employee's duty to co-operate with the employer in carrying out health and safety duties under the Act and at common law. It is of course in the long term interest of the employer to prevent injuries thereby avoiding payment of substantial compensation to his injured employees and also reducing the incidence of sickness and absenteeism.

The employer's duty at common law to take reasonable care to safeguard the employees against the reasonable foreseeable possibility of harm arising from work related disorders is paralleled by the duties laid down in the Health and Safety at Work Act 1974 and the regulations under it.

Effect of failures by the employer

Failure by the employer to take reasonable care of the the employee's health, safety or welfare could result in the following actions by the employee:

- Action for breach of contract of employment.
- Action for negligence, where the employee has suffered harm; the employee could also use as evidence breach of specific health and safety regulations.
- Application in the employment tribunal for constructive dismissal, if it can be shown that the employer is in fundamental breach of the contract of employment.

Case: Crushed thumb[25]

A Senior 11 Radiographer had her left thumb crushed between a fire door and imaging equipment at Epsom NHS trust Hospital where she worked. The accident occurred in December 1997 when she was pushing an imaging intensifier out of the X-ray theatre. The fire doors in the hospital are slow release and then snap shut but as she put her hand out to stop the door hitting her, it snapped trapping her thumb between the equipment and the door, breaking two bones. A similar accident had happened six months before, when the door snapped shut against a colleague's ankle. A door-stop costing £1 could have prevented the problem but nothing had been done. The Trust pointed out that an accident form had not been completed and initially only offered £800 compensation. Eventually £2000 plus losses and expenses incurred was paid.

Special areas

Violence

Unfortunately, there are more and more reports of attacks on health service employees, not just from strangers in the streets but also from carers and even patients. The rules relating to the terms of service of GPs have recently been changed to enable them to arrange for the removal from their list of any patient who threatens violence to them. There have been reported cases of serious harm to health professionals. Thus, in a case in 1983[26], a voluntary patient at a mental hospital was charged with assault occasioning actual bodily harm to an occupational therapist employed at the hospital. Another occupational therapist was killed by a mentally ill patient in the Edith Morgan Unit at Torbay with an inquiry set up following this death[27].

At the Society of Radiography conference in 1999 a motion was put to urge managers to provide adequate funding for security and guidance for radiographers in dealing with potentially dangerous situations. Michael Mackrill of Llandough NHS trust stated that:

'Managers do not provide effective preventative measures because it costs too much. CCTV and self-defence training are no good. Radiographers need more effective security procedures, and to be trained to recognise signs of abusive behaviour.'[28]

At the Annual Conference of Radiographers in 2000 the issue of assaults on health-care workers whilst on duty was debated. One of the speakers gave an example of a person who had physically and verbally assaulted a member of the local ambulance staff being merely bound over to keep the peace, the court officer describing it as part of the risk of the job[29].

It is of course a criminal offence to assault anyone. However securing a successful prosecution may not always be easy and sometimes the Crown Prosecution Service decides that a public prosecution is not maintainable on the evidence, so the individual would have to resort to a private prosecution or to civil action. It was reported in October 1998[30] that North West Durham Health Care Trust are to meet the full legal costs and provide emotional and professional support for all health care staff who take court action against an assailant in cases where the Crown Prosecution Service fails to pursue the offender. If a radiographer is involved in violence or witnesses a violent incident, she should make sure that a report and statement are completed.

The employer has a duty to take reasonable care of the radiographer in relation to reasonably foreseeable violence. A risk assessment would therefore be required of this possibility and as a result any reasonable means to protect the employee should be adopted. The following questions should be asked:

■ Is it possible to remove the risk altogether?

If the answer is yes, but only by providing armed guards in X-Ray and oncology departments, then avoiding the risk completely would not seem to be reasonably practicable.

■ What preventive action or protective measures can be taken?

The answer to this might include the provision of CCTV and two-way radios, personal alarms or, in very dangerous areas, asking the police for assistance. Protective measures may include more staffing, higher levels of supervision of difficult to manage patients and special security measures.

■ Review the situation to ascertain if the nature of the risk has changed.

   For example has the overall level of violence in the hospital increased? Are there more drunken and abusive patients attending? What is the extent of the success of the measures taken to prevent harm to radiographers? Are any further measures necessary?

This type of analysis will relate not only to the radiographers and oncologists but could be part of a wider assessment of all health professionals into which the radiographers and oncologists could have an input.

Reference should be made to the guidance prepared by the Health and Safety Commission[31]. This gives practical advice for reducing the risk of violence in a variety of settings and emphasises the importance of commitment from the highest levels of management.

Monitoring of potentially violent situations is essential and the radiographer should play her full part to bring any concerns to the attention of the management and ensure that action is taken. Lucinda King analysed the research conducted in a large teaching hospital on violence in the workplace[32]. There was evidence of 92.1% of radiographers responding to the survey having been verbally abused. The Society of Radiographers has published guidance on violence at work[33].

Stress

Concern with stress at work is now recognised as part of the employer's duty in taking reasonable care of the health and safety of the employee. The extent of stress amongst therapists was shown in a survey carried out by *Therapy Weekly*. It commenced a Stress Check campaign in October 1992 and attracted a massive response. Simon Crompton analysed the results in a Stress Check booklet[34] and showed that over half of the respondents had considered leaving work within the past year. The factors most likely to affect respondents were:

- having too much to do
- concern at changes in NHS/social services
- inadequate resources
- interruptions.

The following case was the first where the courts recognised that the duty of the employer at common law to take reasonable care of the health and safety of the employee included care for his mental health.

Case: *Walker* v. *Northumberland County Council*[35]

A social worker obtained compensation when his employer failed to provide the necessary support in a stressful work situation when he returned to work following an earlier absence due to stress. The employer was not liable for the initial absence, but that put the employer on notice that the employee was vulnerable and its failure to provide the assistance he needed was a breach of its duty to provide reasonable care for his health and safety as required to do under the contract of employment.

The HSE has funded research into occupational health and in May 2000 announced the preliminary findings[36]. It estimated that 5 million workers suffer from high levels of stress. A Bristol study[37] found that there was an association between reporting being very stressed and a range of job factors, such as having too much work to do or not being supported by managers. There was also an association between reporting being very stressed and a range of health outcomes such as poor mental health, and back pain and health-related behaviours such as drinking alcohol and smoking.

A recent Court of Appeal case may make it more difficult for employees to obtain compensation for stress. The Court of Appeal has laid down the components which an employee has to establish in his claim and emphasised the need to establish reasonable foreseeability and causation[38].

A survey of job stress and satisfaction among clinical radiologists[39] was carried out by J Graham *et al*. They found that the most stressful aspect of work for radiologists was work overload. Inadequacies in current staffing and facilities and concerns about funding were also major sources of stress, as were impositions made on radiologists by other clinicians. A greater proportion of radiologists than other specialists felt insufficiently trained in communication skills.

Reference should also be made to Chapter 14 on negligence and Chapter 17 on equipment issues.

Sexual and other harassment

It is essential that practitioners are sensitive to the dangers of sexual harassment and make every effort to avoid potentially difficult situations. On the one hand they must be aware of the Sex Discrimination laws (see Chapter 22) and must ensure that they do not discriminate either directly or indirectly. On the other hand they must ensure that they are chaperoned in any situation which could lead to accusations of harassment by the radiographer or where the radiographer is herself (or himself) at risk. The patient's privacy and dignity should be respected at all times. Treatment areas should provide privacy, security and comfort with curtaining/screening provided to ensure visual privacy for patients and a room for individual examinations, interviews or treatments of a particularly personal nature.

The Protection from Harassment Act 1997

The Protection from Harassment Act 1997 can also provide some protection in the workplace if an individual considers that they are subject to unreasonable unwanted attention. The Act creates:

- A criminal offence of harassment (section 1) which is defined as a person pursuing a course of conduct which amounts to harassment of another and which he knows or ought to know amounts to harassment of the other. (The reasonable person test is applied.)
- A civil wrong whereby a person who fears an actual or future breach of section 1, may claim compensation including damages for anxiety and financial loss.
- The right to claim an injunction to restrain the defendant from pursuing any conduct which amounts to harassment.
- The right to apply for a warrant for the arrest of the defendant – if the injunction has not been obeyed.
- An offence of putting people in fear of violence – where a person causes by his conduct another person to fear on at least two occasions that violence will be used against them.
- Restraining orders can be made by the court for the purpose of protecting the victim of the offence or any other person from further conduct amounting to harassment or to fear violence.

Certain defences are permitted in the Act including that an individual is preventing or detecting crime.

Bullying at work

One of the reasons for stress at work may be bullying. Managers of departments should be sensitive to the possibility that an individual member of staff is being bullied. Bullying includes offensive, abusive, intimidating, malicious or insulting behaviour or abuse of power, which makes the recipient feel upset, threatened, humiliated or vulnerable, undermines their self-confidence and may cause them stress. In certain circumstances public sexual bullying at the workplace can amount to the criminal offence of indecent assault[40].

In a recent case £100,000 was accepted in an out-of-court settlement by a teacher who alleged that he had been bullied by the head teacher and other staff, when he was teaching in a school in Pembrokeshire[41]. Dyfed County Council denied negligence. He suffered a minor breakdown in October 1996 and was returned to the same school although he had asked for a transfer. He claimed that he was isolated, ignored and subjected to a series of practical jokes. He then suffered a second nervous breakdown. It was claimed that a support plan worked out for him by the council was not properly implemented. In a second case a home help supervisor who claimed that her co-workers had been beastly to her received £84 000 in an out-of-court settlement with Liverpool Council[42]. The lessons for managers from these cases are obvious.

The Society of Radiographers has published guidelines on bullying and harassment at work and the issues were considered in *Synergy* June 1999[43]. The European Health and Safety Framework Directive requires employers to institute coherent overall prevention policies to maintain employees' mental and social well-being. This obviously includes protection from bullying.

Legal remedies for bullying include:

● Personal injury claims
● Constructive dismissal claims
● Use of the sex, racial and disability discrimination legislation
● Use of the Protection from Harassment Act 1997
● Criminal prosecution for indecent assault

In correspondence to *Synergy News*[44] Stephanie McWilliam described the success of using an advocate who is prepared to act on behalf of colleagues who are troubled by harassment or bullying. All staff are informed of the advocate, to whom they can go in confidence, and they are assured that they will not be named in any action nor will they be required to speak to anyone other than the advocate.

The Society of Radiographers has published guidance on harassment and bullying in the work place and on sexual harassment[45].

Repetitive strain injury (RSI)

This condition is now also known as Occupational Overuse Syndrome (OOS). At the Society of Radiographers Conference in 1999 it was stated that the Society had seen a number of claims related to alleged RSI but the evidence was not conclusive; a programme of research was needed to identify the problem and to identify how to take action. Radiographers should be aware both for themselves and for their patients the legal implications of RSI. An analysis of the legal issues in RSI has been undertaken by Karen Barker[46] who discussed the dramatic increase in the reported incidence of Work Related Upper Limb Disorder (WRULD). Even though in an early case a judge was quoted out of context as declaring that repetitive strain injury has no place in medical books[47], RSI has been recognised for the purpose of compensation in health and safety cases. Thus in the case of *Bettany* v. *Royal Doulton UK Ltd*[48] the High Court found that repetitive work causing only pain with no other associated symptoms could be classed as an overuse injury caused by the plaintiff's work. (Although on the actual facts of the case the employers were found not to be in breach of the duty of care which they owed to their employees. The employers had warned of the dangers, had introduced a system of reporting problems and had moved the claimant to lighter work.)

A later House of Lords decision, however, may make it more difficult to obtain compensation for RSI.

Case: RSI claim rejected[49]

On 25 June 1998 the House of Lords rejected claims by Ann Pickford, a secretary who was sacked after she developed a form of repetitive strain injury, to sue her employers. It overruled the Court of Appeal decision that she should be allowed to make a claim against Imperial Chemical Industries. The Court of Appeal had found that ICI was negligent in failing to warn her of the need to take breaks during her work using a word processor and gave her the right to take her case back to the High Court for an assessment of damages, which she estimated at £175 000.

In a majority judgment (4 to 1) the House of Lords decided that ICI did not need to warn her about the dangers of repetitive strain injury because typing took up only a maximum 75% of her workload. The House of Lords also questioned whether she had proved that the pain was organic in origin. She had been sacked in 1990 after taking long periods off work because of pain in both hands. She claimed that the injury had been caused by the very large amount of typing at speed for long periods without breaks or rest periods. The House of Lords said that it could reasonably have been expected that a person of her intelligence and experience would take rest pauses without being told.

It also held that RSI as a medical term was unhelpful. It covered so many conditions that it was of no diagnostic value as a disease. PDA4 (Prescribed disease A4) had however a recognised place in the Department of Health and Social Security's list for the purposes of industrial injury, meaning a cramp of the hand or forearm due to repetitive movements such as those used in any occupation involving prolonged periods of handwriting or typing.

An industrial radiographer has been successful in claiming compensation for RSI[50].

Case: *Hunter* v. *Clyde Shaw plc*

Hunter was an industrial radiographer aged 48 years who suffered from lateral spicondylitis (tennis elbow) from moving castings, mainly of between one and five tonnes, on a turntable at work. Although he complained of pain in his right arm in late 1990, he was left to operate the turntable alone from March 1991 until he ceased work and consulted a doctor for pains in his arm in June 1991. He was made redundant in December 1991. As a result of operations to his left arm in October 1992 and his right arm in March 1993, he was left with weakness and pain on squeezing and gripping both arms. His ability to garden, drive and write were impeded and he was unable to assist his wife with lifting and shopping. His ability to play darts and bowls was also restricted.

An expert hand surgeon stated for the defendants that it was not scientific to assert that this tennis elbow was work related as the condition arose constitutionally but could be aggravated externally. However Hunter's claim succeeded and he was awarded £8000.

Ian Arrowsmith has analysed the reasons why radiographers suffer work-related upper limb disorders[51]. He concluded that over 70% of the radiographers responding to his study suffered work related upper limb disorders (WRULD) and that the demographic factor which has most effect on the likelihood suffering from such a disorder was age, with those over 36 years most likely to experience the symptoms. The working conditions likely to produce WRULD are heavy workload, poor equipment design, lack of training and awareness of both staff and management. All these are factors which could be overcome.

David Chapman-Jones has analysed the problem of musculo-skeletal injury (MSI) for sonographers[52] and concluded that existing research of the incidence of MSI did not take account of their life styles outside work and there was probably a lower incidence which was directly attributable to the work of sonographers. He did however consider that 'the symptoms that the sonographers are presenting with could be reduced or eliminated if working practices, primarily, and lifestyle are modified to accommodate such diversion from our natural state'. He recommended that there should be serious review of working practices to avoid a flood of occupational induced musculo-skeletal disorder compensatory claims.

Manual handling

Back injuries have been recognised as a major reason for sickness and staff retiring early on grounds of ill health. Radiographers are vulnerable to the possibility of back injury because of the work which they undertake in the movement of clients and the lifting of equipment. In a relatively recent case[53] Carol Makin, a radiographer, was awarded £80 000 because of a back injury.

Case: Makin Case

Carol Makin injured her back at work when trying to lift a patient from a wheelchair onto an X-ray table. She tried to continue working but her condition was diagnosed as Spondylolithesis. Eventually she was unable to lift anything and had to retire at the age of 49. Following legal advice she sued her employers who defended the case on the grounds that the condition would have developed anyway. Her answer to this was that the accident may have caused it or have accelerated the condition. She was awarded £80 000 on the basis that she will never be able to return to work as a radiographer.

It is essential therefore that radiographers should have a good understanding of the regulations relating to manual handling and the duties of the employer and of themselves. Legal duties are placed upon employers in relation to manual handling by the Manual Handling Regulations, and also as a result of the duty of the employer under the contract of employment to take reasonable care of the health and safety of their employees.

The Manual Handling Regulations and guidance

Regulations were introduced in 1992 as a result of the EC directive (see Figure 15.4). Figure 15.10 sets out a summary of the Regulations. The Royal College of Nursing and the National Back Pain Association in their *Guide to the Handling of Patients*[54] point out that there are discrepancies between the EC Framework

---

Figure 15.10   A summary of the key Manual Handling Regulations.

(4)   Duties of employers
    (1)(a)   Avoidance of manual handling
      (b)(i)   Assessment of risk
        (ii)   Reducing the risk of injury
        (iii)   The load – additional information
    (2)   Reviewing the assessment
(5)   Duty of employees
(6)   Exemption certificates

Schedule 1: Factors to which the employer must have regard and questions he must consider when making an assessment of manual handling operations.

Directive[55] and the UK Regulations and that the former imposes a higher duty on employers, closer to that of 'practicality' rather than the 'reasonable practicability' of the Regulations. The Society of Radiographers has also published guidance on the manual handling regulations[56].

Guidance on manual handling is given by the Health and Safety Executive[57]. The guidelines are not themselves the law and the booklet advises that they

> 'should not be regarded as precise recommendations. They should be applied with caution. Where doubt remains a more detailed assessment should be made.'

A working group set up by the Health and Safety Commission produced a booklet on *Guidance on Manual Handling of Loads in the Health Services*[58]. This document is described as

> 'an authoritative document which will be used by health and safety inspectors in describing reliable and fully acceptable methods of achieving health and safety in the workplace.'

This is useful health services specific guidance material.

The employer's duty under the regulations can be summed up as follows:

- If reasonably practicable avoid the hazardous manual handling.
- Make a suitable and sufficient assessment of any hazardous manual handling which cannot be avoided (guidance given in Schedule 1).
- Reduce the risk of injury from this handling so far as is reasonably practicable.
- Give both general indications of risk and precise information on the weight of each load; and the heaviest side of any load, where the centre of gravity is not positioned centrally.
- Review the assessment.

Schedule 1 is set out as shown in Figure 15.11

Figure 15.11   **Schedule 1 of Manual Handling Regulations 1992.**

Factors to which the employer must have regard and questions he must consider when making an assessment of manual handling operations.

Column 1	Column 2
Factors	*Questions*
1. The tasks	e.g. do they involve holding or manipulating loads at a distance from the trunk?
2. The loads	e.g. are they: heavy; bulky or unwieldy etc.?
3. The working environment	e.g. are there space constraints preventing good posture; uneven slippery or unstable floors etc.?
4. Individual capability	e.g. does the job require unusual strength, height etc.?
5. Other factors	e.g. is movement or posture hindered by personal protective equipment or by clothing?

Management check-list

Appendix 2 of the Regulations gives an example of an assessment check-list:

- Section A covering the preliminary stages
- Section B the more detailed assessment where necessary; and
- Section C identifying the remedial action which should be taken.

The duty which is owed by the employer is owed not only to employees but also to temporary staff such as agency or bank staff who are called in the assist. All such employees are entitled to be included in the risk assessment process since, as has been seen, the assessment must take into account the individual characteristics of each employee. Radiographers who are unusually small in height or not as strong as the average might require special provision in relation to manual handling.

Lifting Operations and Lifting Equipment Regulations 1998

These regulations (LOLER 1998) came into force for all lifting equipment on 5 December 1998 as a result of the lifting provisions of the Amending Directive to the Use of Work Equipment Directive[59]. They are to be read in conjunction with the Provision and Use of Work Equipment Regulations 1998 (PUWER)[60]. They apply to all equipment, including second-hand or leased equipment, old and new equipment. The duty holders have had to comply with all the requirements from 5 December 1998[61]. Some of the pertinent LOLER regulations for radiographers are discussed below.

The definitions make it clear that 'lifting equipment' means work equipment for lifting or lowering loads and includes its attachments used for anchoring, fixing or supporting it. Although principally designed for other types of workplace LOLER does apply to hospital settings. 'Load' includes a person. Paragraph 29 of the guidance on LOLER gives examples of the types of equipment and operations covered by the regulations and includes a bath hoist lifting a resident into a bath in a nursing home. Equipment used by radiographers for positioning patients for diagnostic and therapeutic radiography would therefore come within the regulations. Paragraph 47 of the guidance explains how the guidance applies to hoists:

> 'As hoists used to lift patients e.g. from beds and baths, in hospitals and residential homes are provided for use at work and are lifting equipment to which LOLER applies, the duty holder, e.g. the NHS trust running the hospital or the owner of the residential home, must satisfy their duties under LOLER.'

In practice of course the NHS trust would delegate the day to day responsibilities under the Regulations to the head of each diagnostic and clinical department.

Duties under the Regulations include in regulation 4:

> 'every employer shall ensure that:
> (a) lifting equipment is of adequate strength and stability for each load, having regard in particular to the stress induced at its mounting or fixing point;
> (b) every part of a load and anything attached to it and used in lifting it is of adequate strength.'

Regulation 7 requires machinery and accessories for lifting loads to be clearly marked to indicate their safe working loads. Lifting equipment which is designed for lifting persons should be appropriately and clearly marked to this effect and lifting equipment which is not designed for lifting persons, but might in error be used for such a purpose, should be marked accordingly.

Regulation 8 concerns the organisation of lifting operations and is set out in Figure 15.12.

Figure 15.12   Regulation 8 LOLER.

(1) Every employer shall ensure that every lifting operation involving lifting equipment is
   (a) properly planned by a competent person;
   (b) appropriately supervised; and
   (c) carried out in a safe manner.
(2) In this regulation 'lifting operation' means an operation concerned with the lifting or lowering of a load.

Regulation 9 requires the employer to carry out a thorough examination and inspection before the equipment is first used unless it has not been used before and there is an EC declaration of conformity with the Lifts Regulations. The regulations require further inspections to be carried out at specified times.

Regulation 10 provides for the person who makes the thorough inspection under Regulation 9 to notify the employer of any defect which in his opinion is or could become a danger to persons, sending a report to the enforcement agency if there is a risk of serious personal injury. Schedule 1 specifies the information which should be included in the report.

Regulation 11 requires the employer to keep copies of reports of inspections and the time limits for which they should be held.

Enforcement

What action can be taken if the employer ignores these regulations? The regulations are part of the health and safety provisions which form part of the criminal law. Infringement of the regulations can lead to prosecution by the health and safety inspectorate. The inspectorate has the power to issue enforcement or prohibition notices against any corporate body or individual. A health authority no longer enjoys the immunity from the criminal sanctions which it once did as a Crown Authority and therefore these enforcement provisions are available against it. Similarly an NHS trust is subject to the full force of the criminal law.

What if the carer or patient refuses to use a hoist?

If a risk management assessment for manual handling for a patient indicates that a hoist is necessary to prevent harm to any carer/professional, then the professional can insist that the patient uses a hoist. If the patient refuses to be placed in a hoist, he must be advised that the only way of safely moving him is by a hoist, and, if the patient continues to refuse, then he can be told that support and assistance will not be provided if it endangers the health and safety of the professionals.

Compensation for injuries from manual handling

Section 47 of the Health and Safety at Work Act 1974 prevents breach of certain duties under the Act being used as the basis for a claim in the civil courts. Breach of the regulations can, however, be the basis of a civil claim for compensation unless the regulations provide to the contrary. Even where what is alleged is a breach of the basic duties, a radiographer who suffered harm as a result of the failure of the employer to take reasonable steps to safeguard her health and safety could sue in the civil courts on the basis of the employer's duty at common law.

The statutory duty to ensure the Act is implemented is paralleled by a duty at common law placed upon the employer to take reasonable steps to ensure the employee's health and safety (see above).

Training in manual handling

This is essential to ensure that staff have the understanding to carry out the assessments and to advise on lifting and the appropriate equipment. Regular monitoring should take place to ensure that the training is effective and the policies for review are in place. There is also a duty on the employer to ensure that staff who are not expected to be regularly involved in manual handling are aware of the risks of so doing.

Case: *Colclough v. Staffordshire County Council*[62]

Mrs Colclough was employed as a social worker in the elderly care team. Her duties consisted largely of assessing clients for residential placement and other needs. She was called out to an elderly man's home after referral from his GP. When she arrived she gained access with a neighbour, only to find the man halfway out of his bed. He was in a very distressed state and she felt it was important for him to be lifted back into the bed as she was worried about him being injured. The neighbour, who had some nursing experience, told the social worker how to lift the man. As both of them attempted to lift the man, who weighed around 15 stone, the social worker sustained a lumber spine injury.

She sued on the grounds that the employers had failed to provide her with any training and/or instruction in lifting techniques. The employers denied liability on the ground that it was not a normal part of a social worker's duties to undertake any lifting tasks. The employers alleged that she should have summoned some assistance from the emergency services.

The judge held that it was reasonably foreseeable that the plaintiff would be confronted with emergency situations when working as a social worker in the elderly care team. Although the situation which arose was most unusual, the employers were under a duty to warn her that she should not lift in such circumstances. This duty did not go so far as to impose upon the employer in these circumstances a duty to provide a long training course but certainly to bring to the notice of social workers the risks of lifting. Her claim succeeded without a finding of contributory negligence.

The implications of this decision are that even staff who are not expected to undertake manual handling as part of their work must be trained in risk awareness in order to protect them and the employer should they ever be in the situation where they could be endangered through manual handling.

Lifting extremely heavy patients

This is of considerable concern to radiographers. An extremely heavy person is defined by E. Fazel[63] as 25 stone (130 kgs) or over. In a case study of the problems encountered following an emergency admission, the author analyses the possible action which could be taken, including reviewing the equipment which is available. The implications for other services such as the Fire Brigade, funeral directors etc. are considered and a protocol for the safe handling of extremely heavy patients is supplied. The legal issues arising are considerable. Staff cannot cease to provide services for such persons, but the consequences in terms of costs and effort in minimising the risk of harm are considerable.

Human rights and manual handling laws

There are potential conflicts between an individual's rights under the Human Rights Act 1998 and the manual handling laws. In the Bouldstridge case[64], a pensioner of 84 was prosecuted after he had attached a length of hose pipe to the exhaust of his car and fed it into his home in an attempt to kill his wife and himself. These actions followed a threat by social services and a private agency to withdraw assistance because he refused to allow a hoist to be used. The assistance he was receiving was of two carers three times a day, seven days a week for help with his wife who was doubly incontinent, completely immobile and suffered from Alzheimers. The judge criticised the prosecution for bringing the case and said that Mr Bouldstridge was 'the victim of cruel and longstanding circumstances' who 'did something which was morally indefensible, although humanly very understandable'. He was sentenced to probation of a year after he had pleaded guilty to the attempted murder of his wife. Unfortunately insufficient information is given about the attempts by social services to persuade him to allow a hoist to be used.

It would be regrettable if the Bouldstridge case were used to support a claim that patients have a right under the Human Rights Act 1998 not to use a hoist. It is hoped that the Manual Handling Regulations are not seen as being in conflict with the Human Rights Act 1998. On the contrary in protecting staff and others from the dangers of manual handling, they support the recognition of staff as human beings to be protected by employers and others. The potential conflict between the human rights of staff and the human rights of patients is still to be considered by the courts.

What will be important in any such dispute is the documentation, which should record clearly the following points:

- What risk assessments were carried out and when and by whom?
- What were the results and recommendations of the risk assessments?
- What information was given to client and carer about the benefits of avoiding manual handling?
- What communications took place? (every visit, telephone conversation, discussions with others etc. must be carefully recorded and dated)
- How suitable was the equipment for the needs of the client?
- What alternative methods of moving were considered?
- Was residential care proposed?
- Were the client and carer offered the opportunity to see a hoist being used on someone else?

All these issues will be extremely important in showing to the court that every reasonable precaution has been taken to recognise, on the one hand the rights of the client and on the other hand the necessity of complying with the Manual Handling Regulations.

Cross-infection

Precautions must be taken to prevent the risk of cross-infection between patients and staff. In serious situations this may necessitate the closure of a department. Patients coming for radiotherapy may often be vulnerable to infections as a result of the immunosuppressive effects of chemotherapy and other treatments and therefore special precautions must be taken to protect them. On the other hand patients may themselves be suffering from infections and liable to spread infections to other patients and to staff. The highest standards of sterile practice and cleanliness are required and can never be relaxed.

Risk assessment and management of cross-infections should be part of the basic philosophy of every department and ward with a clearly identifiable person responsible for ensuring compliance. This would be required by both statutory duties as well as the duties of the employer at common law and as the occupier under the Occupier's Liability Act (see above).

Hospital acquired infection

A recent report by the National Audit Office[65] has raised major concerns about the level of hospital acquired infection (HAI). The Report suggested that HAI could be the main or a contributory cause in 20 000 or 4% of deaths a year in the UK and that there are at least about 100 000 cases of HAI with an estimated cost to the NHS of £1 billion. The NAO drew conclusions on the strategic management of HAI, surveillance and the extent and cost of HAI, and the effectiveness of prevention, detection and control measures. Its recommendations include reviewing the following:

- The value of using an Infection Control Manual should be considered
- The 1995 Guidance on Infection Control should be reviewed
- The cost effectiveness of screening patients and staff and isolation of patients together with standards and guidelines should be considered
- The policies on provision of education and training should be reviewed
- The arrangements for monitoring hospital hygiene and hospital practices should be tightened
- Advice on handwashing should be implemented
- Clinical audit arrangements should be reviewed to ensure infection control is covered
- Isolation facilities should be reviewed
- Guidance on management of HAI outbreaks should be reviewed

The Government has stated that the Commission for Health Improvement (see Chapter 21) and the Audit Commission would conduct ward inspections and be given the right to seek information on HAI and to publish it.[66]

Reference should also be made to the dangers of cross-infection from workers infected with hepatitis who are HIV positive or suffer from other infectious diseases. Recent advice[67] from the NHS Executive on hepatitis B infected health-care workers, adds to previous guidance[68] and recommends

- further testing of all such workers who are e-antigen negative and who perform exposure prone procedures or clinical duties in renal units
- restriction of those who have a viral load which exceeds 1000 genome equivalents per ml from performing exposure prone procedures and
- management of blood exposure incidents for both health-care workers and patients.

Risk management

A risk management strategy is at the heart of any policy relating to health and safety, not just for employees but also for the patients and general public. Guidance is provided by the Health and Safety Commission and is discussed above. Regular monitoring of the implementation of a risk management policy should ensure that harm is avoided and that a quality service is maintained for the public and employees. This should be accompanied by clear, comprehensive documentation. The Health and Safety Executive in 1998 launched a discussion document[69] to reduce the numbers of employees suffering from work related ill-health. The aim was to produce a strategy to be shared with other organisations and to make recommendations to the Health and Safety Commission for Great Britain. This strategy has been announced and published on a dedicated website, www.ohstrategy.net.

Radiation protection for staff

The statutory duties to protect staff and patients outlined in the main legislation and the Regulations are set out in the following chapter. Of key concern in any department of radiography and radiotherapy is to ensure that the requirements on prevention of staff exposure and monitoring levels of radiation and the maintenance and inspection of equipment are strictly implemented. It should be a disciplinary offence if staff fail to ensure that they are appropriately protected at all times and their film badges are always worn in the appropriate place and read at the agreed intervals. A recent case reported in *Synergy*[70] described how a cardiac radiographer had won an appeal to the Medical Appeals Tribunal, which accepted that a benign thyroid tumour she developed four years previously was linked to her exposure to low dose radiation over a period of 23 years. The Industrial Injuries Advisory Committee has included thyroid disease on its list of prescribed diseases. Research in the UK has not yet established a causal connection between thyroid tumours and radiation.

Importance of safeguarding other staff

All staff who work in the vicinity of ionising radiations must be considered as part of radiation protection risk assessment, not just radiographers and radiologists. This would include porters, health-care support workers, nurses and others who regularly visit the department and are at risk. James Plane considers the protection for nurses during radiotherapy[71]. He emphasises that nurses caring for patients undergoing radiation therapy for cancer need to be aware of and follow guidelines on the correct procedures. A combination of measures can be taken to minimise the risk of contamination during treatments. (See Harbison's *Introduction to Radiation Protection*[72])

Conclusions

Constant vigilance is required to ensure that the many risks to health and safety in a radiology and radiotherapy department are assessed and managed. The legal responsibility is upon both the employer (and therefore the manager representing the employer) and also upon each individual member of staff to safeguard the health and safety of employees, patients and others who may visit the department. The law is constantly being updated and guidance revised. Therefore responsibilities for ensuring that the department is kept abreast of all these changes should be clearly allocated and monitored.

✍ **Questions and exercises** _____

1   Undertake a risk assessment of your department.
2   Show the differences between the implementation of the Health and Safety at Work Act by the health and safety inspectorate and a case brought by an employee for compensation because of breach of the duty to care for the health and safety of an employee by the employer.
3   A radiographer reports that the floor of her department is in a dangerous condition. What action should she take if her employer ignores her report?

References

1   *Harris* v. *Evans and Another* Times Law Report, 5 May 1998
2   Reported in *Synergy News* (April 1999) page 3
3   *R* v. *Nelson Group Services (Maintenance) Ltd* The Times Law Report, 17 September 1998
4   Health and Safety Commission (1993) *Management of Health and Safety at Work: Approved Code of Practice* HMSO, London
5   Health and Safety Commission (2000) *Management of Health and Safety at Work: Approved Code of Practice* The Stationery Office, London
6   Council Directive 89/391/EEC
7   Council Directive 91/383/EEC
8   Article 6 and 7 of Council Directive 94/33/EC
9   Council Directive 92/85/EEC
10 Royal College of Radiology (1995) *Risk Management in Clinical Radiology* (BFCR(95)6 RCR)
11 Department of Health (1993) *Risk Management in the NHS* London NHS Executive (EL(93)111)
12 Society of Radiographers News Item *Synergy News* (March 2001) page 3
13 Enquiries can be made to: Health and Safety Executive Information Centre, Sheffield Tel. 0114 2892345, Fax 0114 2892333
14 HSE Press Release E023:00 16 February 2000 *HSE wins funding for Central Incident Reporting Scheme*, HSE Sheffield
15 Control of Substances Hazardous to Health Regulations 1999, SI No. 437 of 1999
16 Health and Safety Executive (1993) *A step by step guide to COSHH assessment* HMSO London; *Guidance and Code of Practice on COSHH*, Stationery Office, London
17 Occupational asthma: how it affects you *Synergy* (March 1999) page 14
18 Massive £150,000 Compensation for radiographer *Synergy News* (September 2000) page 1
19 J. Wall (1999) Beware Latex – Be Latex aware *Synergy* (November 1999) page, 16–7
20 Latex Allergy Support Group PO Box 36 Cheltenham, Glos GL52 4WY; Helpline 7pm–10pm 07071 225838
21 Conference Report *Synergy News* (June 2000) page 7
22 Health and Safety Commission (2000) *Proposals for reducing the incidence of occupational asthma* (HSC 164)
23 Society of Radiographers *Occupational Asthma and Sensitivity to Chemicals* (no date)
24 *Ogden* v. *Airedale Health Authority* [1996] 7 Med LR 153
25 News item *Synergy News* (April 2000) page 4
26 *R* v. *Lincolnshire (Kesteven) Justices, ex parte Connor* [1983] 1 All ER 901 QBD

27 L. Blom-Cooper, H. Hally, & E. Murphy. *The Falling Shadow – One patient's mental health care 1978–1993*, London 1995 (Report of an Inquiry into the death of an Occupational therapist at Edith Morgan Unit, Torbay 1995)
28 Conference Report *Synergy News* (May 1999)
29 Conference Report *Synergy News* (June 2000) page 7
30 A. Frean (1998) Funds for Nurses who prosecute violent patients *The Times* 1 October 1998
31 Health and Safety Commission (1997) *Violence and Aggression to staff in health services* HSE Books, Sheffield
32 L. King (2001) Violence at work: are you at risk *Synergy* (May 2001) pages 22–4
33 Society of Radiographers *Violence at Work* (no date)
34 C. Harris (ed.) (1996) *Stress Check* published by *Therapy Weekly*
35 *Walker* v. *Northumberland County Council* Times Law Report, 24 November 1994; [1995] 1 All ER 737
36 HSE Press release E080:00 18 May 2000 *HSE publishes new research on occupational stress*
37 A. Smith (2000) *The Scale of Occupational Stress: The Bristol Stress and Health at work Study* HSE, Sheffield
38 *Sutherland* v. *Hatton* Times Law Report, 12 February 2002 CA
39 J. Graham and others (2000) Job stress and satisfaction among clinical radiologists *Clinical Radiology* (March 2000) **55**, 3, 182–3
40 *R* v. *Wakefield*; *R* v. *Lancashire* The Times Law Report, 12 January 2001
41 V. Fletcher (1998) Teacher 'bullied by staff' wins £100,000 *The Times* 17 July 1998
42 J. Clarkson (1999) These stress payoffs are enough to make you sick *The Sunday Times* 11 July 1999
43 Workplace bullying – a real issue. *Synergy* (June 1999) pages 16–18
44 Letter on Workplace bullying from S. McWilliam *Synergy News* (August 1999) page 12.
45 Society of Radiographers *Harassment and Bullying in the Workplace*; Society of Radiographers *Sexual Harassment* (no date)
46 K. L Barker (1995) Repetitive Strain Injury: a review of the legal issues *Physiotherapy* (February 1995) **81** 2, 103–6
47 *Mughal* v. *Reuters Ltd* [1993] IRLR 571
48 *Bettany* v. *Royal Doulton UK Ltd* (1994) reported in *Health and Safety Information Bulletin* 'Unidentifiable ULD/RSI can be occupationally caused', HSIB 219 20
49 *Pickford* v. *Imperial Chemical Industries Plc* The Times Law Report, 30 June 1998
50 *Hunter* v. *Clyde Shaw Plc* [1995] SLT 474; [1994] SCLR 1120
51 I. Arrowsmith (2001) Why do radiographers suffer work-related upper limb disorders? *Synergy* (March 2001) pages 6–9
52 D. Chapman-Jones (2001) Musculo-Skeletal injury: is it a problem for sonographers? *Synergy* (April 2001) pages 14–15
53 *Synergy News* March 2000 page 1
54 The Royal College of Nursing and the National Back Pain Association (1997) *Guide to the Handling of Patients* (4th edn.) RCN, London
55 EC Directive 90/269/EEC on the Minimum Health and Safety Requirements for the Manual Handling of Loads (4th individual directive within the meaning of Article 16(1) of Directive 89/391/EEC)
56 Society of Radiographers *Watch Your Back* (no date)
57 Health and Safety Executive (1992) *Manual Handling Guidance on Regulations* HMSO, London
58 Health and Safety Commission (1992) *Guidance on Manual Handling of loads in the Health Services* HMSO, London

59 AUWED 95/63/EC

60 Provision and Use of Work Equipment Regulations 1998 (SI No. 2306 of 1998)

61 HSC (1998) *Safe use of lifting equipment: Approved Code of Practice and Guidance* HSE books, Sheffield

62 *Colclough* v. *Staffordshire County Council* (June 30 1994) *Current Law* No 208 October, 1994

63 E. Fazel (1997) Handling of Extremely Heavy Patients *National Back Exchange Journal* Issue 9 (2 April 1997) pages 13–6

64 H. Johnstone (2000) Man, 84, tried to kill sick wife *The Times*, 7 June 2000; P. Kelso (2000) He only wanted to end his wife's pain. *The Guardian*, 7 June 2000

65 National Audit Office (2000) *The Management and Control of Hospital Acquired Infection in Acute NHS Trusts in England*, Stationery Office, London

66 DoH Press Notice, 12 June 2000; J. Sherman (2000) Infections caught in hospital to be exposed *The Times* 13 June 2000

67 NHS Executive (2000) *Hepatitis B Infected Health Care Workers* HSC 2000/020 DoH, London

68 *Protecting health care workers and patients from hepatitis B* HSG (93)40 and its addendum EL(96)77

69 HSE (1998) *Developing an Occupational Health Strategy for Britain* HSE Books, Sheffield

70 News Item: Victory for radiographer in landmark case *Synergy News* (June 2001) page 1

71 J. Plane (1999) Protection for nurses during radiotherapy *Professional Nurse* (December 1999) vol **15**, 3, 168–171

72 M. A Harbison (1996) *An Introduction to Radiation Protection* Chapman and Hall Medical, London

Chapter 16
Radiological Regulation

The aim of this chapter is to set out the basic statutory provisions for radiological protection and provide an indication of the sources of government and professional guidance. Unfortunately it is not possible in a work of this nature to cover the detail of this guidance and any commentary on it would be both inappropriate and superficial. (The guidance on the 1999 Ionising Regulations is over 200 pages.) Readers are referred to the volumes of documents published by the National Radiation Protection Board.

The international and national context

This country works within the context of many international and national organisations which aim to safeguard the use of radioactive substances. The European Community has enacted Directives which member states are obliged to implement. The UK has implemented these as statutory instruments (see Chapter 2)

International organisations concerned with standard setting and radiation protection include:

- International Commission on Radiological Protection
- International Commission on Non-Ionizing Radiation Protection
- United Nations Scientific Committee on the Effects of Atomic Radiation
- World Health Organization
- International Atomic Energy Agency
- European Atomic Energy Community (Euratom)

Nationally there are:

- United Kingdom Atomic Energy Authority
- National Radiological Protection Board
- Medical Research Council

The statutory framework under which departments of radiology, radiotherapy and medical and nuclear physics operate is summarised below:

- Medicines Act 1968
- Radiological Protection Act 1970
- Health and Safety at Work etc. 1974 (see Chapter 15)
- Radioactive Substances Act 1993
- The Medicines (Administration of Radioactive Substances) Regulations 1978

- The Radioactive Materials (Road Transport) (Great Britain) Regulations 1996
- Ionising Radiations Regulations 1999
- Ionising Radiation (Medical Exposure) Regulations 2000

The Radiological Protection Act 1970

Under this legislation, the Secretary of State for Health is empowered to appoint members of the National Radiological Protection Board and to give directions to the Board. He also has power, after the appropriate consultation, to make orders conferring on the Board new functions or terminating or varying existing functions.

National Radiological Protection Board (NRPB)

The Board is an independent statutory body set up under the Radiological Protection Act 1970 on 1 October 1970. It took over the Radiological Protection Service (which was previously provided by the Medical Research Council) and other functions and is under the direction of the Health Ministers.

The Board consists of a chairman and not fewer than seven nor more than 12 members who are appointed by the Secretary of State for Health after consultation with the UK Atomic Energy Authority and the Medical Research Council.

Powers and functions
The remit of the NRPB is set out in Figure 16.1.

Figure 16.1 **Powers of the National Radiological Protection Board.**

- By means of research and otherwise to advance the acquisition of knowledge about the protection of mankind from radiation hazards
- To provide information and advice to persons, including governing departments, with responsibilities in the UK in relation to the protection of the community as a whole or of particular sections of the community from radiation hazards
- To provide technical services to persons connected with radiation hazards and dangers
- To make charges for such services and for providing information and advice in appropriate circumstances

In carrying out its functions the NRPB is required to act in consultation with the Health and Safety Commission. It can, if required by the Secretary of State, enter into agreement with the Health and Safety Commission to carry out on its behalf its (the Commission's) functions relating to ionising or other radiations (including those which are not electromagnetic). The Health and Safety Commission is required to consult the NRPB before making proposals on electromagnetic radiations to the Secretary of State.

The NRPB disseminates its advice through a series of formal 'Documents'.

The Board provides various services that the public, companies and individuals, can call upon. These may be charged for.

- *Radiation Protection Review Service*: This gives a systematic audit of a company's radiological protection infrastructure to assess the level of compliance with the regulations, including the Management of Health and Safety at Work Regulations 1992 (see Chapter 15)
- *Personal Monitoring Services*: The NRPB provides a range of approved personal dosimetry services for assessing occupational exposure to ionising radiations in the UK and a dose record keeping service. The Central Index of Dose Information, a national database, is maintained on behalf of the Health and Safety Executive (HSE).
- *Dental X-ray protection Services*: The NRPB provides services to dental practitioners and to companies that manufacture, supply, install and maintain dental X-ray equipment. The aim is to ensure that unnecessary radiation doses to patients and to staff are avoided. It assists dentists in meeting the guidelines on radiology standards in primary dental care provided by the NRPB and the Royal College of Radiologists.
- *Training*: NRPB also runs courses to meet all levels of need. There are courses for radiation protection supervisors and other ad hoc courses to meet specific needs.

Work of the NRPB on medical exposures

The NRPB has initiated a study of X-ray examinations in order to provide itself with up-to-date estimates of the magnitude of this major contribution to population exposure and to identify those areas of diagnostic radiology where radiological protection measures can be most effectively directed. It is looking first at paediatric radiology because of the higher lifetime radiation risks to those exposed at a young age. The NRPB is preparing guidance on the optimisation of protection to children undergoing X-ray and nuclear medicine examinations.

Work is also progressing internationally on guidelines on image quality and patient dose criteria for relatively high dose fluoroscopic and computed tomography (CT) examinations on children.

Non-ionising radiation services of the NRPB

The NRPB acts as Laser Protection Adviser to hospitals and other users. The NRPB's work in this field is concerned mainly with

- electromagnetic fields (principally from power lines and radiofrequency sources such as mobile phones)
- levels and effects of ultraviolet radiation (principally from the sun) and
- emissions from lasers and infrared sources.

NRPB's advisory group on Non-ionising Radiation has set up a subgroup on ultraviolet radiation (UVR) with the aim of reviewing recent developments relevant to the effects of UVR on human health in terms of experimental and epidemiological studies and health hazard assessment.

A second subgroup has been set up to give advice on the effects of UVR, lasers and infrared radiation on the eye.

Future developments

In January 2002 the Chief Medical Officer of Health announced that the NRBP is to be part of a new government agency known as the National Infection Control and Health Protection Agency. This new agency will draw together a number of the bodies with expertise in health protection, including the NRBP and the Public Health Laboratory Service.

Other statutory provision

The Radioactive Substances Act 1993

This Act regulates the keeping and use of radioactive material on premises which are used for the purposes of an undertaking and makes provision as to the disposal and accumulation of radioactive waste. Provision is made for the registration of users of radioactive material and for the registration of mobile radioactive apparatus, subject to certain exemptions. The Secretary of State for the Environment has powers under the Act to appoint inspectors, including a Chief Inspector, to assist in the implementation of the Act. He has powers to make regulations and orders and to provide, or arrange for the provision of, additional facilities for the safe disposal or accumulation of radioactive waste and to dispose of such waste.

No radioactive material of any description may be kept or used on any premises unless those premises are registered for that purpose or there is specific exemption. Mobile radioactive apparatus can be used on unregistered premises if it is itself registered or exempted from registration.

Any application for registration in respect of premises, and the keeping and use thereon of radioactive material is made to the Chief Inspector. The application must specify:

- the premises to which the application relates
- the undertaking for the purposes for which those premises are used
- the description of the radioactive material which it is proposed to be kept or used and the maximum quantity likely to be kept or used at any one time
- the manner in which it is to be used

and any other information specified.

The Chief Inspector sends a copy of the application to each local authority in whose area the premises are situated. There is a right of public access to local authority records relating to documents sent to the authority in connection with applications for registration[1].

The Chief Inspector has the power to register the application or refuse the application. The registration can be subject to specified conditions as he thinks fit, but the applicant has a right of appeal to the Secretary of State. On registration, the applicant is furnished with a certificate containing all the material particulars of the registration. Separate provisions relate to the registration of mobile radioactive apparatus. There are regulations relating to the cancellation or variation of registration and appeals to the Secretary of State. Further information is available on the website[2]. See also Technical Notes provided by the Environmental Agency[3].

Medicines Act 1968

A licence is required from the Secretary of State for the importation or exportation of all radioactive substances[4]. The Medicines Act 1968 provides a statutory framework for the regulation of medicinal products (see Chapter 20). The Secretary of State has applied the provisions of this Act to radiopharmaceutical kits, generators and precursors[5].

The Medicines (Administration of Radioactive Substances) Regulations 1978

These regulations prohibit the administration of radioactive medicinal products except by doctors and dentists holding a relevant certificate or by persons acting under the directions of such a doctor or dentist. They have to be administered in accordance with any specifications in that certificate as to the products and the purposes for which they are administered[6]. Notes for the guidance on the clinical administration of radiopharmaceuticals and the use of sealed radioactive sources is provided by the Administration of Radioactive Substances Advisory Committee December 1998.

The Radioactive Material (Road Transport) Act 1991

The regulations enacted under this Act are intended to prevent any injury to health, or any damage to property or the environment, being caused by the transport of radioactive material and to give effect to such international regulations for the safe transport of radioactive material as may be published by the International Atomic Energy Agency. Guidance is provided by the IAEA[7].

Regulations on radiation and ionising radiation

The European Directive (OJ No. L180, 9.7.97) was implemented in the UK by regulations in 1999 and 2000 widening the scope of the previous regulations they replaced. These two statutory instruments are now the key legislation governing the protection of workers and the use of radiation in a medical context.

Ionising Radiations Regulations 1999

These Regulations[8] were enacted to protect the general public and workers against the dangers of ionising radiation, in the exercise of the powers conferred under the European Communities Act 1972.

The regulations and the schedules make detailed provisions for the protection of workers from the initial risk assessment, to control of the working environment, to personal dosimetry in the event of accidents and medical surveillance after such an event. The full text of the regulations is available from the internet.

An approved *Code of Practice* and guidance has been provided by the HSE[9]. The Institute of Physics and Engineering in Medicine has also prepared medical and dental guidance notes on these regulations. It issued a draft and completed an extensive consultation exercise upon it with the final document being issued at the end of 2001. The document can be downloaded from the internet[10].

Ionising Radiation (Medical Exposure) Regulations 2000

These are the second set of regulations[11] enacted to comply with European Directive 97/43/Euratom[12]. The directive lays down:

- Basic measures for the health protection of individuals against dangers of ionising radiation in relation to medical exposure
- Duties on those responsible for administering ionising radiation
- The protection of all persons undergoing medical exposure (whether as part of their own medical diagnosis or treatment, or as part of occupational health surveillance, health screening, voluntary participation in research or medico-legal procedures).

The regulations came into force on 13 May 2000 apart from Regulation 4(1) and (2) on written procedures and protocols which came into force on 1 January 2001 (the delay enabling employers to comply with the requirements on procedures and protocols). Guidance has been provided by the Department of Health and is available on the internet[13]. These 2000 Regulations are wider in scope and more detailed than those which they replace (the Ionising Radiation (Protection of Persons undergoing Medical Examination and Treatment) Regulations 1988 (POPUMET)).

The Explanatory Note to the Statutory Instrument gives a succinct account of the regulations, picking up on the wording of the Directive, and states that:

'These Regulations, together with the Ionising Radiations Regulations 1999 (S.I. 1999/3232) partially implement, as respects Great Britain, Council Directive 97/43/Euratom (OJ No. L180, 9.7.97, p.22) laying down basic measures for the health protection of individuals against dangers of ionising radiation in relation to medical exposure. The Regulations impose duties on those responsible for administering ionising radiation to protect persons undergoing medical exposure whether as part of their own medical diagnosis or treatment or as part of occupational health surveillance, health screening, voluntary participation in research or medico-legal procedures.'

The note goes on to summarise the regulations with emphasis on:

- the wider than usual definition of 'employer'
- adequate training
- the setting up of detailed procedures from referral to clinical audit
- proper evaluation
- screening for those additionally at risk (e.g. pregnant women).

Schedule 1 of the Ionising Radiation (Medical Exposure) Regulations 2000 lists the written procedures which must be drawn up by 'employers'. They include procedures:

(a) to identify correctly the individual to be exposed to ionising radiation
(b) to identify individuals entitled to act as referrer or practitioner or operator

(c)   to be observed in the case of medico-legal exposures

(d)   for making enquiries of females of childbearing age to establish whether the individual is or may be pregnant or breastfeeding

(e)   to ensure that quality assurance programmes are followed

(f)   for the assessment of patient dose and administered activity

(g)   for the use of diagnostic reference levels established by the employer for different categories of radiodiagnostic examination specifying that these are expected not to be exceeded for standard procedures

(h)   for implementation of the regulations and precautions specific to biomedical and medical research

(i)   for the giving of information and written instructions

(j)   for the carrying out and recording of an evaluation for each medical exposure including, where appropriate, factors relevant to patient dose

(k)   to ensure that the probability and magnitude of accidental or unintended doses to patients from radiological practices are reduced so far as reasonably practicable.

Under Schedule 2 of the Ionising Radiation (Medical Exposure) Regulations 2000 training requirements are stipulated (see Chapter 13).

The Ionising Radiation (Medical Exposure) Regulations 2000 apply to GPs and other clinical staff who request X-rays as well as to radiologists and cardiologists; there is a new obligation on all clinical staff who refer patients for X-rays or other medical exposures to provide sufficient clinical information about the patient to enable an assessment of whether the procedure is justified.

A briefing note is provided on the Regulations by the College of Radiographers[14].

The implementation of the regulations is considered in an article following a presentation by Stewart Whitley at the Imaging and Oncology Science meeting in Birmingham in May 2000[15]. He recommended an action plan for the implementation of the Regulations with working groups established to develop major tasks.

- A Standards Group to look at written procedures and Diagnostic Reference Levels (DRLs)
- A QA Group to establish examination protocols and exposure charts
- A Clinical Audit Group to develop a directory of imaging tests and referral criteria
- A Child Focus Group to specifically look at exposure to children
- A Directorate Group to oversee work and progress

He identified the responsibilities of the employer in preparing procedures covering over 11 different activities. DRLs are to be set up for each standard radiological investigation and also for interventional procedures, nuclear medicine investigations and radiotherapy planning procedures.

It is suggested that written protocols should be compiled for every type of standard radiological practice for each piece of equipment. The unidentified authors quote the template used at the Blackpool Victoria Hospital. The form used includes the following:

- Which examination is involved
- The valid reasons for examination
- Patient preparation
- List of standard projections
- Additional projections that may be necessary
- Film/screen speed system
- Standard exposure factors
- The Diagnostic Reference Level (DLR)
- Aftercare of the patient
- Date/review date and authorisation signature

Key themes of the regulations

Being able to provide justification for exposure and ensuring optimal levels of exposure are central requirements of the 2000 regulations and guidance on justification has been provided by the Royal College of Radiologists[16]. The *Guide* explains the critical roles and responsibilities in justification of individual exposures of the employer, the referrer, the practitioner and the operator. It also explains the process of justification and suggests that the process of justification in individual departments should draw heavily upon the RCR's *Guidelines* on referral[17]. The scope of professional practice and justification is considered in Chapter 27.

Another key feature of the Regulations is the duty placed upon the employer, which is widely defined, to ensure that training is in place and that protocols and procedures are drawn up and implemented to ensure safe practice and the carrying out of quality audit and inspections.

Controversy has surrounded the definitions of some of the key personnel who are identified as having responsibilities under the regulations. For example the definition of practitioner in the regulations is 'a registered medical practitioner, dental practitioner or other health professional who is entitled in accordance with the employer's procedures to take responsibility for an individual medical exposure'. There are uncertainties as to which health professionals could be included within this definition. (This is further considered in Chapter 27 on the scope of professional practice. The implications of the regulations on delegation and supervision are considered in Chapter 23.)

Radiation protection practice training

The Ionising Radiation Regulations 1999 require employers to appoint and consult suitable Radiation Protection Advisers (RPAs) to advise and assist them in complying with the regulations. To be an RPA an individual may hold a valid certificate of competence from an assessing body recognised by the Health and Safety Executive. This is the RPA 2000, a non profit making company set up by the Society for Radiological Protection, the Institute of Physics and Engineering in Medicine, the Institute of Radiation Protection and the Association of University Radiation Protection Officers. Its purpose is to certify competence in radiation protection practice. It examines the competence of those wishing to practise as RPAs and, where appropriate, issues certificates. Previous certification schemes in RPA have now been amalgamated and RPA 2000 has taken over responsibility for all current certificate holders and the issuing of certificates.

Conclusion

The importance of this area of law for the practitioner cannot be exaggerated and each practitioner should have ready access to all the statutory documents referred to in this chapter. The guidance material provided by the various organisations should be easily available in each department and regularly updated. Local officers of the Health and Safety Executive are able to provide additional guidance to practitioners and the Health and Safety Executive has a website[18]. Other information is available from the National Radiological Protection Board, the Royal College of Radiologists and the Institute of Physics and Engineering in Medicine.

There should be systematic provision of training by each employer. Employees who are not satisfied with protocols and procedures issued by employers should ensure that constructive criticism is made immediately so that changes can be brought about speedily, if necessary employees should make use of whistle-blowing procedures (see Chapter 22).

 Questions and exercises _____

1   Obtain a copy of the Guidance on the Statutory Instrument 2000 No 1059, The Ionising Radiation (Medical Exposure) Regulations 2000, and consider the extent to which it is fully implemented in your department.
2   Obtain the results of the most recent clinical audit carried out under Regulation 8 of the Ionising Radiation (Medical Exposure) Regulations 2000 and consider the extent to which any lessons arising from this audit have been implemented.
3   Consider the ways in which exposure to ionising radiation by patients can be reduced.
4   You are concerned that one of your colleagues does not appear to wear the personal radiation monitor regularly. You have reminded her of the importance, but your concerns are ignored. What action, if any, should you take? (See also Chapter 15)

References

1   Radioactive Substances Act 1993, section 39
2   http://www.environmental.detr.gov.uk/radioactivity/index.htm
3   Department of the Environment (1995) *Radioactive Discharges from Hospital via patients* Environmental Agency Inspectors Technical Note
4   Import, Export and Customs Powers (Defence) Act 1939, section 1 (as amended); Import of Goods (Control) Order 1954 (as amended) SI No. 23 of 1954
5   Medicine Act 1968 (Application to Radiopharmaceutical-associated Products) Regulations 1992 SI No. 605 of 1992 (reg 1(2)Schedule)

6   Medicines (Administration of Radioactive Substances) Regulations 1978 SI No. 1006 of 1978

7   IAEA Safety Standards, Safety series No 6 *Regulations for the Safe Transport of Radioactive Material* 1990 edition

8   SI No. 3232 of 1999

9   HSE (1999) *Working with Ionising Radiation: IRR 1999 Approved Code of Practice and Guidance* HSE, Sheffield; also HSE information sheets on specific topics

10 http://www.ipem.org.uk/

11 SI No. 1059 of 2000

12 European Directive 97/43/Euratom (OJ No. L180, 9.7.97, p. 22)

13 www.doh.gov.uk/irmer.htm

14 College of Radiographers (2000) *The Ionising Radiation (Medical Exposure) Regulations 2000: Guidance for Radiographers* (February 2000) College of Radiographers, London

15 (Unnamed) IR(ME)R revisited: put it into action *Synergy* (July 2000) pages 17–19

16 Board of Faculty of Clinical Radiology (2001) *A Guide to Justification for Clinical Radiologists* Royal College of Radiologists, London

17 Royal College of Radiologists (1998) *Making the Best Use of a Department of Clinical Radiology: Guidelines for Doctors* 4th edn. RCR, London

18 http://www.hse.gov.uk/hthdir/noframes/iradiat.htm

Chapter 17
Legal Issues Relating to Equipment

This chapter considers the legal issues which arise in the use of equipment in the treatment and investigation of patients. The legal issues relating to telemedicine, teleradiology and PACS are considered in Chapter 24.

Legal rights against the supplier

Common law action in negligence

The law of negligence enables an action to be brought against the manufacture of a defective product if harm has been caused to a consumer or third person. This principle was established in the leading case of *Donoghue* v. *Stevenson*[1]. Actions for negligence are discussed in detail in Chapter 14. It should be noted that in order to succeed the claimant must establish that there was a duty of care, that there has been a negligent breach of this duty, and that, as a reasonably foreseeable result of that breach of duty, harm has been caused. This entire chain may be difficult for the claimant to prove and a contractual claim or the consumer protection legislation may be a preferable cause of action.

Contractual action against supplier

The supplier is under a contractual duty to provide goods in accordance with the contract terms. In addition where the purchaser is a private individual, purchasing from a person in course of business, he or she can rely on the legal rights given under the Sales of Goods and Services legislation, which gives additional protection over and above that contained in the contract documents, by implying certain terms (such as that the goods are fit for their intended purpose and of merchantable quality) into the contract.

Where the purchaser is a large consortium or organisation in its own right, the fact that it could threaten to remove the contract to other suppliers may assist in the performance of the contractual terms without any recourse to legal action.

The Consumer Protection Act 1987

Part 1 of the Consumer Protection Act 1987 makes provision for product liability and covers the sections shown in Figure 17.1

The Consumer Protection Act 1987 enables a claim to be brought where harm has occurred as a result of a defect in a product. It was enacted as a result of the

> **Figure 17.1** **Product liability under the Consumer Protection Act 1987.**
>
> **Section 1**   Purpose and construction of Part I
>
> **Section 2**   Liability for defective products
>
> **Section 3**   Meaning of defect
>
> **Section 4**   Defences
>
> **Section 5**   Damage giving rise to liability
>
> **Section 6**   Application of certain enactments
>
> **Section 7**   Prohibition on exclusions from liability
>
> **Section 8**   Power to modify Part I
>
> **Section 9**   Applications of Part I to the Crown

European Community Directive[2]. It is a form of strict liability in that negligence by the supplier or manufacturer does not have to be established. The claimant will, however, have to show that there was a defect. The supplier can rely upon a defence colloquially known as 'state of the art' i.e. that the state of scientific and technical knowledge at the time the goods were supplied was not such that the producer of products of that kind might be expected to have discovered the defect.

A product is defined as meaning any goods or electricity and includes a product which is comprised in another product, whether by virtue of being a component part or raw material or otherwise.

Who is liable under the Consumer Protection Act?

The producer
Section 2(1) states that 'where any damage is caused wholly or partly by a defect in a product, every person to whom section (2) below applies shall be liable for the damage.'

Section 2(2) includes the following as being liable:

- the producer of the product;
- any person who by putting his name on the product or using a trade mark or other distinguishing mark, has held himself out to be the producer of the product; and
- any person who has imported the product into the EEC in the course of business.

The supplier
In addition to the producers or original importers set out under section 2(2), section 2(3) states that any person who has supplied the product to the person who suffered the damage or to any other person shall be liable for the damage if:

- the person who suffered the damage requests the supplier to identify one or more of the persons who were producers (as set out above);

- that request is made within a reasonable period after the damage occurs and at a time when it is not reasonably practicable for the person making the request to identify all those persons; and
- the supplier fails, within a reasonable period after receiving the request, either to comply with the request or to identify the person who supplied the product to him.

This provision makes it is essential for the practitioner to keep records of the supplier of any goods (including both equipment and drugs) which she provides for the client. In the absence of her being able to cite the name and address of the manufacturer or the company that supplied the goods to her, she may become the supplier of the goods for the purposes of the Act and therefore have to defend any action alleging that there was a defect in the goods which caused harm. Harm includes both personal injury and death and loss or damage of property.

What is meant by a defect?

The statutory definition is shown in Figure 17.2.

Figure 17.2 **Definition of defect: Consumer Protection Act 1987 – section 3.**

(1) Subject to the following provisions of this section, there is a defect in a product for the purposes of [Part 1 of the Act] if the safety of the product is not such as persons generally are entitled to expect; and for those purposes 'safety', in relation to a product, shall include safety with respect to products comprised in that product and safety in the context of risks of damage to property, as well as in the context of risks of death or personal injury.

(2) In determining ... what persons generally are entitled to expect in relation to a product all the circumstances shall be taken into account, including—
(a)   the manner in which, and purposes for which, the product has been marketed, its get-up, the use of any mark in relation to the product and any instructions for, or warnings with respect to, doing or refraining from doing anything with or in relation to the product;
(b)   what might reasonably be expected to be done with or in relation to the product; and
(c)   the time when the product was supplied by its producer to another.

Defences

Certain defences are available under section 4 and are shown in Figure 17.3.

What damage must the claimant establish?

Compensation is payable for death, personal injury or any loss of or damage to any property (including land) (section 5(1)). The loss or damage shall be regarded as having occurred at the earliest time at which a person with an

Figure 17.3 Defences under the Consumer Protection Act 1987 – section 4.

(a) that the defect is attributable to compliance with any requirement imposed by or under any enactment or with any Community obligation; or

(b) that the person proceeded against did not at any time supply the product to another; or

(c) that the following conditions are satisfied, that is to say—

    (i) that the only supply of the product to another by the person proceeded against was otherwise than in the course of a business of that person's; and

    (ii) that section 2(2) above [that the person is the producer or importer] does not apply to that person or applies to him by virtue only of things done otherwise than with a view to profit; or

(d) that the defect did not exist in the product at the relevant time; or

(e) that the state of scientific and technical knowledge at the relevant time was not such that a producer of products of the same description as the product in question might be expected to have discovered the defect if it had existed in his products while they were under his control; or

(f) that the defect—

    (i) constituted a defect in a product (the subsequent product) in which the product in question had been comprised; and

    (ii) was wholly attributable to the design of the subsequent product or to compliance by the producer of the product in question with instructions given by the producer of the subsequent product.

interest in the property had knowledge of the material facts about the loss or damage (section 5(5)). Knowledge is further defined in section 5(6) and (7).

There have been few examples of actions being brought under the Consumer Protection Act 1987 in health-care cases and only a handful of cases brought under it have been reported. One reported in March 1993[3] led to Simon Garratt being awarded £1400 against the manufacturers of a pair of surgical scissors which broke during an operation on his knee, with the blade being left embedded. A second operation was required to remove it.

In a more recent well publicised case[4] patients who had contracted hepatitis C from blood and blood products used in blood transfusions were able to succeed in a claim brought under the 1987 Act. This decision may well lead to greater use of the Consumer Protection Act where personal injuries are caused as a result of defective products, since negligence does not have to be established under the Consumer Protection Act 1987, only that there was a defect in the product which has caused the harm.

The National Consumer Council has published a report[5] on how the Act works.

Medical Devices Agency and warnings

The Medical Devices Agency (MDA) was established in September 1994 to promote the safe and effective use of devices. In particular its role is to ensure that whenever a medical device is used, it is:

- suitable for its intended purpose
- properly understood by the professional user and
- maintained in a safe and reliable condition.

What is a medical device?

The definition used by the MDA is based upon the European Directive definition[6]:

'"Medical device" means any instrument, apparatus, appliance, material or other article, whether used alone or in combination, including the software necessary for its proper application intended by the manufacturer to be used for human beings for the purpose of:
   - diagnosis, prevention, monitoring, treatment or alleviation of disease,
   - diagnosis, monitoring, treatment, alleviation of or compensation for an injury or handicap,
   - investigation, replacement or modification of the anatomy or of a physiological process,
   - control of contraception,
and which does not achieve its principal intended action in or on the human body by pharmacological, immunological or metabolic means, but which may be assisted in its function by such means...'

Annex B to safety notice 9801 from the MDA gives examples of medical devices[7]. It covers the following:

- equipment used in the diagnosis or treatment of disease and monitoring of patients (e.g. syringes and needles, dressings, catheters, beds, mattresses and covers, and other equipment)
- equipment used in life support (e.g. ventilators, defribilators)
- *in vitro* diagnostic medical devices and their accessories (e.g. blood gas analysers) (Regulations came into force in 2000 on *in vitro* diagnostic devices)
- equipment used in the care of disabled people (e.g. orthotic and prosthetic appliances, wheelchairs and special support seating, patient hoists, walking aids, pressure care prevention equipment)
- aids to daily living (e.g. commodes, hearing aids, urine drainage systems, domiciliary oxygen therapy systems, incontinence pads, prescribable foot-wear)
- equipment used by ambulance services (but not the vehicles themselves) e.g. stretchers and trolleys, resuscitators;

Other examples of medical devices include condoms, contact lenses and care products and intra-uterine devices.

Essential requirements

The regulations[8] required that from 14 June 1998 all medical devices placed on the market (made available for use or distribution even if no charge is made) must conform to 'the essential requirements' required by law, and bear a CE marking as a sign of that conformity. Although most of the obligations contained in the regulations fall on manufacturers, purchasers who are positioned further down the supply chain may also be liable – for example, for supplying equipment which does not bear a CE marking or which carries a marking liable to mislead people[9].

This CE marking is the requirement of the EC Directive[6]. The manufacturer who can demonstrate conformity with the regulations is entitled to apply the CE marking to a medical device.

The essential requirements include the general principle that a device 'must not harm patients or users, and any risks must be outweighed by benefits'. Design and construction must be inherently safe and, if there are residual risks, users must be informed about them. Devices must perform as claimed, and not fail due to the stresses of normal use. Transport and storage must not have adverse effects. Essential requirements also include prerequisites in relation to the design and construction, infection and microbial contamination, mechanical construction, measuring devices, exposure to radiation, built-in computer systems, electrical and electronic design, mechanical design, and the function of controls and indicators.

Exceptions to these regulations include the following:

- *in vitro* diagnostic devices (covered by a separate directive)
- active implants (covered by the Active Implantable Medical Devices Regulations[10])
- devices made specially for the individual patient ('custom made')
- devices undergoing clinical investigation
- devices made by the organisation ('legal entity') using them.

In January 1998 the MDA issued a device bulletin[9] giving guidance to organisations on implementing the regulations. The MDA has powers under the Consumer Protection Act 1987 to issue warnings or remove devices from the market.

Devices are divided into three classes according to possible hazards, class 2 being further subdivided. Thus class 1 with a low risk (e.g. a bandage), class 2a medium risk (simple breast pump), class 2b medium risk (ventilator), class 3 high risk (intraortic balloon).

Any warning about equipment issued by the Medical Devices Agency should be acted upon immediately. Failure to ensure that these notices are obtained and acted upon could be used as evidence of failure to provide a reasonable standard of care.

Adverse incident reporting procedures

In 1998 the MDA issued a safety notice[7] requiring health-care managers, health-care and social care professionals and other users of medical devices to establish a system to encourage the prompt reporting of adverse incidents relating to medical devices to the MDA. The procedures should be regularly reviewed, updated as necessary, and should ensure that adverse incident reports are submitted to MDA in accordance with the notice.

What is an adverse incident?

The safety notice defines this as 'an event which gives rise to, or has the potential to produce, unexpected or unwanted effects involving the safety of patients, users or other persons'. They may be caused by shortcomings in:

- the device itself
- instructions for use, servicing and maintenance
- locally initiated modifications or adjustments
- user practices including
  - training
  - management procedures
  - the environment in which it is used or stored
  - incorrect prescription.

The 'effects' are where the incident has led to or could have led to the following:

- death
- life threatening illness or injury
- deterioration in health
- temporary or permanent impairment of a body function or damage to a body structure
- the necessity for medical or surgical intervention to prevent permanent impairment of a body function or permanent damage to a body structure
- unreliable test results leading to inappropriate diagnosis or therapy.

Minor faults or discrepancies should also be reported to the MDA.

Liaison officer

The safety notice suggests that organisations should appoint a liaison officer who would have the necessary authority to:

- ensure that procedures are in place for the reporting of adverse incidents involving medical devices to the MDA
- act as the point of receipt for MDA publications
- ensure dissemination within their own organisation of MDA publications
- act as the contact point between MDA and their organisation.

Keeping up to date

All health professionals are required by their Codes of Professional Conduct and by their registration bodies and by the duty of care which they owe to their patients in the law of negligence to ensure that they keep up to date in relation to the developments within equipment and technology.

Professional warnings

Practitioners have a professional duty to be aware of any information which can affect their safe practice. The practitioner must be alert to any warnings issued by the Medical Devices Agency and must in turn ensure that she completes the appropriate forms for feedback on any dangers or hazards which come to her attention.

MDA publications

The Medical Devices Agency publications include the *Diagnostic Imaging Review* and *Diagnostic Imaging Market Reports*. It also carries out evaluations and reviews of X-ray equipment, magnetic resonance scanners, diagnostic ultrasound units and related equipment.

Inspection and maintenance of equipment

It follows that as a result of the regulations relating to medical devices there should be clear procedures over the maintenance and servicing of any equipment. When equipment is installed, there may be no clarity over who has the responsibility of ensuring that the equipment is regularly checked and, if necessary, serviced or maintained. It is essential that there should be procedures to determine this responsibility when the equipment is first supplied. Some equipment must by law be regularly serviced, for example lifts. When this equipment is installed, an agreement for the future inspection and servicing of the lift should be arranged.

Responsibility for the maintenance would normally reside with the owner of the equipment. If the NHS trust or the social services authority remains the owner and the equipment is loaned to a patient/client, then the trust/authority should set up an appropriate system for inspection and maintenance. This system should also take into account the avoidance of cross-infection.

The MDA guidance[9] suggests the use of a computer system to identify equipment in terms of:

- whether it is simple
- whether it requires:
  - assembly
  - fixing
  - that a prescribing professional be present
  - special instructions for the end-user
- the time and personnel needed to ensure successful and safe delivery, installation and end-user training.

Inventory

Each department should ensure that they keep a list of all equipment, including any which is given out for use in clinics in the community, and that information is kept on the dates for servicing. There should also be a regular review to ensure that the equipment is still in use or whether it should be recalled. The inventory should have details of:

- Nature of the equipment
- Date issued
- Name of patient
- Name of practitioner

- Item(s) issued
- Manufacturer/model/number
- Labelling of equipment
- Date of service.

Situation: old equipment

A patient suffering from the terminal stages of cancer is given a syringe driver for the administration of pain relief. Relatives are concerned that the patient seems to be in intolerable pain and insist upon a senior doctor examining the patient. It is then discovered that the syringe has been wrongly set. It was of an old type with different calibration to the new ones which are used now and the nurse clearly did not understand how to set it correctly. What action can the relatives take?

In the above situation there has been clear negligence by the practitioner in setting the syringe. The employers would be vicariously liable for her negligence. However such a situation is unlikely to lead to civil action, though it could lead to a formal complaint being made. It is hoped that at the very least it would lead to an investigation by the managers and either the withdrawal of the old equipment from the wards and departments or retraining of staff to ensure that they understand how to set both old and new equipment.

Ultrasound units

The responsibility for ensuring that equipment is regularly maintained and inspected should be clearly defined.

As an example, Dr Stephen Pye[11] discusses the calibration and performance of ultrasound physiotherapy machines with reference to current national and international standards, current practices and published surveys of machine performance. He concludes that 'gross faults – resulting in either immediate injury or totally ineffective treatment – can be present in new, factory-checked machines'. He emphasises that all machines require a vigorous programme of testing and calibration in order to deliver outputs within 20% or 30% of that indicated by the front panel. The records of the tests are essential to prove that the practitioner has taken all reasonable care to ensure that the machines are safe and effective. He spells out some important recommendations both for the individual practitioner and for the practitioner educators.

The output of an ultrasound unit must be checked on a weekly basis to see that it is working and giving the correct output. Other tests would measure the treatment time, the treatment frequency, and pulse timing. In addition every year there should be checking on a precision measurement device that is traceable to nationally recognised standards.

Maintenance of hospital equipment

There is a danger that, in these days of increasing pressure on resources, some of the equipment used in the department is not systematically serviced and maintained and unacceptable risks are taken.

Situation: On the blink

One of the hydraulic mechanisms for a table in an X-ray department was malfunctioning on an intermittent basis. A new table was on order, but in the meantime radiographers made do with the existing equipment. On one occasion, when a patient was being moved into position, the table suddenly dropped, causing the patient to fall onto the floor, as a result of which he suffered a broken pelvis.

One cannot imagine any possible defence being offered in the above situation. There is clearly negligence on the part of the practitioners and the employer will be vicariously liable for the harm. There would also be failure on the part of the manager of the department who failed to ensure that a safe system was in operation. Unfortunately there is anecdotal evidence that staff within the NHS appear to make do with equipment which fails on a regular or irregular basis. There are clear dangers in such a practice and under the new national reporting system of adverse incidents (see Chapter 21) and risk management processes within each Trust failures of equipment should be reported. An absence of appropriate management response to such a report could eventually lead to a whistle blowing situation (see Chapter 22).

Statutory provisions under the Ionising Regulations

Under regulation 10 of the Ionising Radiation (Medical Exposure) Regulations 2000[12] 'equipment' is defined as:

'equipment which delivers ionising radiation to a person undergoing a medical exposure and equipment which directly controls or influences the extent of such exposure.'

Regulation 10 requires the employer to draw up, keep up-to-date and preserve at each radiological installation an inventory of equipment at that installation and, when so requested, to furnish it to the appropriate authority.

This inventory has to contain the following information:

- name of manufacturer
- model number
- serial number or other unique identifier
- year of manufacture
- year of installation.

Employers need to ensure that equipment at each radiological installation is limited to the amount necessary for the proper carrying out of medical exposures at that installation.

The provisions of these regulations can be enforced under powers set out in the Health and Safety Act 1974 and guidance[13] has been provided by the Health and Safety Executive on the fitness of equipment used for medical exposure to ionising radiation.

Conclusions

Liability for the supply of equipment which causes harm, has been clarified over recent years and the work of the Medical Devices Agency makes the legal responsibilities of practitioners clear. To keep up to date with technical developments in equipment is becoming a heavy burden for practitioners, but specialisation and clear allocation of responsibilities should ensure that all are supported in keeping up to date within their own specialist areas and that the patients are safe.

 ## Questions and exercises

1 Review the procedure you follow in ensuring that the equipment in your department is always properly maintained and inspected.
2 What action would you take if a patient complains to you that a wheelchair in the X-ray department is faulty?
3 A patient is considering bringing a claim against manufacturers because of faulty equipment. What advice could you give him about his rights?
4 A recently received item of equipment is broken. What actions lie against the manufacturers?

References

1 *Donoghue* v. *Stevenson* [1932] AC 562
2 European Directive No 85/374/EEC
3 B.C. Dimond (1993) Protecting the consumer *Nursing Standard* (3 March 1993) **7**, 24, 18–19
4 *A and Others* v. *National Blood Authority and Another* The Times Law Report, 4 April 2001
5 National Consumer Council (1995) *Unsafe Products: How the Consumer Protection Act works for consumers* National Consumer Council
6 European Union Directive 93/42/EEC concerning medical devices
7 MDA (1998) *Reporting Adverse Incidents Relating to Medical Devices* (January 1998) SN 9801
8 Medical Devices Regulations 1994 SI No. 3017 of 1994 came into force 1 January 1995, mandatory from 14 June 1998; Directive 93/42/EEC
9 MDA Bulletin (1998) *Medical Device and Equipment Management for Hospital and Community based Organisations* (January 1998) MDA DB 9801
10 Directive 90/385/EEC (came into force 1 January 1993 and is mandatory from 1 January 1995)
11 S. Pye (1996) Ultrasound Therapy Equipment – Does it Perform? *Physiotherapy* (January 1996) **82**, 1, 39–44
12 The Ionising Radiation (Medical Exposure) Regulations 2000 SI No. 1059 of 2000
13 HSE Guidance note PM 77 from the HSE (currently being revised)

Chapter 18
Records, X-rays, Statements, Reports and Evidence in Court

The principle purpose of record keeping is to support the quality of care provided for the patient, to facilitate communication between professionals and to maintain a record of the diagnosis, treatment and future plans for the patient. A good standard for documentation would be to ensure that, if any health professional were to be called away in an emergency, their colleagues would be able to provide continuity of care on the basis of full, comprehensive and clear records.

Record keeping is considered in this section because the standard of record keeping is most likely to come to the fore when litigation commences, a prosecution is initiated or a complaint is made. The increase in litigation where patients are seeking compensation for harm also makes it more likely that the practitioner may be called to give evidence in court. In addition many practitioners are developing their role as expert witnesses. This chapter therefore also covers the giving of evidence in court and also looks at some of the rules of evidence and the terminology which is likely to be encountered.

Reference should also be made to Chapter 5 on confidentiality and to Chapter 6 on computerised records, the Data Protection principles and access by the patient and others to personal and health records. The legal issues arising from Picture Archiving and Communication Systems (PACS) are considered in Chapter 24.

Record keeping

Principles of record keeping and standards of practice

Patient care requires a high standard of documentation to record the diagnosis, treatment and future plans, so that all practitioners can share in this knowledge to the benefit of the patient. It should also be clear from the Chapter 14 on litigation that the documentation can play a significant part in any court hearing and it is essential therefore that clear principles on the content, style, clarity, comprehensiveness and accuracy should be followed. Many civil cases may be contested several years after the events to which they relate and the records are therefore extremely important. Some of the basic principles which are shown in Figure 18.1 are taken from the NHS Training Directorate booklet *Just for the Record*[1].

***Figure 18.1*   Principles of clinical record keeping.**

Documents related to the central care plan should:

- Assess and identify a patient's or client's problems/needs
- Plan the expected outcome and the treatment/interventions/care required to achieve it
- Show the planned treatment/interventions/care being put into practice
- Evaluate the actual outcome with the expected outcomes, so care or treatment can be changed where required.

Guidelines to follow in the actual recording

Figure 18.2 sets out some of the basic points to remember in writing the actual records.

***Figure 18.2*   Principles to follow in record keeping.**

- Records should be made as soon as possible after the events which are recorded
- They should be accurate, comprehensive and clear
- They should be written legibly and be jargon-free
- They should avoid opinion and record the facts of what is observed
- They should be signed and dated by the maker
- They should not include abbreviations (unless they are taken from an approved list)
- They should not be altered, unless the changes are made so that the original entry is clearly crossed out, but still readable
- Any change should be signed and dated

What if there is no change in the care of the patient?

Practitioners often ask about what should be recorded when there is no change in the patient's condition and they simply continue the usual treatment. Many may write 'as above' to indicate that treatment has continued to plan. Is this sufficient? It is important that it is clear from the records what interaction there has been between patient and practitioner and if there are any changes in the patient's condition or the treatment plan. It is important that a record should be made each time the practitioner sees the patient. Increasingly there is a tendency to interpret an absence of a record as meaning that there was no activity or interaction: 'If it's not written down, it didn't happen'. This is not in fact an inexorable rule of the courts, but clearly a witness is in a much stronger position in giving evidence if there is a comprehensive record.

Transmitting records

It is essential that if personal information is to be communicated by fax machines, care must be taken to preserve the confidentiality of the information and to ensure that a designated person is appointed to receive it. In 1997 it was reported that a girl died after a fax error at hospital[2]. She suffered from giant cell hepatitis and fell ill on a visit to Middlesborough and her records were faxed from her home in Crawley. Unfortunately they were sent to a fax in a locked room to which no one had access over the weekend. Doctors, unaware of her medical history, gave her an overdose of drugs.

The Consumers' Association in its '*Health Which*' April 1998 noted that in the chains of walk-in surgeries opening in stations and shopping centres GPs are failing to keep records and are not passing on relevant information to the patient's home GP[3] with potentially serious consequences.

Illegibility

Several court cases have arisen as a result of illegible handwriting, especially in writing prescriptions (see Chapter 20). In a coroner's inquest relating to the death of a woman following a routine hysterectomy[4], evidence was given that the junior doctor misread the consultant's prescription of 3 mg of diamorphine to be given by epidural as 30 mg.

Documentary evidence contemporary to the events in issue is an important part of any court case (see below). If a record cannot be read, potentially important facts cannot be proved and any witness would lose credibility if, looking at records they made years previously, they have to say that they are guessing at what some words are.

Abbreviations

It is preferable if the use of abbreviations can be avoided. However realistically abbreviations and symbols can save time, but precautions must be taken to prevent mistakes. There are advantages in each NHS trust or organisation agreeing a list of approved abbreviations with one specific meaning which can be used in that unit. A printed list of these abbreviations would then be provided in each set of records and accompany the records if they were sent to outside agencies. It could be made a disciplinary offence if abbreviations not on the approved list were used or if they were used for a different meaning. In this way the following ambiguities could be avoided:

PID   Pelvic Inflammatory Disease or Prolapsed Intervertebral Disc?
BID   Brought in Dead or Twice?
MS   Multiple Sclerosis or Mitral Stenosis?
NFR   Not For Resuscitation or Neurophysiological Facilitation of Respiration?

and so on.

All that has been said about abbreviations also applies to the use of symbols and signs and other hieroglyphics. Their use can certainly assist record keeping but there should be a clearly approved list available for both patients and health professionals to access.

Reference should also be made to the publications of the NHS Training Authority on standards for record keeping[5]. The UKCC guidelines *Standards for Records and Record Keeping* is also of value to all health professionals[6].

Changing records

Records should not be altered. If the writer discovers that the wrong information was recorded it would be possible to put a line through that information and initial this and then write the correct information. Any attempt to cover what was previously written by tippex or heavy blocking out will arouse suspicions. What was erroneously recorded should still be legible.

It was reported in the *Times* newspaper on 7 November 1995[7] that a casualty nurse who told the parents of a sick baby that he probably had a sniffle, and told them to take him to the family doctor, altered the notes when the baby died one hour later. She changed the words 'extremely pale' to 'quite pale' and added a pulse reading, although she had not taken his pulse. Even though an independent inquiry found that her actions probably had no bearing on the child's outcome, she faced internal disciplinary proceedings which could lead to her dismissal and also professional conduct proceedings which could lead to her being struck off the register of the UKCC.

Whilst the first aim of record keeping is the care, treatment and diagnosis of the patient, it is important to ensure that the records will also protect the practitioner in the event of any litigation, complaint or any investigation into the care. Paul Butt[8], in his advice to radiologists as a result of his work in litigation, states that

> 'It is quite sensible to write a detailed report at the time that something goes wrong because one knows well that six years down the line memories will be blurred. It is important to be sure that critical points are entered into that report.'

The standards set by the CNST

The Clinical Negligence Scheme for Trusts has identified hospital records as one of its core standards (see Chapter 14). The criteria for this standard, their level and the weight attached to them are set out in Figure 18.3.

X-Rays are not specifically included in the guidance of the CNST, but are the subject of guidance issued by the NHS Executive[9]. Section 8 of HSC 1999/053 covers non-paper records. It notes that the provisions of the Data Protection Act 1998 apply to photographs of identifiable individuals as well as to other personal records. In the case of *Hammond* v. *West Lancashire* (see Chapter 14) it was held than X-rays are part of a patient's medical records.

Marking of X-rays

In November 2000 the Commission for Health Improvement reported on its investigation into Prince Hospital in Llanelli where a patient had died following the removal of the wrong kidney[10]. It found that the current system of marking X-rays had the potential for confusion and inconsistency of approach. It made the following recommendation in relation to the marking of X-rays.

> 'The method of marking X-rays should be reviewed to establish whether a trust-wide system of hole punching X-rays "L" and "R" as a routine measure would enable consistency of approach and provide an additional safeguard in reporting'

Figure 18.3 Standard 6: Health Records.

A comprehensive system for the completion, use, storage and retrieval of health records is in place. Record keeping standards are monitored through the clinical audit process.

	Detailed criteria	*Level*	*Weight*
6.1.1	There is a unified health record which all specialities use.	1	H
6.1.2	Records are bound and stored so that loss of documents and traces are minimised for in-patients and out-patients.	1	M
6.1.3	The health record contains clear instructions regarding filing of documents.	1	M
6.1.4	Operation notes and other key procedures are readily identifiable	1	M
6.1.5	CTG and other machine produced recordings are securely stored and mounted.	1	M
6.1.6	There is a computer system, or other, for identifying and retrieving x-rays.	1	L
6.1.7	The storage arrangements allow retrieval on a 24 hour/7 day arrangement.	1	L
6.1.8	There is clear evidence of clinical audit of record keeping standards for all professional groups in at least 25% of specialities, including any high risk specialities, within the 12 months prior to the assessment.	1	H
6.1.9	There is a mechanism for identifying records which must not be destroyed.	1	L
6.2.1	A&E records are contained within the main record for patients who are subsequently admitted.	2	L
6.2.2	There is a system for ensuring that the GP is sent a copy of the A&E record.	2	L
6.2.3	Nursing, medical and other records (e.g. physiotherapy notes) are filed together when the patient is discharged.	2	M
6.2.4	There is a system for measuring efficiency in the recovery of records for in-patients and out-patients.	2	L
6.2.5	The health record contains a designated place for the recording of hyper-sensitivity reactions, and other information relevant to all healthcare professionals.	2	H
6.2.6	There is clear evidence of clinical audit of record keeping standards for all professional groups in 50% of the specialities, within the 12 months prior to the assessment.	2	H
6.3.1	An author of an entry in a health record is clearly and easily identifiable.	3	H
6.3.2	There is clear evidence of clinical audit of record keeping standards for all professional groups in all of the specialties, within the 12 months prior to the assessment.	3	H
6.3.3	There is a computer based Patient Administration System.	3	L

The storage of records and time for which they should be kept

Records should be kept so that they are easily accessible to those who require to access them but at the same time with efficient controls to prevent unauthorised access and disclosure. The Audit Commission in its report on hospital records[11] considered that patients were being put at risk because their medical records are not kept carefully and are sometimes lost. Failure to find records led to consultations being cancelled and to operations being postponed. It recommended that hospitals set up one main records library with good security.

Suggested storage times for different categories of records are given by the NHS Executive[9]. Clearly this guidance would be subject to checking through the material to ensure that records which are potentially the subject of litigation or complaints are kept for longer. The suggestion in the circular is that X-ray films (including formats for all imaging modalities) should be the subject of local decisions, with regard to the preservation of these records which are considered to be of transitory nature. X-ray registers should also be the subject of local decisions with regard to their permanent preservation, in consultation with relevant health professionals and places of deposit. X-ray reports (including reports for all imaging modalities) should be considered as part of the permanent patient record and subject to the same guidance as hospital patient case records. X-ray request cards are not mentioned in the guidance of the NHS Executive, but if this is the only record of the reason for doing an examination, the way the examination was done and the reasons why the examination might have been modified then there would be good reasons to keep this request card together with the X-ray report.

Where litigation is being contemplated, reference should be made to the time limits within which action can be brought which are discussed in Chapter 14. In such circumstances, where there is a likelihood of litigation, it would be extremely unwise to destroy any records.

In other circumstances, records could be destroyed according to the advice given by the Department of Health[9] unless the records are so old as to amount to historical documents when the Public Records Act 1958 comes into play and legal advice should be taken. The general time recommended for retention is eight years from completion of treatment. Children's records should be kept until the patient's twenty-fifth birthday, or twenty-sixth if the young person was 17 at the conclusion of treatment, or eight years after the patient's death if the death occurred before the eighteenth birthday. For oncology patients, the recommended time is eight years after conclusion of the treatment, especially where surgery only was involved. The Royal College of Radiologists has recommended the permanent retention on a computer database when patients have been given chemotherapy or radiotherapy[12]. For maternity records the recommended time for retention is 25 years. This would clearly be subject to an exception where it is apparent that a baby has suffered brain damage which could be the subject of a claim, since there is no time limit on an action for compensation being sought where the person is under a mental disability until the person dies, at which point a three year time limit comes into being (see Chapter 14 on limitation of time).

Implementing lifetime records

The record of a patient's lifetime exposure to X-radiation may soon be implemented as a consequence of the Ionising Regulations (Medical Exposure) Regulations[13]. National reference levels for exposure have been set and are continuously monitored. However work in establishing the standardisation of breast radiotherapy (START) project reported by Amanda Deighton showed that data on simulator and treatment verification radiation exposure varies considerably from department to department[14]. Screening time is recorded in half of the departments and the number of localisation films is recorded in three quarters. The simulator log book was the most common form of record keeping. Half of the departments do not take verification films for breast patients, and those that do, with the exception of one, take a single verification film/image, usually on the first day of treatment.

What if records are lost by the practitioner?

It may be that the records are misfiled, thrown out with rubbish in an untidy office, or they are lost between hospital departments. Clearly the failure to take reasonable care of records would be a disciplinable offence. Once the records are lost, there may be little which can be done to retrieve them. It may be possible to create a new patient file from parallel records held by other departments.

Process of destruction

Even though any critical time limits have been passed, most departments would prefer to transpose records onto microfilm rather than destroy them completely. However this is expensive and time consuming and might not always be justifiable. Whether the decision is taken to transfer the records or that they can be destroyed, it is important to prevent any breach of confidentiality during the process. There have been scandals where health records have been found still legible on a public dump.

The ownership and control of records

NHS records are owned by the Secretary of State and responsibility is delegated to the statutory health authorities. This also applies to the NHS records kept by general practitioners as part of their terms of service. Under the new arrangements since April 1996 the new health authorities are responsible for arranging the transfer of the records to a new general practitioner where the patient has indicated his wish to transfer and for collecting the records from a general practitioner where a patient has died.

For NHS trusts the ultimate decision on disclosure to others rests with the chief executive officer of the health authority or NHS trust. Thus statutes such as the Data Protection Act 1998 give to the holder of the records the ultimate decision on whether access should be permitted. The holder should however consult the health professional who cared for the patient (see Chapter 6).

Situation: Destruction on request

> A practitioner is treating a patient who is suffering from mental illness. In one session the patient became very aggressive and this was noted by the practitioner in the records. The next session she was very apologetic and asked if the practitioner would delete the record of her outburst since it was so uncharacteristic and she was extremely contrite. What is the legal situation?

The practitioner should be very clear that the records cannot be changed. There is a statutory process by which a patient can request access under the Data Protection Act 1998 and ask for records to be amended if they are incorrect (see Chapter 6), but this does not apply here. In July 1998 a GP who allowed a patient to destroy part of her records was found guilty of serious professional misconduct by the GMC[15]. He had allowed the patient, who was involved in an acrimonious property dispute with her children, to remove a letter in which she was described as 'bad tempered' and another document which referred to her drinking.

In the private sector the patient records and X-rays would normally be owned by the private practitioner unless she is working under a contract with a private hospital or centre where the contract stated that the records were in the ownership of the private hospital. It would be open to private practitioner and private patient to include in their contract provision for access, ownership, and who holds the records. It would not, however, be advisable or necessarily in the patient's best interests for it to be agreed that the patient has actual ownership of the records.

Unified system of record keeping

The development of a unified system of record keeping is on the agenda of many NHS trusts and community units. The aim is that all members of the multi-disciplinary team keep their patient records in the same patient folder to ensure that maximum cooperation and multi-disciplinary planning in the care of the patient takes place.

This development is to be applauded, but some practitioners may fear the loss of control over the records. They may therefore be tempted to provide an additional set of records in case the main set goes missing. The danger of this cautionary practice is that neither set may be complete or it may be assumed that there is only one set and that the fact that there are records retained in another set is not known. If as a consequence of a dual system of record keeping, significant information was not in the set of records used by a practitioner and, as a result of this ignorance, harm was caused to the patient, then there could be a successful claim for compensation. Clearly the employer would be vicariously liable for any negligence on the part of the practitioners caring for the patient and also directly liable for the failure to establish a safe practice of record keeping.

Client held records

Many different professionals are increasingly allowing clients to hold their own records. There are some fears associated with the patient acting as custodian of the records, the main one being that records could be lost if the health professional ceases to be in control of the care of the records. This leads to the setting up of a second system of record keeping at a central point. The dangers of this dual system are that neither might be complete and there might not be consistency on what was recorded in each place. There is also a fear that if records in the custody of the client go missing and litigation is commenced, then the professional will be at a disadvantage in defending herself. The burden is however on the claimant to establish negligence on a balance of probabilities, and this may be difficult to do if the documentation is missing and the claimant is responsible for that loss. The introduction of the patient electronic health record for every person by 2005 should ensure that every person has a patient held record (see below).

Litigation and evidential value of records

It will be apparent from Chapter 14 on accountability and the discussion on times within which an action can be brought, that in many cases witnesses would be unable to remember any details and will be completely dependent in giving evidence on the records that were kept. Staff who have been involved in litigation, disciplinary proceedings and other hearings should share the lessons which they have learnt with their colleagues, and illustrate the significant role which documentation played in their giving evidence.

Records include evidence from radiographs and there are many early cases where X-rays were used in evidence. Many of these cases in which radiographic evidence is referred to are Workman's Compensation cases. For example in a New South Wales case[16], as early as 1936 radiographic evidence was discussed in a dispute over whether the disease was attributable to work in the mine. The radiograph showed pneumoconiosis, there being a mottling on the lungs which meant fibrosis and fine particles of dust, and that the condition observed might be brought about by silica dust or other dusts. Early reference to X-rays in evidence is also seen from a case reported in 1939[17], where a workman at a colliery was injured when loading a load of dirt when he was crushed between two tubs and his pelvis was fractured.

Incomplete or missing records

Case: *Skelton* v. *Lewisham and North Southwark HA*[18]

> The claimant who suffered from Williams' Syndrome was operated upon for repair of supra valve aortic stenosis. He sustained severe brain damage in the perioperative period. The claimant sued the health authority alleging that the anaesthetists were negligent. The judge found that the anaesthetic notes were below the standard acceptable in 1983 and the significance of the poor note taking was not that it was indicative of negligence in the legal sense, but that it was indicative of an unexplained carelessness. The judge found that the anaesthetists has negligently failed to observe and respond to a hypotensive episode early enough.

If records have been deliberately destroyed and are not therefore available as evidence in court, there is a presumption *omnia praesumuntur contra spoliatorem*[19] i.e. there is a presumption against those who caused the loss. Where the records are lost accidentally, then the judge can determine in the light of other evidence available any inferences which are appropriate.

Legal status of records and evidential value

When does a record become a legal record? This is a question often asked and the answer is that any record, any information, however recorded, can be ordered to be produced in a court of law if it is relevant to an issue which arises in the proceedings and if it is not privileged from disclosure. (Reference should be made to Chapter 5 on confidentiality and the powers and limitations of the court in requiring the production of witnesses and documents.)

It does *not* follow that what is contained in any record is necessarily accurate or true. It is possible for a completely fictitious account to be recorded. In determining the weight to be attached to the records and to determine the evidential value, the judge would listen to the makers of the records being cross-examined and in the light of those answers determine how much value can be placed upon the records.

Adverse incident reporting and statements

If there is an adverse incident (see Chapters 15 and 17), statements should be written up by all concerned as soon as possible after the event. These may be needed for any internal enquiry, disciplinary hearing or, in extreme cases, a criminal prosecution. They would also be needed if civil proceedings arise out of the event. The same principles apply as for statements prepared by witnesses of fact in civil proceedings (see below).

Electronic health records

Some Trusts have made considerable progress with the computerisation of patient data and record keeping, but in other areas records are still kept in completely manual form. The then Secretary of State for Health, Frank Dobson, announced on 24 September 1998 that there would be £1 billion investment to put all medical files on computer[20]. The initiative will take place over seven years enabling records to be available for access on a 24 hour basis across the country and also permitting patient access in his own home. The initiative will link in an NHS website and an expansion of NHS Direct which offers the public a 24-hour telephone advice service on non-urgent health matters. £40 million is to be spent connecting GPs to the NHS Net.

In 4 February 2001 the Department of Health issued a press release that, by March 2005, every person in the country will have her own electronic health record (EHR)[21]. The electronic health record is defined by the Department of Health as holding summarised key data about patients, such as name, address, NHS number, registered GP and contact details, previous treatments, ongoing conditions, current medication, allergies and the date of any next appointments. It is intended that it will be securely protected, created with patient consent, with individual changes made only by authorised staff. The timetable for the electronic health record envisages that 5 million people will have their own lifelong EHR by 2003, rising to around 25 million by 2004 and then everyone by March 2005.

Whilst the computer will avoid problems of illegibility, considerable care will still have to be taken. In August 1998 it was reported[22] that a student, suffering from meningitis, may have died as a result of her name being wrongly spelt on a computer. The omission of the letter 'P' in her surname (Simpkin) meant that her records could not be accessed and an inquiry found that she might have lived if vital results of blood tests, entered into the computerised records under the wrong name, had been seen by staff.

Picture Archiving and Communication Systems (PACS) are considered in Chapter 24.

Conclusions on record keeping

The importance of high standards of record keeping cannot be over-emphasised as part of the professional duty of care to the patient. If this duty is met then the records should also provide essential evidence in the event of litigation or other court hearing or inquiry. Regular audit is essential to ensure that high standards are maintained. The work of the CNST in standard setting will continue to place record keeping standards at a central place in risk management and the prevention of litigation.

The General Medical Council's guidelines[23] state:

'In providing care you must keep clear, accurate and contemporaneous patient records which report relevant clinical findings, the decisions made, the information given to patients and any drugs or other treatment prescribed. You must keep colleagues well informed when sharing the care of patients.'

Report writing

Report writing to the radiologist will have a very different meaning from report writing to an expert witness. Both areas will be covered in this section.

Reporting on X-rays

This is also discussed in Chapter 27 on the scope of professional practice. In terms of the actual preparation of the report, the writer would be required to follow the accepted standards of report writing. For example in its guidance on the use of computed tomography in the initial investigation of common malignancies[24], the Council of the RCR sets out certain conditions which should be fulfilled by diagnostic radiologists. They state:

'Although there is a great variation in style of reporting, it is good practice to provide a succinct conclusion, paying attention to answering the specific clinical question posed. Recommendations regarding follow-up, biopsy and alternative radiological studies should also be made in the conclusion.'

The RCR *Good Practice Guide for Clinical Radiologists*[25] states:

'The written radiology report constitutes the legal record of the imaging investigation. It is therefore vital that the information contained within this record is accurate, explicit, understandable and informative. It should be unambiguous with a level of confidence either clearly implied or explicitly stated. Where uncertainty exists, this should be made clear within the text of the report. The report should include clear patient identification, the name of the clinical radiologist and of the secretary where appropriate and advice or information given to the patient at the end of the procedure. It should include documentary evidence of drugs/contrast used during the procedure and advice of post-procedural care.'

The RCR has published further advice specifically on reporting[26] and in the joint publication of the RCR and the ScoR[27], it states that reporting has two elements:

- a description of the finding – the descriptive report
- a medical interpretation and/or opinion – the medical report.

Practitioners are referred to these works for more detail.

Reports by expert witnesses

Expert witnesses will normally be asked to prepare a report by a solicitor representing one of the parties to the case. This report is vital since, if it is unfavourable to the party seeking it, the outcome may be that the case is settled or even withdrawn. On the other hand, if a party proceeds on the basis of a report that paints too rosy a picture of the case and the expert witness fails to justify it under cross-examination, that party could lose the case or be awarded less compensation than had previously been offered in settlement and so be heavily penalised in having to pay the other side's legal costs as well as their own.

Principles to be followed in report writing

These are helpfully set out in the Code of Guidance[28] published by the Expert Witness Institute, paragraphs 15 and 16 of which state:

'Information

15) All experts' reports should contain the following information:
- a) the expert's academic and professional qualifications;
- b) a statement of the source of instructions and the purpose of the advice or report;
- c) a chronology of the relevant events;
- d) a statement of the methodology used, in particular what laboratory or other tests (if any) were employed, by whom and under whose supervision;
- e) details of the documents or any other evidence upon which any aspects of the advice or report is based;
- f) relevant extracts of literature or any other material which might assist the court in deciding the case; and
- g) a summary of conclusions reached.

Content of report

16) In providing a report experts:
- a) must address it to the court and not to any of the parties;
- b) must include a statement setting out the substance of all instructions (whether written or oral). The statement should summarise the facts

and instructions given to the expert which are material to the opinions expressed in the report or upon which those opinions are based;

c) where there is a range of opinion in the matters dealt with in the report, give
   (i)   a summary of the range of opinion; and
   (ii)   the reasons for his own opinion.

d) must express any qualification of, or reservation to, their opinion;

e) if such opinion was not formed independently, should make clear the source of the opinion;

f) must declare that the report has been prepared in accordance with this Code and the requirements of the Civil Procedure Rules; and

g) must include a statement of truth, as required by Part 35, Practice Direction 1.3.'

As can be seen this takes into account the requirements of the Civil Procedure Rules.

Common mistakes in report writing

- Lack of clarity
- Too complex a style for reader
- Use of inappropriate jargon
- Use of misleading abbreviations
  - Inconsistency
  - Ambiguities
- Inaccuracies
  - Lack of dates within the report
  - Wrong names included
- Failure to follow a logical order
  - Confusing account
  - Mix of evidence and sources
  - Opinion without facts
- Failure to cite facts to support statements
- Failure to give conclusions
- Failure to base conclusions on the evidence
- Lack of signature and/or date
- Failure to ask someone else to read it through.

Good report writing

For most purposes the style likely to be of greatest use is one of simplicity – with short sentences, clear paragraphing and sub-paragraphing, and avoidance of jargon and meaningless clichés. The report should begin with the statement as to its purpose, the person(s) to whom it is addressed, and the name and status of the writer. If it is confidential this should be highlighted at the beginning. Other documents which are relevant should be carefully referenced. If it is for court purposes it should scrupulously follow the format and contain the information required by the CPR and Practice Direction.

Giving evidence

Statement making

Witnesses can refer to any contemporaneous records and contemporaneous statements in giving evidence and therefore since it takes many years for some court hearings to take place, it is vital that comprehensive clear records have been kept and statements made. Before preparing a statement a health professional should have advice from a senior colleague and if possible a lawyer. The elements shown in Figure 18.4. should be contained in a statement.

Figure 18.4   **Elements to include in a statement.**

- Full name, position, grade and location of maker
- Date and time the statement was made
- Date and time of the incident
- Full names of any persons involved e.g. patient, visitor, other staff
- A full and detailed description of the events which occurred
- Signature
- (Any supporting statements or documents should be attached)

The statement writer should ensure that the statement is:

- accurate
- factual
- concise
- relevant
- clear
- legible (usually typed)

Hearsay, i.e. repeating what another person has said, should be avoided. Other people could be asked to provide their own statements if they have relevant information relating to the subject.

The statement maker should read it through checking on its overall impact and whether all the relevant facts are included. A copy should be kept. Advice should be sought on its clarity and comprehensiveness and it should not be signed unless the maker is completely satisfied that it records an accurate, clear account of what took place. Many years later the statement could be used in evidence in court and it is an easy point for cross-examination (see below) if the witness contradicts in court what she put in her statement.

Witness of fact

Any one who can give evidence on a matter relevant to an issue before the court can be summoned to appear. The only grounds for refusing to attend and give evidence is if the evidence is protected against disclosure in court by legal professional privilege or if, on grounds of national security or other public interest, a minister of state has signed a public interest immunity certificate that the information should not be disclosed. (Legal professional privilege is considered in Chapter 5 on confidentiality.)

Importance of records and other documentary evidence

Inevitably after a lapse of time the value of a practitioner as a witness will depend significantly upon the clarity and comprehensiveness of any records which she kept and/or contemporaneous statement she made. Documentary evidence may include reports from pathology, X-Rays, and any other relevant information, in whatever form it is held. All this information would have to be made available to the other side during the process known as disclosure. This equality of access to all available records is very important.

Case: *Cunningham* v. *North Manchester HA*[29]

Frank Cunningham alleged lack of care by medical staff as a result of which he lost his leg following a motorcycle accident. A retrial was ordered when it was discovered that the claimant's expert had only had access to miniaturised copies of the original X-Rays and arteriograms, whereas the defendants' experts had seen the originals.

Mr Cunningham subsequently accepted an offer of £325 000. He was a litigant in person, that is he was not represented by a lawyer.

Giving evidence of facts

As a witness of fact the practitioner may be required to give direct evidence over a matter with which she has been involved. In giving evidence she should ensure that she keeps to the facts and does not offer an opinion. In some cases she may be asked to pronounce upon the prognosis of the client: she should not magnify the extent of the disability and the poor prognosis in order to obtain more compensation for the client. The practitioner has to ensure that her professional standards are maintained and she tells the client honestly the nature of the prognosis as she sees it. She may need guidance and training in how to respond to cross-examination. It is vital that she does not give facts which are outside her knowledge. Thus which ever party calls her as witness, she should not alter the facts or emphasis to support that party but should give evidence according to professional standards of integrity.

Key points for witness of fact

Preparation

- Ensure that the records are available. Identify with stickers significant entries, but do not mark or staple or pin anything to the records. Read them through so that you are familiar with them;
- Try to obtain assistance from a lawyer or senior manager in preparation for the court hearing, so that you are prepared for giving evidence in chief and answering questions under cross-examination.
- Try to visit the court in advance to familiarise yourself with its location, car-parking, toilet facilities etc.

At the court before the hearing

- Be prepared for a long wait and take work to do or something to occupy yourself with.
- Dress appropriately and comfortably but not too casually.
- Try to relax.

While giving evidence

- Keep calm.
- Give answers clearly and without exaggeration.
- Tell the truth.
- Do not feel that you are there to represent only one side; you must answer the questions honestly even though it might put the side cross-examining you in a good light.
- Take time over your answers and do not make up replies if you are unable to answer the question raised.
- Do not answer back or allow yourself to be flustered during the cross-examination.
- If you do not understand any legal jargon which is used, ask for an explanation.
- Keep to the facts and do not express an opinion.
- Ask for time to refer to the records if this is necessary.

Cross-examination

This is the term applied to the opportunity of the one side (A) to question the witnesses called by the other side (B) (and vice versa). There are two distinct objectives in cross-examination. The one is to discredit witnesses or show that their evidence is irrelevant to the point being established. The other is to use the witness to strengthen the case of the cross-examining party.

Preparation is essential to be able to handle cross-examination and most health professionals would now be able to obtain expert advice from the solicitors for their NHS trust before attending court on behalf of the employer.

Expert witness

An expert witness is invited to give evidence of opinion on any issue which is subject to dispute. It might be what would be the appropriate standards of care which would have been expected according to the Bolam test (see Chapter 14), it may be an opinion on the interpretation of an X-ray, a failure to diagnose cancer or the correct positioning of a patient for an X-ray to be taken.

It used to be the case that where an expert had prepared a report for a solicitor in anticipation or in the course of litigation, that report and any correspondence connected with it were protected by legal professional privilege and it could not be ordered to be disclosed in court nor the expert compelled to appear. Once the report was disclosed, it lost its professional privilege (although this continued to attach to any correspondence between the parties which had not been disclosed). For example an expert might have prepared a report on request but in the covering letter advised the solicitor that his client was likely to lose the case. Both the report and the letter were privileged from disclosure. However as a result of the changes in civil procedure following the Woolf reforms (see Chapter 2) where an expert's report is used in evidence, all amendments and changes to that report and the relevant correspondence must also be disclosed.

An expert witness should not change views according to the side which calls her. The expert may be asked to edit the report to make it more favourable to the side asking for the opinion. Any amendments should only be agreed if the expert is satisfied that the changed report accurately represents her professional opinion and can be supported by oral evidence in court.

One useful rule for the practitioner to follow is to give an honest reasoned opinion whichever side call her. She must not be partisan, nor should she exaggerate or belittle the amount of compensation. If she always gives an honest and professional view, she will be respected by the solicitors who will know that they will be able to trust her to withstand cross-examination as an expert witness and will know her to be reliable. She will not see the court battle personally as involving her and thus whichever side wins, she will be able to feel that she has given an honest report to the court. A carefully prepared, well substantiated report, can reduce the length of a court hearing and enable many matters to be agreed by the parties, thus saving court time.

Duty of expert witness to the court

In a reported case[30] the court held that the expert witness had a responsibility to approach the task of giving evidence seriously and an expert should not be surprised if the court expressed strong disapproval if that was not done. The expert in his report had stated that 'as far as I am aware no other previous seal manufacturer had used such a system'. In fact it became apparent not only that that system was used by others in the trade, but that the witness neither knew what systems were used by such others nor had made any effort to find out. The lesson from this is that an expert must not express an opinion unless it is clearly based on fact and where possible on established authorities or research. A further lesson is that the expert should know and keep within her field of competence.

The House of Lords in the *Bolitho* case[31] has emphasised that expert witnesses must be able to show that the body of opinion which they are supporting had a logical basis (see Chapter 14).

Where there is a variety of practice and opinion, which will be particularly the case in medical negligence issues, the expert must have a broad-minded approach. Rigid adherence to practices unsupported by research-based evidence will help neither the client not the court. In *Sharpe* v. *Southend Health Authority and Bloomsbury and Islington Health Authority*[32] the judge stated that:

'In relation to medical negligence cases ... an expert witness should make it clear in his/her report that, although the expert would have adopted a different approach/practice, he/she accepts that the approach/practice adopted by the defendant was in accordance with the approach/practice accepted as proper by a responsible body of practitioners skilled in the relevant field. Had this guideline been followed in the present case, it is likely that the allegations against the defendant's clinician would not have been advanced in the first place (as opposed to being withdrawn in the claimant's counsel's final speech)'

The reforms to civil procedure, which are considered below, stipulate that the first duty of the expert is to the court.

The court to evaluate expert evidence

In a case concerning a missed fracture[33] the claimant brought an appeal on the following grounds:

- The judge failed to evaluate the evidence of the parties' experts and to make clear findings as to what part of the evidence of each he accepted and what part he rejected.
- The complaints of 'gross' pain by the claimant to the doctor were inevitably indicative of the need for X-ray.
- The judge erred, having rejected the defendant's expert's view that there had been no fracture, not rejecting the expert's support for the management and decision-taking by the doctor.

The Court of Appeal decided that it was not incumbent on a judge to explain at great length why he has found the expert contribution perhaps partisan and unhelpful and all the issues were issues of fact which were for the judge to decide and he did so. No flaw was demonstrated in his reasoning or in the consistency of the findings which he made.

Opinions on the standard of care, causation and quantum

Expert evidence may be required on how the standards of care which were provided matched up with the reasonable standard which could have been expected and whether there was a causal link between any failure to follow the reasonable standard of care and the harm which was suffered. Expert evidence, although probably not from radiographers or radiologists, might also be required on quantum, i.e. the amount of compensation which the claimant is seeking. The expert must have clear factual evidence as to how she arrives at her estimate of needs of the patient and the cost of meeting these.

Paul Butt in the article referred to above[8] discusses some of the moral dilemmas which are faced by the expert.

- Even if there is no apparent negligence by the radiologist for whom he is providing a report, does the expert advise the claimant's solicitor that there is evidence that the general care was grossly deficient?
- If there is evidence of practice by a radiologist which is so dangerous as to amount to a criminal act does the expert tell the instructing solicitor to inform the police?
- Is there a duty on an expert who becomes aware of extremely dangerous unprofessional practice by a specific clinician to inform the GMC?

Some of these dilemmas may perhaps be resolved in practice by the new Civil Procedure Rules introduced in 1999 where it has been made clear that the first duty of the expert is to the court. Reporting to the police and GMC may be justified in the public interest and be seen as a professional duty on the part of the expert (see Chapter 5). (See also the Public Interest Disclosure Act 1998 and whistle blowing considered in Chapter 22.)

New Civil Procedure Rules for experts

Lord Woolf published, following an interim report and a consultation paper, a final report, *Access to Justice* in July 1996[34]. This was implemented in April 1999. This is discussed more fully in Chapter 2. One of the consultation papers relates to the use of expert evidence. Lord Woolf considered that the uncontrolled adversarial nature of the previous system of civil litigation was the main cause of excessive cost, delay and complexity. He therefore recommended a new system in which the courts would have an active role in case management, including control over the use of expert evidence. He recommended a fast track for cases below £10 000 where experts would normally be jointly appointed by the parties and would not be required to give oral evidence in court. Cases above £10 000 would be allocated to a multi-track, in which the court would have wide powers to define the scope of expert evidence and prescribe the way in which experts should be used in particular cases. His proposals on expert evidence included the following:

- Appointment of court experts and expert assessors
- A clearer role for experts and guidance which emphasises their independence and their duty to the courts
- Appropriate choice and use of experts
- Better arrangements for expert evidence at trial.

Since the implementation of the new Civil Procedure Rules there has been a case on the question of a joint expert being imposed upon the parties by the court[35]. The solicitors to both parties were specialists in the field of medical negligence and before the case management conference they had agreed directions. In spite of that agreement the district judge directed that they should jointly instruct a causation expert. The appeal against this decision was successful on the grounds that the judge should have taken into account the fact that it was a complex case and the solicitors had agreed directions.

However in another case the Court of Appeal upheld the principle that the expert's duty was to the court rather than to the party who had instructed him[36]. The Court of Appeal upheld the judge's decision to debar an expert from giving evidence where it was clear that he had no concept of the requirements placed upon him in this respect by the Civil Procedure Rules.

Conclusion

There are considerable fears about giving evidence in court and it is vital that any witness, whether expert or witness of fact, should be properly prepared for the occasion. Even though they are not on trial themselves, their professional standing and integrity is being put to the test and it is therefore essential that they follow the highest standard of professional practice.

Questions and exercises _____

1   With some colleagues carry out an audit of the standards of record keeping amongst yourselves. Imagine that you were having to answer questions on the records in ten years time. How robust would the records be in protecting your practice?

2   What abbreviations do you consider could be usefully used in record keeping by radiographers? What steps would you take to ensure that there was no confusion arising from their use?

3   Consider ways in which the keeping of radiography records could be made more efficient.

4   You have been asked to appear as a witness in a case. Draw up a list of your fears and try to work out ways in which these fears could be resolved.

5   Try to attend a court hearing and analyse the way in which it operates, the procedure followed and the actions of judge, jury (if present), barristers, solicitors, court clerk, court usher, witnesses and any other person taking part in the court proceedings.

6   Prepare a protocol for the preparation of a report as an expert witness.

References

1   NHS Training Directorate (1994) *Just for the Record: A guide to record keeping for health care professionals.* NHS Training Directorate; NHS Executive (1999) HSC 1999/053 *For the Record* DoH, London

2   News item *The Times* 16 December 1997

3   I. Murray (1998) Walk-in-surgeries fail to keep records *The Times* 7 April 1998

4   D. Kennedy (1996) Hospital blamed in report on overdose death *The Times* 3 July 1996

5   NHS Training Directorate (1994) *Just for the Record*; NHS Training Directorate (1992) *Keeping the record straight*

6   United Kingdom Central Council (1993) *Standards for Records and Record Keeping* (April 1993) UKCC

7   P. Wilkinson (1995) Notes on dead baby altered by nurse *The Times* 7 November 1995

8   P. Butt (1998) Radiological Negligence *Newsletter of the RCR* (Summer 1998) Issue No 52 page 14

9   NHS Executive (1999) HSC 1999/053 *For the Record* DoH 1999

10   www.doh.gov.uk/chi/carmar.htm

11   Audit Commision (1995) *Setting the Records Straight: A Study of Hospital Medical Records* (June 1995) HMSO, London

12   Royal College of Radiologists (1996) BFCO(96)3

13   The Ionising Radiation (Medical Exposure) Regulations 2000 SI No. 1059 of 2000

14   A. Deighton (2000) Screening, Record Keeping and Checking films *Synergy* (December 2000) pages 14–5

15   P. Forster (1998) GP allowed patient to tamper with records *The Times* 7 July 1998

16   *Metropolitan Coal Co Ltd* v. *Pye* [1936] 1 All ER 919

17   *Llay Main Collieries* v. *Jones* [1939] 1 All ER 8

18   *Skelton* v. *Lewisham and North Southwark HA* (1998) Lloyds Law Reports Medical, 324

19   *Malhotra* v. *Dhawan* [1997] 8 Med LR 319

20   M. Henderson (1998) £1bn scheme will put all medical files on computer *The Times* 25 September 1998
21   Department of Health *Patients to gain access to new at-a-glance Electronic Health Records* 4 February 2001
22   H. Johnstone (1998) Spelling mistake may have cost student her life *The Times* 28 August 1998
23   General Medical Council (1998) *Good Medical Practice* GMC, London
24   Council The Royal College of Radiology (1995) *The use of Computed Tomography in the initial investigation of common malignancies* (RCR(95)1) RCR, London
25   Board of Faculty of Clinical Radiology (1999) *Good Practice Guide for Clinical Radiologists* (BFCR(99)11) RCR, London
26   Royal College of Radiologists (1995) *Statement on Reporting in Departments of Clinical Radiology* (BFCR(95)1) RCR, London
27   RCR and the ScoR (1998) *Inter-professional roles and responsibilities in a Radiology Service* RCR, London
28   Expert Witness Institute (2001) *Code of Guidance on Expert Evidence: A Guide for Experts and those Instructing them* EWI, London (www.ewi.org.uk)
29   *Cunningham v. North Manchester Health Authority* [1997] 8 Med LR 135
30   *Autospin (Oil Seals) Ltd v. Beehive Spinning (A firm)* Times Law Report, 9 August 1995
31   *Bolitho v. City and Hackney Health Authority* [1997] 3 WLR 1151
32   *Sharpe v. Southend Health Authority and Bloomsbury and Islington Health Authority* [1997] 8 Med LR 299
33   *Lakey v. Merton, Sutton and Wandsworth HA* [1999] Lloyd's Rep. Med. 119
34   Lord Woolf (1995) (1996) *Access to Civil Justice Inquiry: Interim Report* (June 1995) and *Consultation Paper* (January 1996) Lord Chancellor's Office (1996) *Final Report: Access to Justice* (July 1996) HMSO, London
35   *S(a minor) v. Birmingham Health Authority* (9 July 1999) QBD
36   *Stevens v. Gullis* (1999) *The Times*, 6 October 1999; [2000] All ER 527

Chapter 19
Handling Complaints

Introduction

The Hospital Complaints Act 1985 started the process of complaints procedures being a statutory requirement. The recommendations of the Wilson Committee for dealing with hospital and primary care complaints have been implemented by the establishment in 1996 of a complaints procedure which is discussed below. In addition in the National Plan[1] the Government stated that it was to establish:

- a full mandatory reporting scheme for adverse health-care events (see Chapter 21)
- improved professional regulatory mechanism for doctors and other health professionals (see Chapter 12) and
- a new patient advocacy service.

Complaints relating to hospital and community health services

There is a statutory duty under the Hospital Complaints Act 1985 for each health authority to establish a complaints procedure. Guidance required authorities also to establish a procedure in relation to community health services. In addition, as part of the Patient's Charter initiative, local charters covering the handling of complaints are also required of other providers of health-care. Such requirements are included in the NHS agreements between health authorities and those who provide services.

The Wilson Report

In the early 1990s the system for dealing with complaints relating to health services was seen to be confusing, bureaucratic, slow and inefficient. The report of the review committee chaired by Professor Alan Wilson[2] reviewed the current situation and set objectives for any effective complaints system. The principles it identified are set out in Figure 19.1.

Figure 19.1 **Principles of an effective complaints system.**

(1) Responsiveness
(2) Quality enhancement
(3) Cost effectiveness
(4) Accessibility
(5) Impartiality

(6) Simplicity
(7) Speed
(8) Confidentiality
(9) Accountability

The report recommended that these principles should be incorporated into an NHS complaints system.

The areas covered by its recommendations are shown in Figure 19.2

Figure 19.2 **Recommendations of the Wilson report on the review of complaints procedures.**

(1) There should be a common system for all NHS complaints
(2) The complaints procedure should not be concerned with disciplining staff
(3) Staff should be empowered to deal with complaints informally
(4) There should be training of staff
(5) Support should be provided for complainants and respondents
(6) The degree of investigation should relate to the complainant's required degree of response
(7) Conciliation should be made more widely available
(8) Time limits should be set
(9) Deadlines should be set for
    (a) the acknowledging of complaints (two working days)
    (b) the response to the complaint (three weeks)
    (c) further action and response (two weeks)
(10) Confidentiality should be preserved and complaints filed separately
(11) There should be a system for recording and monitoring
(12) Impartial lay people should take part in the system
(13) Key aspects of the system should be set by the Department of Health but detailed implementation and operation should be left to individual organisations
(14) Threefold procedures:
    stage 1 – immediate first line response
    stage 2 – investigation/conciliation
    stage 3 – action by HA officer or chief executive officer for trusts (a panel being set up to consider those complaints which cannot be resolved in the earlier stages)
(15) There should be training in communication skills
(16) Oral and written complaints should be treated with the same sensitive treatment
(17) Community service staff should have particular training in responding to complaints
(18) Purchasers should specify complaints requirements in their contracts with non-NHS providers.

Continued

Figure 19.2 **Continued.**

(19) Complaints about policy decisions should be referred to the Health Service Commissioner if they cannot be resolved locally by the purchasers
(20) Where more than one organisation is involved it should be the organisation which receives the complaint which makes sure that a full response is sent
(21) Community care (there should be close liaison with local authorities and the Government should consider further integration of NHS and local authority complaints procedures)
(22) Stage 2 procedures (there should be a screening officer)
(23) The jurisdiction of the HSC should be extended to GPs and the operation of the FHSA service committees
(24) Recommendations on implementation.

The 1996 complaints procedure

This came into effect on 1 April 1996 and implements the majority of recommendations contained in the Wilson Report. Three stages are recognised.

First stage – local resolution

The complaint should be dealt with speedily and often an oral response will suffice. Where investigation or conciliation is required an initial response should be made within two working days and a final response within four weeks. Chief executives should personally approve and sign the response to all formal complaints. In family health services, practices will be expected and encouraged to set up their own practice based complaints procedure, using independent persons to assist in resolving the dispute at local level.

Second stage – independent review

Consideration of an application for independent review
If complainants remain dissatisfied after the first stage, they can apply for further consideration by an independent panel. This request will be considered by a non-executive director of the Trust or health authority to whom the complaint was made. This non-executive director is known as the convenor and will have the decision as to whether the complaint should be referred to an independent review panel. The circumstances in which it is not recommended that there should be an independent review are shown in Figure 19.3.

   Where the convenor refuses to refer the complaint for independent review, the complainant must be informed of his right to complain to the Ombudsman.

Independent review panels
All panels have an independent lay chairman.

● For non-clinical complaints, the panel comprises a non-executive director of the relevant health authority, or, where appropriate, a GP fundholder.
● For family health service complaints, the panel is comprises the convening health authority non-executive director and an independent lay person.

Figure 19.3 **Situations where there will be no independent review.**

- Where legal proceedings have commenced or there is an explicit indication by the complainant of the intention to make a legal claim against:
  ○ a Trust or health service authority or
  ○ one of their employees or
  ○ against a family health services practitioner.
- It is considered the Trust/health authority has already taken all practicable action and therefore establishing a panel would add no further value to the process. However, consideration of the cost of instituting an independent review is not an appropriate reason for refusing to proceed.
- Further action as part of local resolution is still believed to be appropriate and practicable – for example conciliation – so that referral back to the chief executive is considered preferable to instituting the independent review process.

- For clinical complaints, the panel is advised by two independent clinical assessors following advice from the relevant professional bodies.

The panel is established as a committee of the Trust/health authority and the assessors are appointed by the Trust/health authority to advise the panel.

Third stage – Health Service Commissioner (HSC) (Ombudsman)
The final option for unresolved complaints will be recourse to the Ombudsman. The legislation which came into force on 1 April 1996 widened his jurisdiction to cover complaints relating to the exercise of clinical judgment and those about family practitioners. Disciplinary matters, however, are still not included in his jurisdiction. (The role of the HSC is considered in more detail below.)

Time limits

A time limit for making a complaint is six months from the event giving rise to the complaint; or six months from the complainant becoming aware of the cause for complaint up to a maximum of one year after the cause for complaint arose. There is a discretion to extend this time limit where it would be unreasonable in the circumstances of a particular case for the complaint to have been made earlier and where it is still possible to investigate the facts of the case.

Complaints and the Community Health Councils (CHCs)

Community Health Councils have had a significant role to play in both the representation of their community at large and also in facilitating any complaint by an individual. The NHS Plan envisaged that CHCs would cease to function, and Clause 20 of the NHS Reform and Health Care Professions Bill 2002 abolishes CHCs in England. They are to be replaced by Patient Forums which will have powers of inspection.

The role of the Ombudsmen

If a complainant is not satisfied with the response of the authority to a complaint, he can apply to the Health Service Commissioner (Ombudsman) for further investigation of complaints about the NHS. The powers and jurisdiction of the Health Service Commissioner is set out in the Health Service Commissioners Act 1993. In April 1996 the jurisdiction of the Health Service Commissioner was extended to include the investigation of matters concerned with the exercise of clinical judgment and the investigations of complaints about family practitioner services[3]. The HSC has a duty to prepare a report which is submitted to Parliament under section 14(4) of the Health Service Commissioners Act 1993. The Select Committee of the House of Commons has the power to investigate further any complaint reported by the HSC, if necessary summoning witnesses to London for questioning. The HSC is completely independent of the NHS and the government and has the jurisdiction to investigate complaints against any part of the NHS about:

- a failure in service;
- a failure to purchase or provide any service an individual is entitled to receive; or
- maladministration (administrative affairs).

Other quality assurance methods

NICE and CHI

Individuals who have complaints about the services provided in the NHS do not have any contractual right to bring an action before the court for breach of contract. If harm has been suffered as a result of a failure or omission, they may have a successful claim in the law of negligence (see Chapter 14) or if a service has not been provided they may be able to bring a case of breach of statutory duty for failure to provide that service (see Chapter 3). Otherwise they must rely upon the complaints procedure.

There are however many other mechanisms to ensure the maintenance of high standards of health care although these cannot be directly accessed by the patient. The White Paper in 1997[4] put forward a strategy for improving quality assurance and its mechanisms. These mechanisms included a National Institute of Clinical Excellence (NICE), a Commission for Health Improvement (CHI) and a framework for national standards. The establishment of Clinical Governance whereby chief executives of trusts are held accountable for the clinical performance of their organisations provides more evidence to the patient about the standards of care locally. (These matters are considered in Chapter 21.)

Audit and monitoring

Under complaints procedures both the NHS trusts and the health authorities have a duty to monitor the handling of complaints. This would include audit of the times taken for the procedures to be completed and any feedback from

Independent Review Panel (IRP) reports and from the Ombudsman. It is of considerable value if this audit and monitoring process can take place not only at Board level but also at departmental level, so that all employees can learn from the lessons arising from any complaint.

Practitioners should expect to take part in quality assurance and audit initiatives as part of their routine work in ensuring standards are set and maintained.

Patient advocacy service

In the NHS Plan[1] it is stated that:

> By 2002, an NHS-wide Patient Advocacy and Liaison Service (PALS) will be established in every trust, beginning with every major hospital, with an annual national budget of around £10 million.

It is explained that patients need an identifiable person they can turn to if they have a problem or need information while they are using hospital and other NHS services. The intention is that patient advocates will act as an independent facilitator to handle patient and family concerns, with direct access to the chief executive and the power to negotiate immediate solutions. It also envisages that the PALS will be able to steer patients and families towards the complaints process where necessary and will take on the roles which CHCs currently fulfil of supporting complainants. Additional support for complainants would be obtained from the Citizens Advice Bureaux.

Section 12 of the Health and Social Care Act 2001 implements these provisions by placing a duty upon the Secretary of State 'to arrange, to such extent as he considers necessary to meet all reasonable requirements, for the provision of independent advocacy services'.

Independent advocacy services are defined as services providing assistance (by way of representation or otherwise) to individuals making or intending to make:

- a complaint under a procedure operated by a health service body or independent provider
- a complaint to the Health Service Commissioner
- a complaint of a prescribed description which relates to the provision of services as part of the health service.

The Secretary of State may make such other arrangements as he thinks fit for the provision of assistance to individuals in connection with health service complaints. He should have regard to the principle that the provision of services should 'so far as practicable, be independent of any person who is the subject of a relevant complaint or is involved in any investigating or adjudicating on such a complaint' (section 12(5))

Inevitably at present a complaint may be the first stage in the process of litigation and some claimants may use the complaints procedure to obtain information which will assist them in a future claim.

Future developments

It is dangerous to assume that an absence of complaints is indicative of a satisfactory service, or that many complaints show that an organisation is worse than one with fewer complaints. The reasons why people do not complain, even when there is a perceived reason to complain, are many and it could be that the organisation with no complaints is so appalling that patients consider that complaining would be a waste of time. Any league tables should, however, highlight the speed and efficiency with which complaints are handled. The House of Commons Select Committee considered the NHS complaints procedure in 1998–9[5], noting that there was a government funded project currently carrying out research into the effectiveness of the existing Complaints Procedure. The Select Committee made significant recommendations for reform.

In the light of the results of research commissioned into the present complaints system the Department of Health published a document suggesting a number of ways to improve the current procedure[6]. The Department of Health has also issued a consultation document[7] on which feedback is invited at the time of writing. It is likely to lead to significant changes to the present complaints system in 2002.

In the NHS Plan it is noted that Government will act on the evaluation of the NHS complaints procedure and reform it to make it more independent and responsive to patients. It states that:

> Making the complaints procedure less adversarial should result in fewer clinical negligence claims against the NHS.

It is in the interests of all health professionals to ensure that any complaints relating to the provision of health services are resolved as speedily as possible informally without requiring the complainant to make use of the formal procedure. Practitioners should have the confidence to realise that complaints can be a useful way of monitoring and improving the services to patients, that it takes courage to make a complaint, especially where the patient suffers from a chronic condition, and that improvements can be made if patients are prepared to discuss with the health professionals ways in which the services could be enhanced. Every complaint should be dealt with objectively and no assumptions made about the genuineness or grounds for the complaint until it has been effectively and thoroughly investigated. Complaints should be seen as only a small part of the quality assurance mechanisms in every organisation.

 ## Questions and exercises _____

1   Draw up a procedure for the handling of complaints in your department which includes how the lessons learnt from them could be implemented.
2   A client tells you that he is not happy with the care provided by another health professional. What action do you take and what advice do you give?
3   In what way could the handling of informal complaints be improved?
4   To what extent do you consider that the number of complaints is a useful device for monitoring the quality of service provided by your department. What other methods for quality assurance would you recommend?

5 How would you envisage the new Patient Advocacy and Liaison Service could operate effectively in your department?

References

1 DoH (2000) *The NHS Plan: a plan for investment, a plan for reform* Cm 4818–1 (July 2000) Department of Health, London

2 A. Wilson (1994) *Being Heard.* (The Report of a review committee Chaired by Professor Wilson on NHS complaints procedures) Department of Health, London

3 Health Service Commissioners (Amendment) Act 1996

4 DoH (1997) White Paper *The New NHS modern – dependable* HMSO, London

5 House of Commons Select Committee on Health Procedures Related to Adverse Clinical Incidents and Outcomes (HC 549–1 Session 1998–9)

6 DoH (2001) *The NHS Complaints Procedure: National Evaluation* (September 2001) Department of Health, London

7 DoH (2001) *Reforming the NHS Complaints Procedure: a listening document* (September 2001) Department of Health, London

Chapter 20
Medicinal Products

This chapter reviews the law relating to the prescribing, administration and supply of medicines and its implications in the field of radiography and radiology. The control of radioactive substances, whilst it comes under the Medicines Act 1968, is considered in Chapter 16.

Legislative framework for medicines

The 1968 Medicines Act provided a statutory framework for the supply and control of medicines. Figure 20.1 shows the basic contents of the Act. The Misuse of Drugs Act 1971 and subsequent legislation regulates the supply of specified controlled drugs referred to below. These statutes have been supplemented by Statutory Instruments providing more detailed regulation. The Medical Control Agency has the function of monitoring the safety and quality of medicines. Its website provides detailed information for health professionals, members of the public, academics, the pharmaceutical industry and journalists[1]. It also operates a Defective Medicines Report Centre.

Figure 20.1 **Framework set up by the 1968 Act.**

(1) An administrative system
(2) A licensing system
(3) Controls over the sale and supply of drugs to the public
(4) Retail Pharmacies
(5) Packing and labelling of medicinal products
(6) British Pharmacopoeia

Classification of drugs

Under the legislation all licensed drugs fall within one of the following categories:

- general sales list
- pharmacy only products
- prescription only list.

Any procedure for dealing with medicines in hospitals or in a community home, whether residential care, nursing or mental nursing, should ensure that the specific requirements for these different classes of drugs are met.

The general sales list covers drugs which are sold through a variety of outlets and a registered pharmacist does not have to be present. Pharmacy only products are those drugs which can only be purchased under the supervision of a registered pharmacist or given out by a dispensing doctor (i.e. one in a remote area who is authorised to dispense medicines).

Prescription only drugs can only be obtained from a registered pharmacist and only if duly prescribed (see below).

Guidance[2] issued by the College of Radiographers

A joint sub-committee of the Standing Medical, Nursing and Midwifery, and Pharmaceutical Advisory Committees was formed in 1986 under the chairmanship of Professor Duthie. Its task was to revise and consolidate guidance to health authorities/boards on the safe and secure handling or medicines. It reported in 1988[3]. The College of Radiographers has made recommendations based on the Duthie Report.

- A senior pharmacist shall be appointed as responsible for organising, monitoring and reporting on a system for ensuring the safe and secure handling of medicines. This person shall ensure that whenever responsibility for medicines is transferred from one individual to another it is on a defined and documented basis.
- A designated person (who shall be a professional) shall control access to the medicines within the department and have responsibility for ensuring that a system of security of the medicines is maintained. (The College of Radiographers supports the practice of designating a named radiographer in those departments where this would be practicable, provided it is negotiated in liaison with the appropriate parties.)
- Keys should be personally handed over to the next person who will retain responsibility, or placed in a secure place in the hospital which is manned 24 hours such as the hospital security office or switchboard.
- The authorisation of a suitably qualified practitioner must be obtained prior to the administration of medicines to patients. The authorisation must be obtained:
  ○ following a written instruction by a medical practitioner or on the basis of an official chart; or
  ○ in accordance with locally agreed procedures.
- The administration of medicines may be by either:
  ○ a suitably qualified practitioner, or
  ○ an authorised nurse in accordance with authorisation by an appropriate practitioner or on their own responsibility within local guidelines (see below under Patient group directions).
- Replenishment of medicines outside of normal working hours should be in accordance with a locally agreed policy that ensures that stocks of controlled drugs are maintained at a minimum level and replenished immediately after use.

- It is the responsibility of the senior pharmacist to arrange periodical security checks and an audit of controlled medicines in the Radiography/Radiotherapy department on a regular basis, and at least every three months.

Prescribing

Apart from exceptions in relation to the supply of medicinal products in hospitals, a request for prescription only drugs must be written in the specified form and presented to a registered pharmacist for dispensing unless the general practitioner has dispensing rights.

Nurse prescribing in the community

Following the first Crown Report[4] the powers of prescribing were extended to nurses and health visitors where the patient is not necessarily going to be seen by a doctor. The Medicinal Products (Nurse Prescribing etc.) Act 1992 enables a registered nurse, either health visitor or district nurse, who has the requisite additional training to prescribe those medicinal products contained in a Nurse's Formulary (set out in a schedule to the Prescription Only Medicines Order[5]). Section 58 of the Medicines Act 1968 (as amended by the 1992 Act) enables an appropriate practitioner to provide a prescription to be dispensed by a registered pharmacist.

Nurse prescribing in the community has a clear statutory basis and can take place within certain clearly defined parameters[6]. In February 2000 an amendment by Statutory Instrument[7] added nurses employed by a doctor whose name is included in a medical list (i.e. practice nurses) and those nurses in a Walk-in Centre (defined as a centre at which information and treatment for minor conditions is provided to the public under arrangements made by or on behalf of the Secretary of State) to the group of nurses who are recognised as being able to prescribe after the appropriate training had been given.

Prescribing in hospitals by non-doctors and non-dentists

Prescribing by nurses and other health professionals in hospital Trusts has developed on an ad hoc, quasi-legal basis. Clinical nurse practitioners or nurse specialists, working to locally devised protocols, have in certain Trusts been given powers to supply prescription only medication to patients where the doctor has not personally seen the patient. Radiographers, in certain circumstances, particularly those working in the therapeutic field, may have agreed protocols which enabled them to prescribe against an agreed list of medications. The Medicines Act 1968 required prescription only medicines in hospitals to be given on the written instructions of the doctor. A protocol could be seen as the written instruction of a doctor and this vagueness therefore enabled non-doctors to prescribe medicines against such a protocol. It could be said that the actual wording of the Act was complied with but not its spirit.

The second Crown Report

The uncertainties about prescribing in hospitals by health professionals other than doctors required investigation and Dr Crown was appointed in 1997 to chair a committee to review prescribing, supply and administration of medicines. Its terms of reference included the development of a consistent policy framework to guide judgments on the circumstances in which health professionals might undertake new responsibilities with regard to prescribing, supply and administration of medicines. The committee was also asked

- to advise on likely impact of any proposed changes
- to consider possible implications for legislation, professional training and standards and
- to advise on prescription etc. under group protocols and on any appropriate safeguards.

Its initial report was published in 1998 and was concerned with prescribing, supply and administration under group protocols[8]. It recommended that the majority of patients should continue to receive medicines on an individual basis. However current safe and effective practice using group protocols which are consistent with criteria defined in the Report should continue. The law should be clarified to ensure that health professionals who supply or administer medicines under group protocols are acting within the law and all group protocols should comply with specified criteria (see below under Patient group directions).

The final Report of the Crown Review was published in March 1999[9] and covers the other three terms of reference. The recommendations of this final report are shown in Figure 20.2.

Other recommendations are made in respect of training.

Independent and dependent prescribers

The recognition that there should be independent and dependent prescribers is central to the recommendations of the Final Crown Report.

'(i) independent prescribers – professionals who are responsible for the initial assessment of the patient and for devising the broad treatment plan, with the authority to prescribe the medicines required as part of that plan;
(ii) dependent prescribers – professionals who are authorised to prescribe certain medicines for patients whose condition has been diagnosed or assessed by an independent prescriber, within an agreed assessment and treatment plan.'

The final recommendation of the Crown Report is to individual practitioners:

'All legally authorised prescribers should take personal responsibility for maintaining and updating their knowledge and practice related to prescribing, including taking part in clinical audit, and should never prescribe in situations beyond their professional competence.'

Figure 20.2   **Recommendations of Final Report of Crown Review.**

(1)   The legal authority in the UK to prescribe should be extended beyond currently authorised prescribers.
(2)   The legal authority to prescribe should be limited to medicines in specific therapeutic areas related to the particular competence and expertise of the group.
(3)   Two types of prescribers should be recognised: the independent prescriber and the dependent prescriber.
(4)   A UK-wide advisory body (provisionally entitled the New Prescribers Advisory Committee) should be established under section 4 of the Medicines Act to assess submissions from professional organisations seeking powers for suitably trained members to become independent or dependent prescribers.
(5)   Newly authorised groups of prescribers should not normally be allowed to prescribe specified categories of medicines, including controlled drugs.
(6)   The current arrangements for the administration and self-administration of medicines should continue to apply. Newly authorised prescribers should have the power to administer those parenteral prescription only medicines which they are authorised to prescribe.
(7)   Repeatable prescriptions should be available on the NHS, with limits on the number of repeats and the duration of its validity.
(8)   There should be an evaluation of likely costs and benefits to the NHS in specific areas before general adoption of the recommendations takes place.
(9)   There should be primary legislation which permits ministers through regulations to designate new categories of dependent and independent prescribers for the purpose of the Medicines Act, defining what classes of medicines they could prescribe.
(10)   The new arrangements should be subject to evaluation and monitoring.

The implications for the scope of professional practice for radiographers

The Crown Report has in a sense given its approval to a controlled development of professional competence in areas formerly the sole reserve of medical and dental staff. However clear checks are to be in place to ensure that these developments take place with well defined precautions to secure patient safety and also to secure efficient use of resources. Whilst nurses are likely to be the most numerous group to develop prescribing skills, other professionals such as physiotherapists, radiographers, orthoptists, dietitians, speech therapists and many others will also find that the new legislation will facilitate professional development or at least validate activities already taking place. The need to obtain a doctor's personal attendance on a patient in order that a specific drug could be prescribed has placed an unnecessary obstacle in the advancement of professional practice for many health professionals and this will now be lifted.

In an article[10] written by Mary Embleton, Professional Officer of the Society of Radiographers, the Crown Recommendations were welcomed:

'It is desirable that highly trained health professionals should be able to use their full range of skills in the interests of patient care. By placing the responsibility of prescribing with the person responsible for the continuing care of the patient there is provision for more timely initiation of treatment and better communication with the patient, leading to a more convenient seamless service.'

Following the publication of the final Crown Report, the Society of Radio-graphers set up a working party to consider the implications for the profession[11]. It was noted that some radiographers are already supplying and administering medicines under group protocols.

The areas the Society identified as suitable for the radiographer being authorised to prescribe are:

- Radiotherapy (medicines prescribed for treatment related toxicity)
- Contrast radiography (radiographic contrast media)
- Gastro-intestinal radiography (muscle relaxants)
- Renography (diuretics)
- Nuclear medicine (radiopharmaceuticals)

The Society has asked for information from members on instances where:

- Patients experience long waits while a doctor is found to sign a prescription
- Under group protocols radiographers are selecting the specific medication for a particular patient
- Radiographers are initiating prescriptions, e.g. asking the doctor to 'write up' a patient for a particular medicine
- Radiographers are asked for their opinion as to what should be prescribed
- Medical practitioners not specifically trained in radiology may be prescribing substances, such as contrast media, without the specific knowledge that a radiographer may have.

The working party is also considering details of education and training requirements and systems of registration, regulation and audit to enable radio-graphers to become independent prescribers. In the light of this information, the New Prescribers Advisory Committee would take decisions on whether radio-graphers could be recognised as independent or dependant prescribers in various specialist areas.

An interim report[12] by the working party outlined its terms of reference and work to date. In 2001 the Society and College of Radiographers published its statement of policy on prescribing by radiographers[13].

Patient Group Directions

As a consequence of the Crown Report on group protocols new regulations[14] came into force on 9 August 2000. These provide for Patient Group Directions to be drawn up to make provision for the sale or supply of prescription only medicines in hospitals in accordance with the written direction of a doctor or dentist. To be lawful the Patient Group Directions must cover the particulars which are set out in Part 1 of Schedule 7 of the Statutory Instrument. These particulars are shown in Figure 20.3.

***Figure 20.3*   Particulars for a Patient Group Direction.**

(a) the period during which the Direction shall have effect
(b) the description or class of prescription only medicines to which the Direction relates
(c) whether there are any restrictions on the quantity of medicine which may be supplied on any one occasion and, if so, what restrictions
(d) the clinical situations which prescription only medicines of that description or class may be used to treat
(e) the clinical criteria under which a person shall be eligible for treatment
(f) whether any class of person is excluded from treatment under the Direction and, if so, what class of person
(g) whether there are circumstances in which further advice should be sought from a doctor or dentist and, if so, what circumstances
(h) the pharmaceutical form or forms in which prescription only medicines of that description or class are to be administered
(i) the strength, or maximum strength, at which prescription only medicines of that description or class are to be administered
(j) the applicable dosage or maximum dosage
(k) the route of administration
(l) the frequency of administration
(m) any minimum or maximum period of administration applicable to prescription only medicines of that description or class
(n) whether there are any relevant warnings to note and, if so, what warnings
(o) whether there is any follow up action to be taken in any circumstances and, if so, what action and in what circumstances
(p) arrangements for referral for medical advice
(q) details of the records to be kept of the supply or the administration of medicines under the Direction

---

The classes of individuals by whom supplies may be made are set out in Part III of Schedule 7 and include the following:

- Ambulance paramedics (who are registered or hold a certificate of proficiency)
- Pharmacists
- Registered health visitors
- Registered midwives
- Registered nurses
- Registered ophthalmic opticians
- State registered chiropodists
- State registered orthoptists
- State registered physiotherapists
- State registered radiographers

The person who is to supply or administer the medicine must be designated in writing on behalf of the authorising person (see below) for the purpose of the Patient Group Direction. In addition to compliance with the particulars set out in Figure 20.3, a Patient Group Direction must be signed on behalf of the authorising person. This is defined as the Common Services Agency, the (Special) Health Authority, the NHS trust or Primary Care Trust.

Legislation implementing the Final Crown Report is contained in section 63 of the Health and Social Care Act which amends the Medicines Act 1968. It amends section 58 of the Medicines Act to enable 'other persons who are of such a description and comply with such conditions as may be specified in the order' to be eligible to write prescriptions for medicinal products. Section 63(3) lists those persons who are eligible as including persons who are registered by a board established under the Professions Supplementary to Medicine Act 1960. This includes state registered radiographers. The list also includes 'persons who are registered in any register established, continued or maintained under an Order in Council under section 60(1) of the Health Act 1999 (see Chapter 11). Section 63(3) also requires the conditions under which any appropriate practitioner can prescribe to be specified. The Order specifying these conditions is awaited.

The role of the National Institute of Clinical Excellence (NICE)
It is hoped that the publications of NICE will assist in the professional knowledge of non-medical prescribers. As the work of this organisation, established on 1 April 1999, progresses information will be provided to health personnel and organisations on the effectiveness of certain drugs and procedures and newly eligible prescribers will be aided by this research. (See Chapter 21 where the role of NICE is considered.)

Implications for staff
Whilst the Crown Report anticipated that the majority of patients should continue to receive medicines on an individual basis, it recognised that there is likely to be a continuing need for supply and administration under group protocols in certain limited situations. It could well be that these situations will increase in number. The eventual impact of this on the traditional role of the doctor as the person who is central to the health care of the patient in hospital may however be considerable.

Liability and medicines

The basic principles of accountability and liability apply to all aspects of medication, whether the practitioner is prescribing, supplying or administering medicines. Clearly, however, as the role of the radiographer expands to include prescribing as an independent or dependent prescriber, the responsibilities will increase. The patient is entitled to receive the same standard of care, whoever is responsible.

There are many cases, where compensation has been paid out because of errors in relation to the prescribing, dispensing and administration of medicines. The following are just two examples.

Case: *Prendergast* v. *Sam & Dee Ltd*[15]

The doctor prescribed amoxil (an antibiotic) for the patient which, because of bad handwriting, was misread as daonil (a drug used by diabetics) by the pharmacist. As a consequence of the wrong medication the patient suffered from severe hypoglycaemia and brain damage from oxygen shortage in the blood. The doctor was held 25% to blame and the pharmacist 75%. The latter should have been alerted to the misreading because of the dosage and the fact that the patient paid for the prescription. £119,302 was paid out in compensation.

Case: Failure to heed manufacturers' dosage[16]

The doctor prescribed Migril but failed to heed the manufacturers warnings and instead of limiting the dose to not more that 12 tablets in the course of one week and not more than one every four hours, prescribed 60 tablets to be taken as two tablets every four hours. The pharmacist did not spot the error. The patient's condition deteriorated and the mistake was not noticed by another doctor in the practice who visited the patient. Compensation of £100,000 was agreed, 45% payable by the prescribing doctor, 40% by the pharmacist and the remaining 15% by the second doctor who visited. On appeal the second doctor was found not liable and his 15% contribution was accepted by the pharmacist.

At the heart of the issue of negligence is the question of whether the accepted standard of the reasonable professional has been followed. This is known as the Bolam test[17] (see Chapter 14). In the new field of prescribing by health professionals other than doctors, standards will have to be defined, protocols drawn up and procedures agreed to ensure that there are recognised standards for professional practice[18]. However it is clear that the public should not expect a lower standard of care because radiographers have the role of prescribing than the standard which they would have received from a doctor[19].

Determination of the appropriate product

What is the situation if the practitioner fails to diagnose a serious condition or a contradiction to the usual medication?

Clearly the training must ensure that practitioners know their limitations and they know which signs to watch out for and when it is essential that the doctor should see the patient. Initially, the practitioner, particularly if a dependent prescriber, will be limited to a small range of products and any situation for which these products are not appropriate should be reported to the doctor for diagnosis and assessment.

The test which will be applied to the practitioner is 'Would any reasonable practitioner in those circumstances and following the approved accepted standards of the professional have acted as that practitioner did?' If the answer to that question is 'Yes', then the practitioner should not be found liable for negligence. This is the application of the Bolam test.

It is helpful for the practitioner to have a check list when assessing the patient and making the decision whether or not a product should be prescribed.

Patient's failure to communicate

What if the patient fails to tell the practitioner about known allergies or contra-indications? The practitioner should consult the patient's records and have some knowledge of the medical history of the patient. There should therefore be a record of any known allergy. If, however, this is not known to the clinicians but known to the patient and the patient fails to tell the practitioner, then, provided that the practitioner had asked the relevant questions and followed the accepted practice, they would not be held responsible for this ignorance. Where there is fault on the part of the practitioner but also fault by the patient, the patient would be regarded as contributorily negligent. This means that, in the event of his claiming compensation for harm resulting from negligence by the practitioner, the extent of his fault in contributing to his harm would be taken into account and his compensation reduced accordingly. In some cases there could be 100% contributory negligence (see Chapter 14).

Consent and capacity

Issues relating to consent by the patient and the patient's capabilities are considered in Chapter 4 and the general principles should be borne in mind when decisions over prescribing and supplying medicines are being made. If the patient is over 18 years and is incapable of giving a valid consent, then at present no person can give consent on his or her behalf. Health professionals have to act in the best interests of the mentally incapacitated patient according to the accepted approved standard of care (the Bolam test)[20].

Children of 16 and 17 have a statutory right to give consent to surgical, medical and dental treatment and this includes consent to diagnostic and ancillary procedures such as an anaesthetic. The parents also have a parallel right to give consent. Those below 16 can give a valid consent in their own names provided they have the maturity to make the decision, i.e. they are 'Gillick competent'. Their parents can also consent on their behalf provided that the proposed treatment is in the best interests of the child. Where parents refuse treatment or diagnostic procedures necessary to the best interests of the child, then their refusal can be overruled in the interests of the child. If time permits a court order can be obtained (see Chapter 8).

Principles to be followed in making out the prescription

The following are factors which must be taken into account when prescribing.

- Is a prescription really required?
- If so, what is the appropriate drug or medicinal product?
- Are there any contra-indications?
- What is the appropriate dose?
- What is the recommended level?
- What is the age and condition of the patient?
- Has this same product be prescribed before?
- Is a higher than usual dose justified?
- Is there any danger of misuse, e.g. overdosing?
- What should the interval of administration be?
- What is the appropriate route – oral, intramuscular, external use, suppository?

- What is the appropriate length of course of treatment?
- What is the shelf-life of the product?
- When should it be reviewed?

Contra-indications

In determining contra-indications, a practitioner would need to know whether the substance being prescribed is compatible with other drugs which the patient is taking. The practitioner must know the content of the medicinal products which are to be prescribed so that any likely contra-indications are identified.

In a case in 1994, a GP was charged with manslaughter for prescribing beta-blocker tablets to a patient who suffered from asthma and who died after taking one tablet. He was also charged with attempting to pervert the course of justice since it was alleged that he tried to change the computer records, not realising that the information was also held on hard disk[21].

Advice is given by C. Gunn and C.S. Jackson[22] on drugs and radiographic contrast agents. They suggest guidelines for the administration of medicine covering the different sites and procedures for handling controlled drugs. Advice on the use of radiographic contrast agents is also given and they recommend:

'It is important that students understand the contraindications for the various contrast agents and to know why the specific agents are used.'

If there is a reaction, the practitioner should record the type of reaction, the contrast agent: dose and batch number and the drugs given.

Repeat prescriptions

Every care should be taken where the practitioner is writing a prescription for a product that the patient has already been taking, to ensure that the necessity for that particular product to be continued is assessed each time and that there is a regular comprehensive review and monitoring of its effects and value.

The pharmacist may query or challenge the prescription, in which case the practitioner should be able to provide all the information required, since such questions are ultimately in the best interests of the patient[23].

Commercial pressures

Health professionals may occasionally come under pressure from pharmaceutical companies to prescribe or supply a particular product to patients. The sole criteria in deciding what product if any to prescribe must be the patient's best interests.

Record keeping

This is considered in Chapter 18. Practitioners should ensure that all the details relating to the prescribing, supply and administration of medications are clearly documented. This is clearly in the patient's interest as well as being essential for the protection of the practitioner in the event of any later allegations.

Information

Consideration must also be given to the information with which the patient should be provided. The patient is entitled in law to receive information about the possibility of significant risks of substantial harm. (This topic is considered in Chapter 4.) The Bolam test has been applied to the giving of information[24].

> 'The test of liability in respect of a doctor's duty to warn his patient of risks inherent in treatment recommended by him was the same as the test applicable to diagnosis and treatment, namely that the doctor was required to act in accordance with a practice accepted at the time as proper by a responsible body of medical opinion.'

Practitioners have to ensure that they are familiar with the side effects of any treatment or diagnostic techniques and notify the patient of those risks just as any practitioner following the accepted approved practice would do. The information should enable the patient to make a balanced decision on whether to proceed with that treatment or investigation or not.

Clearly the practitioner must take into account the mental capacity of the patient to understand details about the product. However, if it is reasonable for the patient to be given certain information before consenting to have the medicinal product, then this information should be given whether or not questions are asked.

The patient does not have to be given all the information that is available.

Case: *Blythe* v. *Bloomsbury Health Authority*[25]

A patient claimed that she should have been given full information about the possible side effects of the Depo Provera drug and that information which the hospital had through its research should have been made available to her. The Court of Appeal allowed the appeal by the health authority against the award of damages by the High Court for the following reasons.

- There was no obligation to pass on to the plaintiff all the information available to the hospital, i.e. all the information contained in the senior house officer's files.
- What a plaintiff should be told in answer to a general enquiry could not be divorced from the Bolam test any more that when no such enquiry was made.
- Answers given must depend upon the circumstances, i.e. the nature of the enquiry, the nature of the information which was available, its reliability and relevance, and the condition of the patient.
- The extent of the duty to give information was to be judged in the light of the state of medical knowledge at the time.
- There was no rule of law that, where questions were asked or doubts expressed by a patient, a doctor was under an obligation to put the patient in possession of all the information on the subject which may be available in the files of a consultant who may have made a special study of the subject
- The amount of information to be given must depend on the circumstances and it must be governed by the Bolam test.

The practitioner must ensure that she gives to the patient all the information which any other reasonable practitioner would give. This would include instructions about a product's use or application and advice on signs to look for and how long before improvement can be expected, again. The patient is entitled to receive all that he could reasonably be expected to need to know. The practitioner needs to be familiar with any limitations of the patient and have a good understanding of the product and the various forms in which it can be administered. Advice must include what action the patient must take if any side effects appear.

Misuse of medication

Some misuse may occur because the patient fails to understand how the medication is to be used. For example there are accounts of patients putting patches on top of each other, not taking off the wrapping or eating suppositories. If this misuse occurs because of poor instructions by the practitioner, then clearly there is a breach of the duty of care.

If possible the practitioner should double-check to be sure that the patient (or carer) understands the instructions. The practitioner should ensure that she herself is familiar with the packaging and way in which the product should be used.

The difficulties of some elderly patients and those with limited capacity in understanding instructions in relation to medication must be taken into account by the practitioner as part of her decision over what if anything to prescribe.

Administration of the products

It may often be that the practitioner who has prescribed is also the person to administer the product. However, where this is not so, the practitioner should enquire who is to administer the product and ensure if possible that the person understands what is required.

Defects in the medicines

If there is a defect in the product the practitioner would not be liable for that unless she should have known that such a product was not to be recommended. The practitioner would not usually be regarded as a supplier for the purposes of the Consumer Protection Act 1987 (see Chapter 17). If there were any defect in the product which caused harm to the patient, the patient would have a right of action against the seller of the product or the manufacturer. However where the product has been adapted or modified within the department prior to its supply to or use by the patient, then the practitioner may be seen as the supplier under the 1987 Act and her employer therefore liable.

Writing the prescription?

The following are some of the elements which should be taken into account in the writing of a prescription.

- Legibility, in ink or otherwise indelible, dated and signed in ink by the prescriber (with the full name and address).
- Full name and address of patient and hospital number (where appropriate).
- Age of the patient (essential where under 12 or elderly).
- Name of product stated in full (check that the title is approved and to be used on the label).
- Advise the pharmacist whether or not the title should be put on the con-

tainer (in some exceptional situations this information is withheld from the patient).

- Dose and dose frequency must be stated, together with the strength and quantity. (The form of the product should also be set out, e.g. tablet, capsule, liquid.)
  - Use only the abbreviations for dosage and route recognised in the BNF (e.g. 1 gm for one gram, 500 mg for half a gram etc.
  - Cubic centimetres are not used.
  - Always place a zero in front of a decimal point
- Where drugs can be taken as required, the minimum dose frequency should be stated.
- Any instructions about whether the product should be taken before or after meals or with water and similar instructions should be stated.
- State the number of days to be supplied in the box indicated, or the maximum quantity in respect of 'as required' products.
- Where a drug has been withdrawn but is to be prescribed, the prescription should be written personally by hand by the prescriber.
- Any other warnings about the drug should be stated. (For example the drug may cause drowsiness and the patient should be advised not to drive.)

Liability can arise if the writing is such that it is misread and harm occurs to the patient as a consequence. The actual circumstances will determine the extent of contribution between the practitioner prescribing and the pharmacist dispensing.

The BNF gives information relating to computer-issued prescriptions based on the recommendations of the Joint Computing Group of the General Medical Services Committee and the Royal College of General Practitioners.

Training

It will be a statutory requirement for any practitioner to undergo the necessary training in order to be an authorised prescriber. Would it be possible for a practitioner to refuse this expanded role and not undertake the training? The answer depends upon whether it is a reasonable instruction for the employer to require specific practitioners to undertake work as independent or dependent prescribers. If prescribing is seen as central to the role within specific areas of that person's professional responsibility, then it would probably be reasonable for a practitioner to be required to take on this expanded role.

Any practitioner whose role is enhanced to include prescribing would be entitled to obtain from their employer the necessary training to fulfil that duty safely.

Supervision of students
Students are not eligible to prescribe. Any student must be under the supervision of a registered practitioner, and this person would be liable for any inappropriate delegation and supervision.

Myodil

Harm can arise to patients through side effects or allergies to substances used in diagnostic testing. Myodil was used as a dye injected into the spinal cavity prior to X-ray. It was used extensively since the 1940s. However evidence that it may have caused arachnoiditis (inflammation of the membranes covering the nerve roots within the spinal cord) led to its voluntary withdrawal by Glaxo in 1987. They paid an *ex gratia* sum of £7 million in total to the 3600 patients who alleged negligence in the testing of the dye, without any admission of liability[26]. A subsequent case brought by a patient who alleged that he has suffered from Myodil, was struck out on the grounds that the claimant had to be taken as fully compensated by the Glaxo settlement[27], no fresh allegations of negligence were being put forward. In the light of a recent successful case[28] in respect of contaminated blood, patients may seek in the future to bring a class action under the Consumer Protection Act 1987 in respect of alleged defects in diagnostic or medicinal products (see Chapter 17).

Conclusions

The full implications of the Crown reports and the subsequent amendments to the Medicines Act 1968 are at the time of writing not yet apparent. It seems likely that they will lead to significant changes in the professional relationships of radiographers and doctors and other health professionals. Close monitoring of the prescribing, supply and administration of medicines will be essential for the protection of patients and the safe development of professional practice.

 Questions and exercises _____

1 The head of department suggests that you could take on the role of a dependent prescriber for certain medicines. What is meant by this and what preparation would you insist on as essential before taking on this expanded role?
2 You are concerned about the administration of pain medication to a terminally ill patient. What action could be taken in relation to control of medication?
3 You are asked by an oncologist to administer a drug which you consider inappropriate for a particular patient. What action would you take? (Refer also to Chapter 22 and whistle blowing.)

References

1 www.open.gov.uk/mca/mcahome.htm
2 College of Radiographers (1996) *Guidelines for the safe and secure handling of medicines* College of Radiographers, London
3 Department of Health (1988) *Guidelines on the safe and secure handling of medicines* (The Duthie Report) DoH, London

4   DoH (1989) *Report on Nurse Prescribing and Supply* (Advisory Group chaired by Dr June Crown) Department of Health, London

5   Prescription Only Medicines Order 1994 SI No. 3050 of 1994

6   B.C. Dimond (1995) *Nurse Prescribing* Merck Dermatology and Scutari Press

7   The National Health Service (Pharmaceutical Services) Amendment Regulations 2000 SI No. 121 of 2000

8   DoH (1998) *Review of Prescribing, supply and administration of medicines: a Report on the supply and administration of medicines under Group Protocols* (April 1998) Department of Health, London

9   Department of Health (1999) *Final Report on the Prescribing, supply and Administration of medicines* (Chaired by Dr June Crown) (March 1999) Department of Health, London

10 M. Embleton (1999) Prescribed medicines under review *Synergy* (June 1999) pages 8–9

11 Radiographers as prescribers News item *Synergy News* (March 2000) page 6

12 C. Freeman (2000) The Crown Report II – The Working Party *Synergy News* (April 2000) page 9

13 CoR (2001) *Prescribing by Radiographers: A Vision Paper* College of Radiographers, London

14 Prescription only Medicines (Human Use) Amendment Order 2000 SI No. 1917 of 2000

15 *Prendergast* v. *Sam & Dee Ltd* [1989] 1 Med LR 36; *The Independent* 17 March 1988.

16 *Dwyer* v. *Roderick and others* (1983) *The Times* 12 November 1983

17 *Bolam* v. *Friern Hospital Management Committee* [1957] 2 All ER 118

18 B.C. Dimond (1994) *Standards Setting and litigation. British Journal of Nursing* **3**, 5 (10–23 March 1994) 235–238

19 *Wilsher* v. *Essex Area Health Authority* [1988] I All ER 871 (CA)

20 *F* v. *West Berkshire HA (Re F)* [1989] 2 All ER 545

21 *The Times* 15 April 1994

22 C. Gunn & C.S. Jackson (1991) *Guidelines on Patient Care in Radiography* Churchill Livingstone, Edinburgh

23 M.R. Rawlings (1990) Nurse Prescribing: the Pharmacist's point of view. *Nursing Times* 1990, **86**, 55–7

24 *Sidaway* v. *Bethlem Royal Hospital Governors and others* [1985] 1 All ER 643

25 *Blythe* v. *Bloomsbury Health Authority* (1987) *The Times* 11 February 1987

26 I. Kennedy & A. Grubb (2000) *Medical Law* (3rd edn) Butterworths, London

27 *Rawlinson* v. *N Essex HA* (2000) Lloyds Rep. Med. 54

28 *A and Others* v. *National Blood Authority and Another* (2001) The Times Law Report, 4 April 2001; [2001] 3 All ER 289

Section E
Management Areas

Chapter 21
Statutory Organisation of the NHS

Background to the NHS

Set out in the Beveridge Report as part of the scheme to rebuild Britain's infrastructure after the Second World War, the NHS was established on 5 July 1948 under the National Health Service Act 1946. This legislation was re-enacted in the National Health Service Act 1977. Section 1 enshrines the basic principles:

(1) It is the Secretary of State's duty to continue the promotion in England and Wales of a comprehensive health service designed to secure improvement —
(a) in the physical and mental health of the people in those countries, and
(b) in the prevention, diagnosis and treatment of illness,
and for the purpose to provide or secure the effective provision of services in accordance with this Act.

(2) The services so provided shall be free of charge except in so far as the making and recovery of charges is expressly provided for by or under any enactment, whenever passed.

It is the duty of the NHS to meet 'all reasonable requirements' in respect of the specified aspects of health-care. There is no absolute duty to provide services (see Chapter 3).
Part I of the Act covers:

- Hospital accommodation
- Other accommodation for the purpose of any service provided under the Act
- Medical, dental, nursing and ambulance services
- Facilities for the care of expectant and nursing mothers and young children appropriate to the health service.

Part II of the Act (as amended) covers the provision of services by General Practitioners, dental practitioners, pharmacists and others who provide services under a contract for services with the Health Authorities (which took over responsibilities from the Family Health Service Authorities in 1996).
There was a significant change in 1990 when the NHS and Community Care Act 1990 led to the establishment of NHS trusts and Group Fund Holding Practices. The NHS trusts were to be the principal providers of NHS secondary and community health care. Purchasers were either GPs who were approved as fundholders to hold a budget to purchase secondary and community health care services for their patients or health authorities. In this way, the internal market was created and the purchase and provision of

health care was agreed in NHS contracts. In April 1996 health authorities were reorganised – the former district health authorities (DHAs) and family health services authorities (FHSAs) were abolished and in their place were established new health authorities which had the responsibility of commissioning and, in conjunction with GP fundholders, purchasing services from providers as well as carrying out the responsibilities in relation to the primary health care services formerly undertaken by FHSAs.

However this organisation was radically changed following the 1997 White Paper on the NHS[1] and the Health Act 1999.

The White Paper on the new NHS

The White Paper[1] on the NHS envisaged that the internal market would be abolished. The main features of the White Paper on the NHS are shown in Figure 21.1.

Figure 21.1   **Main features of the 1997 White Paper.**

(1)   Abolition of the internal market and GP Fundholding
(2)   Establishment of Primary Care Groups leading to Primary Care Trusts
(3)   Establishment of the National Council of Clinical Excellence
(4)   Establishment of the Commission for Health Improvement
(5)   Setting up of National Service Frameworks
(6)   Introduction of NHS Direct
(7)   Introduction of Clinical Governance

Abolition of the internal market and GP fundholding

The NHS agreements between health authorities or GP fundholders and NHS trusts were replaced by long-term, three year, arrangements for the provision of services. Extra-contractual referrals no longer exist. GP fundholding no longer exists. GPs are expected to participate in the new arrangements for primary health care (in Wales known as local health groups).

Establishment of Primary Care Groups and Trusts

In Chapter 5 of the White Paper proposals were set out for Primary Care Groups. These are to bring together GPs and community nurses in each area to work together to improve the health of local people and would grow out of the range of commissioning models that have developed in recent years. They would have strong support from their health authority and the freedom to use NHS resources wisely, including savings.

The White Paper envisaged that some Primary Care Groups could become Primary Care Trusts, i.e. free-standing organisations. Such trusts could include community health services from existing trusts. All or part of an existing community NHS trust could combine with a Primary Care Trust in order to integrate better services and management support. The White Paper specifically states that these new trusts would not be expected to take responsibility for specialised mental health or learning disability services.

More than 40 PGCs said that they wished to apply for PCT status in October 2000 and there were possibly a further 100 or more applications for trust status in 2001[2]. These are major organisational developments which are still in the process of being reviewed. It is likely that there will be many different models followed and considerable flexibility across the country.

Sections 1 to 12 and Schedule 1 of the Health Act 1999 amend earlier statutes to regulate the establishment of Primary Care Trusts. Schedule 1 to the 1999 Act provides for more detailed regulation, including the Primary Care Trust Orders, their constitution membership and staff, and their powers and duties. Rules also cover the transfer of property and the transfer of staff.

It is a specific requirement of the PCT that, as soon as practicable after the end of each financial year, every PCT shall prepare a report of the Trust's activities during that year and shall send a copy of the report to the health authority in whose area the trust is sited and to the Secretary of State. Official Guidance has been provided by the Department of Health covering the financial framework[3], the arrangements for staff transfer[4] and arrangements for estates and facilities management[5]. All these documents are available from the website[6].

The NHS Confederation provided a briefing note on the Primary Care Trusts[7] and expressed concerns about the lack of clarity of accountability within the Primary Care Trusts and the internal governance arrangements outlined in the Department of Health Guidance. It is likely that when the review of the pilot Primary Care Trusts takes place, this will lead to more robust arrangements for accountability. Further developments in the establishment of Care Trusts are to take place when Part 3 of the Health and Social Care Act 2001 is implemented. Partnership arrangements can be directed under section 46 when it is considered that a NHS body or local authority is failing in the exercise of its functions.

Standards

Following the White Paper there has been greater emphasis on standard setting in the light of research findings on clinical effectiveness and excellence. Standard setting and monitoring will become an even more significant part of the practitioner's professional responsibilities. Standards in relation to the law are discussed in chapter 14 on the law of negligence. The extent to which clinical guidelines, protocols, procedures and practices are enforceable through the courts is considered in a fascinating work by Brian Hurwitz[8].

Introduction of clinical governance

One of the most significant changes envisaged by the Government in its White Paper is the concept of clinical governance. It is defined[9] as:

'A framework through which NHS organisations are accountable for continuously improving the quality of their services.'

The idea of clinical governance is basically simple. In the past, the the Trust board and its chief executive have been responsible for the financial probity of the organisation, there has been no statutory responsibility on the part of the Trust for the overall quality of the organisation. Under the concept of clinical governance the board and its chief executive is responsible for the quality of clinical services provided by the organisation. In theory this could mean that a Board might be removed or a chief executive dismissed if a baby suffers brain damage at birth or the wrong limb is amputated.

In its College Review of Radiology Services[10] the RCR identifies the essential elements of clinical governance as:

- Governance of clinicians by clinicians – local self-regulation
- Support for clinicians by managers – to ensure adequate resources for the maintenance of high standards
- Involvement of clinicians in the management of the NHS.

As an aid to the implementation of clinical governance the RCR has set up a College team which would be available to review the structure and function of any Department of Radiology. As a result of being called in by a Trust the Review team may make recommendations over a wide area:

- Changes to the working environment, support facilities, equipment replacement programmes – not just clinical practice, but communication and management support
- Further training of an individual consultant radiologist(s)
- That the practice of individual radiologists or of departments should be restricted, where the facilities are inadequate for the safe performance of particular procedures; or the numbers of procedures being performed are inadequate to maintain competence
- Disciplinary proceedings or referral to the GMC
- The review and revision by the Trust of its local practice in the light of the Review team's report, published data and evidence from other institutions.

The concept of clinical governance is based on the statutory duty of quality under section 18 of the Health Act 1999.

The duty of quality

For the first time in its history there is a statutory duty on the NHS to promote quality. Section 18 of the Health Act 1999 is shown in Figure 21.2

Figure 21.2 **Section 18 of the Health Act 1999.**

It is the duty of each Health Authority, Primary Care Trust and NHS Trust to put and keep in place arrangements for the purpose of monitoring and improving the quality of health care which it provides to individuals.

The duty falls primarily upon the chief executive of each health authority and NHS trust to implement. In practice, each chief executive designates officers to be responsible for quality or clinical governance in specified areas of clinical practice. Government guidance was published in March 1999[11]. This follows from the original consultation document *A First Class Service: Quality in the new NHS*[12]. The aim is to develop quality within the NHS in three ways:

- setting clear national quality standards
- ensuring local delivery of high quality clinical services and
- effective systems for monitoring the quality of services.

The RCR has provided guidance on carrying out an audit for the purposes of clinical governance and revalidation[13].

Commission for Health Improvement (CHI)

CHI's forerunner – CSAG

The Clinical Standards Advisory Group was set up under the NHS and Community Care Act 1990 as a statutory body to advise UK Health Ministers on standards of clinical care. It was abolished on 1 November 1999 under the Health Act 1999, its duties being taken over by the Commission for Health Improvement. This body has much wider functions and powers than CSAG. Sections 19 to 24 of the Health Act 1999 establish the CHI, set out its functions and powers and make provision for appropriate delegated legislation. It is a body corporate, i.e. it can sue and be sued on its own account.

The Commission for Health Improvement can suggest to the Audit Commission that it joins with it in exercising its functions. This can include conducting and making reports on studies designed to improve economy, efficiency and effectiveness in the performance of NHS functions. However, before the Audit Commission acts with the CHI, the latter must agree to pay the full costs incurred by the Audit Commission in so acting.

The Secretary of State has additional powers under section 23 of the 1999 Act to make regulations allowing authorised persons

- to enter NHS premises to inspect those premises
- to take copies of prescribed documents or require people to produce documents, other information or reports and
- to conduct interviews.

Regulations can also be made (section 23(2)) on the disclosure of confidential information and the identification of a living individual.

There is some protection in that section 24(1) makes it a criminal offence knowingly or recklessly to disclose confidential information obtained by the Commission without lawful authority.

Activities of CHI

One of the earliest tasks undertaken by CHI on the day it was established was to visit Garlands Hospital in Carlisle run by the North Lakeland Healthcare NHS Trust in Cumbria. An independent investigation[14] had found that staff had physically and mentally abused patients. The Chairman of the NHS trust was dismissed by the Secretary of State. The Secretary of State ordered CHI to visit the hospital.

A spokesman for the Commission has stated that its programme for scrutinising NHS trusts could include questions about the resuscitation of older people following complaints that some hospital doctors are ignoring guidelines[15]. CHI has a rolling programme of inspections so that over five years all NHS trusts will be visited and reports published.

Audit Commission

The Commission for Health Improvement will work alongside the Audit Commission supporting its work by inspections and publishing advice to organisations and practitioners. In 1997 the Audit Commission reported on radiology services[16]. Its recommendations are considered in Chapter 23.

National Council of Clinical Excellence (NICE)

This statutory body was established on 1 April 1999 to promote clinical and cost effectiveness. The then Secretary of State stated that its task would be to abolish 'postcode variation' in the country, so that there would be national standards for the provision of health care such as medicines. It would no longer be the case that certain medicines or treatments were available on the NHS in one area but only privately in another.

One of the functions of NICE is to issue clinical guidelines and clinical audit methodologies and information on good practice. The National Institute for Clinical Excellence has a major role to play in the setting of standards of practice, by disseminating the results of research of what is proved to be clinically effective, research-based practice.

One of the results of NICE guidance is that those patients who claim that they have suffered as a result of a failure to provide a reasonable standard of care are able to use evidence of clinical effectiveness and research-based practice to illustrate failings in the care provided to them. It could be argued that failure to follow the recommendations of NICE will be *prima facie* evidence of a failure to follow a reasonable standard of care according to the Bolam test[17].

Impact of NICE and CHI on radiography, radiotherapy and radiology

The implications of NICE and CHI on cancer and radiology services are considered in various guest editorials to *Radiography*.

R James[18] analyses the functions of CHI and NICE and the quality assurance (QA) systems within the NHS and recommended that NICE assessments need to be a dynamic form of process QA involving a group of stakeholders.

Neville Goodman[19] discusses NICE and the new command structure in *Some thoughts on evidence, competence and authority*. He points out that evidence-based medicine (EBM) presents some basic problems. One is that it is derived from statistical data collected from populations and therefore does not provide the information necessary to treat individual patients. Another is that it places too much faith in randomised controlled trials, the conditions of which are often far removed from the conditions of clinical practice. He is concerned that many decisions of NICE will be based on cost-effectiveness and, like the decision on beta-interferon, may be not a medical decision but a political one. He concludes that EBM does not provide evidence robust enough for national guidelines.

Steve Harrison[20] writes on *NICE, CHI, clinical governance and health-care rationing.* He points out that rationing in the NHS is inevitable, that decisions have to be made about *who* will receive *what* care, according to *what* criteria (implicit or explicit) and by *what mechanism* this will be implemented. The effect of the new arrangements is to put the Government (advised by NICE) in the role of decision maker with CHI and clinical governance as the means of implementation.

Setting up National Service Frameworks (NSFs)

The White Paper envisages that there will be evidence-based National Service Frameworks which set out what patients can expect to receive from the NHS in major care areas or disease groups. One of the first National Service frameworks to be published was that for Mental Health[21]. Some of the problems of implementing this framework in the context of traditional professional attitudes and views of organisations are discussed in a research paper by Edward Peck and others[22].

Eventually NSFs will cover most of the main spheres of clinical practice. They will doubtless assist managers and clinicians in obtaining the resources to ensure a reasonable standard of care for their patients. Inevitably, however, they are also likely to support litigation where patients who claim to have suffered are able to compare local facilities unfavourably with the norm laid down in the NSF.

Standards in cancer care
In January 2001 the Government published its standards for care of patients suffering from cancer[23]. This manual sets 426 benchmarks for cancer centres being assessed by a team of inspectors. The worst centres are suspended while they try to improve staffing, facilities or systems. Failure to improve leads to a unit being closed. In the field of radiotherapy the manual sets out 60 specific standards. Priorities include:

- Clear rotas for specialists, including out of hours cover
- Minimum equipment to include two linear accelerators, treatment planning computer with 3-D imaging, simulator, X-ray and electron therapy facilities
- Sufficient consultants to concentrate on two major and two minor tumour types each
- New waiting times – urgent treatment within 48 hours moving to 24 hours, radical treatment within four weeks moving to two weeks
- Access to CT scanners for planning and radical treatments.

Overall standards are set for all cancers including the clinical team, the preparation of written treatment plans for all new patients, a written policy on communicating with GPs and a survey of patients' views. In addition there are specific standards in the following areas:

- Breast cancer
- Colorectal
- Lung
- Gynaecology
- Chemotherapy

- Patient-centred care
- Diagnostic services
- Non-surgical oncology
- Palliative care
- Communication
- Management organisation

The implications in relation to litigation of such standards are considered in Chapter 14.

Evidence based practice and clinical effectiveness

Eventually all clinical procedures and practices within radiography, radiotherapy and radiology will be subjected to testing research on clinical effectiveness. Practitioners will be involved in regular monitoring and review of their functions and outcomes. Stephen Brealey and Anne-Marie Glenny[24] suggested a framework for radiographers planning to undertake a systematic review. The context of their work is the fact that the demand for evidence-based health care is increasing and is equally necessary in both diagnostic and therapeutic practice. The objective of their paper was to delineate a basic framework for carrying out systematic reviews, using essentially the principles developed by the NHS Centre for Reviews and Dissemination (CRD). They used a specific radiography scenario with regard to the reporting of accident and emergency plain films by radiographers to illustrate the application of these principles. The main features of the framework are shown in Figure 21.3.

Figure 21.3 **Features of a framework for systematic review (Brealey and Glenny).**

- Identifying the need for a review
- Formulating the problem and specifying the objectives
- Developing the review protocol
- Literature searching and study retrieval
- Assessing study for inclusion
- Assessing and grading studies on the basis of validity
- Extracting data from the selected studies
- Synthesizing data from the selected studies
- Interpreting the results
- Dissemination and implementing the results

The authors emphasise that systematic reviews also have important implications for the development of a research infrastructure in radiography. A useful glossary of terms adapted from the CRD report accompanies the article.

Dominic Upton[25] reviews the concept of clinical effectiveness from the perspective of how much radiographers knew about it and what they thought of the concept. He found that many in the sample considered that their level of knowledge of clinical effectiveness/evidence-based practice to be low, but a majority considered that clinical effectiveness was a key issue and fundamental to their practice. He concluded that the current underlying culture provides a firm foundation for the necessary education and encouragement required for the fuller implementation of evidence based practice in radiographers.

Organisational changes

NHS Direct

The 1997 White paper on the NHS proposed the establishment of NHS Direct. The Government's stated aim was that by the end of the year 2000 the whole country will be covered by a 24 hour telephone advice line staffed by nurses. The pilot scheme whereby patients could phone direct to a 24 hour phone line and get immediate advice from a registered nurse was followed by the implementation of NHS Direct across the country. NHS Direct was one of the first of the innovations introduced by the Labour Government for the NHS and at the time of writing has been operating for about two years on a restricted basis. The service aims to provide both clinical advice to support self-care and appropriate self-referral to NHS services, as well as access to more general advice and information. Eventually NHS Direct may, through linking up with out of hours services, provide a triage assessment for out of hours visits by doctors. In November 2001 the Department of Health launched an interactive enquiry service for NHS Direct which enables people to make specific requests for information and receive a personal response.

Evaluation of NHS Direct
The Medical Research Unit at Sheffield University undertook an evaluation of NHS Direct. In its interim report published in March 1999[26] it stated that 97% of callers surveyed said that they were satisfied or very satisfied with the service and the service appears to have been of great benefit to parents since about one in four calls is about a child of five or under. However there were some concerns:

> 'There was a small number of callers who expressed some dissatisfaction including the length of time taken to speak to a nurse, and some callers were not happy with the large number of questions asked during the call.'

An early NHS Direct report stated that over the 1998 Christmas period NHS Direct pilot schemes handled 2700 calls[27]. Overall 40% of callers who spoke to a nurse were advised that they could look after themselves. In general around 25–30% of triaged calls over this period were about flu type symptoms and in half of these cases nurses were able to give advice on how patients could look after themselves. In September 2000 the Department of Health[28] announced a new seven year partnership with Axa Assistance to provide a £22 million national computer system for NHS Direct. It would ensure that there is consistency of advice for patients wherever they are telephoning from and would play a key part in developing plans for NHS Direct to work closely with other services, such as out of hours doctors' services and ambulance services.

Walk in clinics

In September 1999 a press announcement[29] publicised the setting up of more direct access clinics run by nurses, to which any person can go for assistance and advice on health care. Seventeen new clinics were announced bringing the number up to 36 in total. Their aim, in the words of the press release, was to

> 'offer quick access to a range of NHS services including free consultations, minor treatments, health information and advice on self-treatment. They are based in convenient locations that allow the public easy access and have opening hours tailored to suit modern lifestyles, including early mornings, late evenings, and weekends. The centres will have close links with local GPs ensuring continuity of care for their patients.'

The advantages to the public are clearly apparent – fast service, no wait, close to work, easy access, immediate advice, speedy prescriptions. Nevertheless there have been concerns about lack of communication with GPs (see Chapter 18 page 235) but many of the clinics are planned to be linked with GP surgeries through effective use of information technology.

In February 2000 the classification of nurses who could have powers to prescribe in the community was extended by statutory instrument[30] to include nurses assisting in the capacity of a nurse in the provision of services in a Walk-in Centre, as defined by the regulation (See Chapter 20).

Criticism by doctors

An adverse effect of both NHS Direct and the Walk in clinics, and one emphasised by critics in the BMA[31], is that they could weaken the role of primary care and the family practitioner and undermine what is seen as one of the most important benefits in our NHS. However it may be that, in the long term and with improved information technology where records are easily accessible, both these services could be linked in with the developing primary care groups. Ultimately they should be able to access records and information from the GP and the GP will receive information about any out of hours services provided, remaining accountable for the patient.

Additional funding of £20 billion

In March 2000 the Chancellor of the Exchequer announced that an additional £20 billion was to be given to the NHS over the next four years. Following this the Prime Minister set up a Cabinet Committee to agree and monitor the standards for performance within the NHS. He identified five areas for improvement.

- All parts of the NHS would be required to work to end bed-blocking and unnecessary hospital admissions.
- They would have to put systems in place to identify and root out poor clinical practice.
- More flexible training and working practices should be introduced and efforts made to ensure doctors do not waste time dealing with patients who could be treated by other care staff.

- Booking systems ensuring that patients with the most serious conditions get treated as quickly as possible should be adopted.
- They should also address prevention, with better health awareness programmes.

National Plan for the NHS

On 22 March 2000 the Prime Minister announced to the House of Commons that there were five challenges to be faced in the NHS. These are shown in Figure 21.4.

Figure 21.4 Challenges for the NHS.

- *Partnership:* making all parts of the health and social care system work better together and ensuring the right emphasis at each level of care
- *Performance:* improving both clinical performance and health service productivity
- *Professions:* increasing flexibility in training and working practices and removing demarcations in the context of major expansion of the health-care workforce
- *Patient care:* which has two components: ensuring fast and convenient access to services and empowering and informing patients so that they can be more involved in their own care
- *Prevention:* tackling inequalities and focussing the health system on its contribution to tackling the causes of avoidable ill-health

---

Following the Prime Minister's announcement, the Secretary for Health announced that he was setting up discussions with key professionals in the NHS to develop a National Plan based on these five challenges. He intended to establish six modernisation action teams with a specific remit to address variations in performance and standards across the care system.

National reporting of adverse health-care incidents

The Government published a press release on 13 June, 2000[32] on the setting up of a national system for the NHS to learn from experience, just like the aviation and other industries' experience of analyzing incidents and 'near misses'. The NHS was to set up a new national mandatory reporting system for logging all failures, mistakes, errors and near misses in health care. The press release announced the publication of a report, *An Organisation with A Memory*[33], written by an expert group chaired by Professor Liam Donaldson, Chief Medical Officer of the Department of Health. The then Health Secretary Alan Milburn gave strong support for the recommendations of the report and Professor Donaldson was to implement them immediately with the new system being in place before the end of 2000.

The recommendations of the report include:

- The introduction of a mandatory reporting scheme for adverse health care events and 'near misses' based on sound, standardised reporting systems and clear definitions
- The introduction of a single overall database for analyzing and sharing lessons from incidents and near misses, as well as litigation and complaints data to identify common factors and consider specific action necessary to reduce risks to patients in the future
- The encouragement of a reporting and questioning culture in the NHS which moves away from 'blame' and encourages a proper understanding of the underlying causes of failures
- Improving NHS investigations and enquiries and ensuring that their results are fed into the national database so the whole NHS can learn lessons.

Research suggests that as many as 850,000 adverse health-care events may occur each year in the NHS hospital sector. The financial cost of adverse events to the NHS is difficult to estimate, but undoubtedly major and probably exceeded £2 billion a year. One example of persistent failure to learn lessons is that of spinal injections. At least 13 patients have died or been paralysed since 1985 because a drug has been wrongly administered by spinal injection.

Target setting to reduce adverse health-care events
An Organisation with a Memory also recommends that the Department of Health should examine the feasibility of setting specific targets for the NHS to achieve in reducing the levels of frequently reported incidents:

- by 2001 reduce to zero the number of patients dying or being paralysed by wrongly administered spinal injections
- by 2005 reduce by 25% the number of instances of negligent harm in the field of obstetrics and gynaecology which result in litigation (these cases currently account for around half the annual NHS litigation bill)
- by 2005 reduce by 40% the number of serious errors in the use of prescribed drugs (these currently account for 20% of all clinical negligence litigation)
- by 2005 reduce to zero the number of suicides by mental health inpatients as a result of hanging from non-collapsible bed- or shower-curtain rails on wards (hanging from these structures is currently the most common method of suicide on mental health inpatient wards).

National Patient Safety Agency
In April 2001 the Department of Health published its proposals for establishing a National Patient Safety Agency which will run the mandatory reporting system for logging all failures, mistakes, errors and near misses across the health services[34]. The Department of Health's publication *Building a Safer NHS for Patients*[35] sets out details of the scheme together with recommendations for an improved system for handling investigations and inquiries across the NHS. It retained the targets set out above.

Implications for radiography and radiology
There are of course a considerable number of statutory requirements for reporting which are considered in Chapters 15 and 16 in relation to health and

safety, medical devices and radiation protection. This new system of national reporting will bring together in a single system all reported occurrences of untoward incidents so that the lessons can be learnt from them. Clearly the first stage would be to ensure that each individual department and directorate has an effective system of reporting which includes not only defective equipment, etc., but also mistakes and negligence by staff. It must be realised that many accidents may be found in the end to be the result of a recognised risk and are not necessarily evidence that there has been any failures in professional practice. Audit and standard setting and advice from professional bodies are considered in Chapter 23.

Bristol paediatric heart surgery inquiry

The Report of the inquiry[36] into the deaths of children during heart surgery in Bristol is likely to have a major impact upon standards and procedures within the NHS. Some commentators have suggested that in future, people will talk about 'before and after Bristol'. The inquiry has made significant and strong recommendations across a wide field of professional practice including:

● Respect and honesty
● A Health Service which is well led
● Competent health-care professionals
● The safety of care
● Care of an appropriate standard
● Public involvement through empowerment
● The care of children

These recommendations are likely to become the starting point for future reform for standards within health-care and the Commission for Health Improvement will have them in mind in carrying out its inspections.

Conclusion

There is no doubt that clinical governance, clinical effective practice, evidence based medicine, and the National Service Frameworks (NSF) will have an increasingly major impact upon health care. The future challenge for the Government is to impose high national standards across the country in the provision of health care but at the same time foster local decision making and local initiatives to ensure high morale and enterprise upon which developments within health care depend.

 Questions and exercises _____

1   To what extent are your professional actions supported by research as being clinically effective?
2   Examine the systems for reporting untoward incidents in your department. To what extent are they effective in ensuring accountability and improvements in the quality of the service?

3   What national standards or Audit Commission reports have been published in relation to your work? To what extent have their recommendations been implemented?

4   Do you consider that litigation and complaints have been reduced as a result of quality monitoring and audit in your department?

5   Obtain a copy of the report of the Bristol Inquiry and identify the extent to which your department has practices in accordance with its recommendations.

References

1   Department of Health (1997) *A New NHS: Modern Dependable* Cmnd 3807 HMSO, London

2   Department of Health Press Announcement (2000/0041) 20 January 2000

3   NHS Executive *Primary Care Trusts: Financial Framework* (December 1999) Catalogue No 10389

4   NHS Executive *Working Together: Human resources guidance and requirements for Primary Care Trusts* (December 1999) Catalogue No. 10390

5   NHS Executive *Primary Care Trusts: A Guide to estate and facilities matters* (December 1999) Catalogue No 10393

6   http://www.doh.gov.uk/coin.htm (or they can be viewed on the internet at http://tap.ccta.gov.uk/doh/coin4.nsf)

7   NHS Confederation Briefing *Primary Care Trusts – new guidance* (February 2000) Issue No 39

8   B. Hurwitz (1998) *Clinical Guidelines and the Law* Radcliffe Medical Press, Oxford

9   Department of Health (1998) *A First Class Service: Quality in the new NHS* DoH, London

10 Board of Faculty of Clinical Radiology (1999) *College Review of Radiology Services* (BFCR(99)4) RCR, London

11 NHS Executive (1999) *Clinical Governance: Quality in the new NHS*, HSC 1999/065

12 NHS Executive (1998) *A First Class Service: Quality in the new NHS.* HSC 1998/113

13 G. de Lacey, R. Godwin & A. Manhire (eds.) (2000) *Clinical Governance and Revalidation* Royal College of Radiologists, London No 250

14 North Lakeland Healthcare NHS Trust (2000) *Report of Independent Inquiry into Garlands Hospital* (March 2000) North Lakeland Healthcare NHS Trust and North Cumbria Health Authority

15 Healthcare Parliamentary Monitor Issue No 250 24 April 2000 page 3

16 Audit Commission (1997) *Improving your image, How to Manage Radiology Services More Effectively* The Audit Commission, London

17 *Bolam* v. *Friern Barnet Hospital Management Committee* [1957] 1 WLR 582

18 R. James (2000) The impact of NICE and CHI on cancer and radiology services *Radiography* (May 2000) Vol 6, pages 71–74

19 N. Goodman (2000) NICE and the new command structure: Some thoughts on evidence, competence and authority *Radiography* (February 2000) Vol 6, pages 3–7

20 S. Harrison (2000) NICE, CHI, clinical governance and health-care rationing *Radiography* (February 2000) Vol 6, pages 9–10

21 Department of Health (1999) *National Service Framework for mental health services* DoH, London

22 E. Peck, B. Grove & V. Howell (2000) Upsetting the Apple Cart whilst pulling it along the road: Implementing the National Service Framework for Mental Health *Managing Community Care* Vol 8, No 2 (April 2000)

23   Department of Health (2001) *The Manual of Cancer Service Standards* (January 2001) DoH, London

24   S. Brealey & A. Glenny (1999) A framework for radiographers planning to undertake a systematic review *Radiography* Vol 5, pages 131–146

25   D. Upton (1999) Clinical effectiveness: how much do radiographers know about it and what do they think of the concept? *Radiography* Vol 5, pages 79–87

26   University of Sheffield (1999) *Evaluation of NHS Direct first wave sites* Interim Report (March 1999)

27   Information leaflet published by NHS Direct (7 October 1999); NHS Direct 0845 4647

28   Department of Health Press Notice (11 September 2000)

29   Department of Health Press Release *Frank Dobson announces more NHS walk-in clinics* (30 September 1999) DoH, London

30   The National Health Service (Pharmaceutical Services) Amendment Regulations 2000 SI No 121 of 2000

31   GPs attack growth of walk-in surgeries *The Times* 1 October 1999

32   Department of Health (2000) *National System for NHS to learn from Experience* 2000/349 13 June 2000

33   Department of Health (2000) *An Organisation with a Memory: report of an expert group chaired by Professor Liam Donaldson Chief Medical Officer*, Department of Health, London (Copies are available from the Stationery Office, PO Box 29, Norwich NR3 1GN or from the Department of Health website http://www.doh.gov.uk.)

34   Department of Health Press release *National patient safety agency to be launched* (April 2001) DoH, London

35   Department of Health *Building a Safer NHS for Patients* (April 2001) DoH, London

36   Bristol Royal Infirmary Inquiry *Learning from Bristol: the report of the public inquiry into children's heart surgery at the Bristol Royal Infirmary 1984–1995* Command paper CM 5207 2001

Chapter 22
Employment Law

This chapter sets out the basic principles of employment law and how they relate to the practitioner.

The employment contract

As soon as an unconditional offer of employment (by the employer) or to be employed (by the employee) has been accepted by the other party, a contract of employment comes into existence. The contract may be subject to conditions, e.g. receipt of satisfactory references or a satisfactory medical examination. If these prove not to be satisfactory, then the contract will either not come into existence, or cease to exist.

As a result of the contract of employment both employer and employee have duties and rights. The source of these are:

- express terms (either agreed by the parties individually or resulting from collective bargaining procedures)
- implied terms
- terms set by statute.

Express terms

Some duties arise by express agreement between the parties. These would include the basic terms of the contract – title of the post, starting date, salary, holidays, sickness, pensions, etc. Some of these terms may have already been part of collective bargaining within the workplace either at national (through the Whitley Council bargaining procedures) or at local level.

An individual employee might also agree specific terms with the employer when commencing, e.g. that a previously booked holiday can be taken or that they can start the day an hour later than usual because of childcare commitments. Such terms are valid and enforceable, but written evidence of the agreement that the term is part of the contract of employment would be of considerable assistance to the employee in a claim that these terms were not being upheld.

Local bargaining

Most practitioners are employed by NHS trusts. A minority are employed in the private sector. Within the NHS the framework of collective bargaining under the Whitley Councils is gradually being dismantled as local bargaining replaces centrally negotiated terms and conditions. Practitioners need to ensure that they understand the principles of contract law and employment law in order to make maximum use of the system of local bargaining.

Implied terms

The law implies into a contract of employment certain terms which are binding upon both parties even though such terms were never expressly raised by the parties. Figure 22.1 lists the terms which would be implied by law as obligations upon the employer and Figure 22.2 lists the terms which would be implied by law as obligations upon the employee.

The basic principle is that where express terms cover the issue, terms will not have to be implied.

Fgure 22.1   Implied terms binding upon the employer.

(1)   A duty to take reasonable care for the health and safety of the employee, including the duty to ensure that the premises, plant and equipment are safe, that there is a safe system of work and that fellow staff are competent.
(2)   A duty to co-operate with the employee to enable him to fulfil his contract of employment.
(3)   An obligation to pay the employee.

Figure 22.2   Implied terms binding upon the employee.

(1)   A duty to obey the reasonable instructions of the employer.
(2)   A duty to act with reasonable care and safety.
(3)   A duty to co-operate with the employer, including the duty to account for profits, to disclose misdeeds and not to compete with the employer.
(4)   A duty to maintain the confidentiality of information learnt during employment.

In the case of a junior hospital doctor it was argued that there was an implied term that an employer would take care of its employees and not ask him to work an excessive amount of overtime[1]. In this case the junior doctor became ill as a result of the excessive amount of overtime he was asked to work.

Statutory rights

The employer does not have complete discretion over what terms he can negotiate with the employee. Various Acts of Parliament require the employer to recognise certain rights, known as statutory rights, to which the employee is entitled. The employer could offer terms which improve upon these rights, but not reduce the rights. Certain qualifying conditions stipulate which employees are entitled to benefit from these statutory rights.

Figure 22.3 sets out the principle rights given by statute.

***Figure 22.3* Statutory rights (Employment Rights Act 1996 and others).**

- Written statement of particulars
- Itemised statement of pay
- Time off provisions:
  ○ to take part in trade union (TU) duties and training
  ○ to take part in TU activities
  ○ to look for job or undergo training if made redundant
  ○ to attend ante-natal clinic appointments
  ○ to act as JP and certain public service duties
- Provisions relating to pregnancy and maternity (including pay)
- Sickness pay
- Health and safety rights
- Rights relating to TU membership and activities
- Bank holidays
- Guarantee payments
- Redundancy payment
- Medical suspension payment
- Rights under the Working Time Directive
- Rights under the Parental Leave Directive
- Rights of part-time workers right not to be treated less favourably

---

The Human Rights Act 1998 raises potentially new issues in the employment field since, in certain circumstances, an employee of a public authority or one exercising public functions may be able to argue that he is being treated in a inhuman or degrading way contrary to Article 3. In addition where civil rights and obligations are in dispute, a person is entitled to have a hearing by an independent and impartial tribunal under Article 6 (see Chapter 3).

Performance of the contract

Both parties under the contract of employment have a duty to fulfil the express, implied and the statutory requirements in the contract of employment. Failure by an employee to fulfil the contractual requirements could result in them facing disciplinary proceedings. Failure by the employer to fulfil its contractual obligations could result in an employee claiming that she has been constructively dismissed by the employer, i.e. the employer has shown an intention of no longer abiding by the contract of employment and this therefore gives the employee the right either to see the contract as ended by this breach of contract or of treating the contract as continuing but being able to claim damages or compensation for this breach of contract. Rights in connection with constructive dismissal are considered below.

It is a basic principle of contract law that one party to a contract cannot unilaterally change the terms of the contract without the consent of the other person. Thus an employer who requires an employee to work in a different capacity or in a different location could be seen as being in breach of the contract if the capacity and the location were express terms in the contract.

Termination of the contract:

A contract of employment can come to an end in the following ways:

- Performance
- Expiry of a fixed term contract
- Giving notice
- Breach of contract by one or other party
- Frustration.

Performance

A contract which specifies a specific service to be provided will come to an end when these services have been given.

Fixed term contract

A fixed term contract will come to an end at the passing of the specified time unless the contract is renewed.

Notice

Under the employment protection legislation the employee is entitled to a minimum length of notice terminating the job. The period depends upon the length of continuous service. However there will usually be agreed in the contract of employment notice provisions which are in excess of the statutory lengths. Where the employer dismisses an employee without regard to the lengths of notice, this constitutes a wrongful dismissal. Giving the correct length of notice to end a contract may still constitute an unfair dismissal by the employer (see below).

Breach of contract

By the employer
If the employer is in fundamental breach of the contract of employment, the employee might see herself as being constructively dismissed and bring an application for unfair dismissal (see below).

By the employee
Where an employee is in breach of contract the employer can, if the circumstances justify, see the contract of employment as at an end and dismiss the employee. The employee does however have the right to claim that the dismissal is unfair if the circumstances do not justify such action (see below).

Frustration

Where an event occurs which was not in the contemplation of the parties at the time the contract was agreed and this makes the performance of the contract impossible, then the contract will end by law without any requirement for the employer to terminate it, i.e. the performance of the contract is 'frustrated'. Each case depends on its own facts and the following events have been seen as frustrating and therefore bringing to an end a contract of employment – death, imprisonment, and blindness (in a pilot).

Protection against unfair dismissal

One of the most important statutory rights has been the right not to be unfairly dismissed. There was a requirement that employees had to have worked continuously for the same employer for two years for at least 16 hours a week, or for five years for at least eight hours a week. This requirement of two years continuous service was challenged and the Court of Appeal[2] ruled that, because fewer women than men could comply with the qualifying period, it was incompatible with the equal treatment enshrined in the Equal Treatment Directive of the European Community[3]. The qualifying period for bringing an unfair dismissal application has since been reduced from two years to one year of continuous service[4].

There are certain dismissal situations where no continuous service requirement exists and an application can be brought even though the employee has worked in that employment for less than a year.

- Dismissal in connection with TU activity and membership
- Dismissal in connection with pregnancy, childbirth, maternity or parental leave
- Dismissal in connection with discrimination
- Dismissal in connection with health and safety
- Dismissal for asserting a statutory right
- Dismissal for exercising a right under the Working Time Regulations or the Part-time Workers Regulations
- Dismissal for making a protected disclosure

Application for unfair dismissal ruling

If an allegation of unfair dismissal arises, and the employee has failed to win an internal appeal, an application to an employment tribunal can be made. The time limit for making such an application is three months from the date of dismissal.

The Advisory, Conciliation and Arbitration Service (ACAS) will contact the employee in an attempt to conciliate between the parties, so that a hearing of the case is unnecessary. ACAS has a general duty of promoting the improvement of industrial relations. It can provide advice on employment legislation and industrial relations and can also assist in the settling of disputes. It has also published a *Code of Practice* on the disciplinary practice and procedures in employment (revised 2000)[5]. From 4 September 2000 employers must comply with the revised Code. This requires that disciplinary rules and procedures are clearly set out and accessible to the employees. Failure by any employer to follow the ACAS guidelines will not make the employer liable to proceedings but this information could be used against the employer in evidence before an employment tribunal.

In new statutory rights which became effective on 4 September 2000, the employee has a right to be accompanied at a disciplinary and grievance hearing[6]. Failure by the employer to allow the worker to be accompanied or to rearrange a hearing (for up to five days) may lead to compensation payable by the employer of up to two weeks' pay.

Where disciplinary proceedings involve medical staff, there are specific guidelines issued by the Department of Health[7]. The Court of Appeal held that an employer disciplining and dismissing a doctor should use the definition of professional conduct set out in the Circular and if there were allegations of professional misconduct then the matter should go to an independent tribunal. Matters of a personal nature could be the subject of internal disciplinary action[8].

The employee must show that there has been a dismissal and not a resignation. A dismissal may be:

- an ending of the contract of employment by the employer;
- a constructive dismissal where the employee is able to regard the contract as ended by the employer's fundamental breach of contract; or
- the failure to renew a fixed term contract.

Defence to an unfair dismissal application

The employer must show the reason for the dismissal and the fact that the reason is recognised in law as capable of being a reason for dismissal. He must also show that he acted reasonably in treating this statutory reason as justifying the dismissal. The statutory reasons that can render a dismissal fair are:

- Conduct
- Capability
- Redundancy
- Going on strike
- Legal impossibility
- Another substantial reason

The factors which are taken into account in determining the reasonableness of the dismissal and the employer's action are

- Consistency
- Following the ACHS Code of Practice
- Clarity
- Hearing the employee's case
- Allowing the employee to be represented
- Giving a series of warnings
- Making a fair investigation of the facts

Case: *Watling* v. *Gloucestershire County Council*[9]

An occupational therapist in the NHS was warned not to engage in private work during his working week. He ignored the warning and continued seeing private clients. He was seen by a manager seeing a private client during his lunch break and was dismissed for gross misconduct. His dismissal was held by the tribunal to have been fair and he also failed in his appeal to the Employment Appeal Tribunal. His defence that he was doing no more than taking an early lunch was rejected on the grounds that lunch hours are for lunch and not for seeing private patients. The Employment Appeal Tribunal was satisfied that the employers has conducted a reasonable and fair enquiry into what had happened and that the decision of the Industrial Tribunal was beyond any sensible criticism.

Employee protection and health and safety

The Trade Union Reform and Employment Rights Act 1993 (now consolidated in the Employment Rights Act 1996) has given to the employee considerable protection against dismissal where the employee is taking action on grounds of health and safety. There is no continuous service requirement placed upon the employee to obtain protection against dismissal or any other action short of dismissal.

The criteria for judging the appropriateness of the employee's actions are 'all the circumstances including, in particular, his knowledge and the facilities and advice available to him at the time' (ERA 1996 section 100(2)).

A defence is available to the employer if the employee's actions were so negligent, that a reasonable employer might have dismissed him as the employer did (section 100(3)).

These provisions should give the employee much greater protection when bringing issues of health and safety hazards to the attention of the employer so that she should not be unfairly dismissed. These provisions have been strengthened by the insertion of new sections (sections 43A to 43L) into the Employment Rights Act as enacted by the Public Interest Disclosure Act 1998 which is considered below under Whistle-blowing.

Rights of the pregnant employee

Statutory rights given to the pregnant employee are:

● Time off to attend for antenatal care
● Maternity leave
● Maternity pay
● Right to return after confinement
● Protection against dismissal on grounds of pregnancy or childbirth
● Right to receive pay during suspension on grounds of pregnancy, recently given birth or breastfeeding.

The above rights are the rights given by statute. Many employers however give far more generous benefits than those given as a statutory right. The employee cannot, however, have both. The Whitley Council conditions are in many ways superior to the statutory rights for those who have been in employment for more than two years.

Parental leave

A new right is given by the Employment Relations Act 1999[10] to enable either parent to be absent from work for the purpose of caring for a child or making arrangements for the child's welfare[11]. The right can be claimed by an employee who has a baby or adopts a child after 15 December 1999 and who has completed one year's continuous service with their employer by the time they wish to take leave. Anyone satisfying the conditions can have unpaid leave of up to thirteen weeks per child. Parental leave can be taken any time up to the child's fifth birthday, or five years after the adoption takes place, or in the case of a child with a disability, living with the parent, up to the child's 18th birthday.

The parent is entitled to return to the same job as before if the leave is for less than four weeks, or a similar job if the leave was for longer than four weeks. Procedures can be agreed between employer and employees for the details of parental leave. An employee who has been refused parental leave can take a case to the employment tribunal.

Time off for dependants

From 15 December 1999, reasonable time off is permitted where it is reasonable for an employee to deal with a domestic incident[12]. This includes when a dependant is ill, gives birth or is injured, when a dependent dies, unexpected disruption of arrangements for the care of the dependant, or an incident at school. The employee must notify the employer of the reason for the absence as soon as is reasonably practicable and how long it is likely to be. 'Dependant' includes a spouse, a child, a parent, a person who lives in the same household as the employee (other than a tenant or lodger) and includes any person who reasonably relies on the employee for assistance when ill or injured. An employer's refusal to give time off for dependants could be followed by an application by the employee to an employment tribunal.

Neither the parental leave right nor that of time off for dependants give a right to paid leave.

Rights in relation to sickness

Employees are entitled to receive statutory sick pay from their employer when they are sick. Those who are not in work or are self-employed may be able to claim state incapacity benefit instead. These include sickness benefit, invalidity benefit, and severe disablement allowance.

Statutory sick pay is payable for up to 28 weeks incapacity. Many employees receive superior sickness benefits under their contracts of employment. In the NHS most employees with the necessary continuous service have, under Whitley Council conditions, had six months full pay and six months half pay to cover sickness.

Hours of work

Working time regulations

These regulations were introduced following EC Directives[13]. Employers are subject[14] to restraint on the maximum average weekly working time and the average normal hours of night workers. There are also requirements on the provision of health assessments for night workers, rest breaks and entitlement to annual leave[15]. There has been criticism that the Directive was not fully implemented in the regulations and in February 2001 the Advocate General of the European Community ruled that the United Kingdom's requirement of a 13 week period of continuous service before there was an entitlement to annual leave was unlawful.

Guidance is provided by the Society of Radiographers on the implementation of the Working Time Directive[16].

Part-time workers

On 1 July 2000 regulations came into force to prevent part-time workers being treated less favourably than full time workers[17], implementing the European Directive[18]. Paragraph 5 of these Regulations gives the part-time worker

'the right not to be treated by his employer less favourably than the employer treats a comparable full-time worker —
(a)   as regards the terms of his contract; or
(b)   by being subjected to any other detriment by any act, or deliberate failure to act, of his employer.'

The right applies only if the treatment is on the ground that the worker is a part-time worker and the treatment is not justified on objective grounds. The part-time worker has to compare himself with full-time workers working for the same employer. The right also applies to workers who become part-time or, having been full-time, return part-time after absence, to be treated not less favourably that they were before going part-time. It does not give an employee the right to insist on having part-time work.

The Regulations (Paragraph 6) also entitle workers who consider that they have been treated in a manner which infringes this right, to request from their employer a written statement giving particulars of the reasons for the treatment. The worker must be provided with a statement within twenty-one days of his request. Failure to provide a statement at all or only in an evasive or equivocal way will enable the tribunal to draw any inference which it considers just and equitable to draw, including an inference that the employer has infringed the right in question. The regulations also protect the part-time worker from unfair dismissal and give a right not to be subjected to any detriment (Paragraph 7).

Workers who considers that their rights have been infringed can present a complaint to an employment tribunal within three months of the day of the matter complained of taking place. This is subject to the right of the tribunal to consider out of time cases if, in all the circumstances, it is just and equitable to do so.

At present employees do not have a right to insist on working part-time, but a task force has been set up by the Government to examine the possibility of introducing legislation to create a qualified right with appropriate defences for employers.

Protection against discrimination

Race and sex discrimination

The main legislation protecting persons against discrimination over race and sex are the Race Relations Act 1976 and the Sex Discrimination Act 1975 and subsequent amendments. The Sex Discrimination Act 1986 equalised the position of men and women in relation to retiring age following a decision of the European Court[19]. The Equal Pay Act 1970 implies an equality clause into any employment contract, that a woman employed on like work to a man is entitled to have similar terms and conditions. The Race Relations (Amendment) Act 2000 strengthens the duty on public authorities to promote equality of opportunity and good race relations.

The basic principles under the race and sex discrimination laws, and these apply both within and outside the employment field, are shown in Figures 22.4 and 22.5.

Figure 22.4 **Principles of protection against discrimination on grounds of race.**

Basic principle
Discrimination on grounds of colour, race, nationality or ethnic or national origins is unlawful.

Direct discrimination
This occurs where one person treats another less favourably on racial grounds than he would treat a person of another race.

Indirect discrimination
This exists when an employer applies a requirement or condition which, although applicable to all people, is such that a proportion of people of one race who can comply with it is smaller that the proportion in another, or where the employer cannot show that the requirement is justifiable on other than racial grounds and it is to the detriment of the complainant because she cannot comply with it.

It is also unlawful to victimise or segregate on grounds of race.

Exempt areas
- Genuine occupational grounds (e.g. the essential nature of the job requires a particular physique and authenticity, like playing the Moor in *Othello*)
- National security
- Charitable trusts

Other provisions
It does not apply to immigration rules, or civil service regulations.

Enforcement
This is through an application to an employment tribunal.

Assistance can be provided by the Commission on Racial Equality (CRE) which has a statutory duty to work towards the elimination of discrimination, to promote equality of opportunities and to keep the Race Relations Act under review. The CRE can itself take action in relation to advertisements which indicate an intention to discriminate. It has the power to seek an injunction to prevent discrimination on racial grounds.

Figure 22.5 **Principles on protection from discrimination on grounds of sex.**

Basic principle
To treat a person less favourably on the grounds of sex than a person of the other sex would be treated is unlawful. It is also unlawful for an employer to discriminate against a person on grounds of marital status.

Indirect Discrimination
This occurs where an employer applies a requirement or condition which, even though it applies equally to all persons, is such that a proportion of people of one sex who can comply with it is considerably smaller that the proportion in the other and where the employer cannot show justification on other than sexual grounds, and is to the detriment of the complainant.
    It is also unlawful to victimise or segregate on grounds of sex.

Exempt areas
● Genuine occupational qualification:
    ○ essential nature of the job requires a person of a different sex
    ○ authenticity, decency and privacy
    ○ personal services
    ○ work abroad which can only be done by a man
    ○ the job is one of two held by a married couple.
● National security
● Work in private households
● Charitable trusts
● Ministers of religion
● Sports and sports facilities
● police and police cadets (in respect of certain terms only)

Enforcement
This is through an application to an employment tribunal
    Like the CRE the Equal Opportunities Commission (EOC) has a duty to work towards the elimination of discrimination and in promoting the equality of opportunities. It keeps the Sex Discrimination Act under review and can bring action itself in the event of advertising which indicates an intention to discriminate unlawfully. It cannot also bring an action for an injunction to prevent a person discriminating unlawfully.

A test case[20] on the Equal Pay Act 1970 was brought by speech therapists who claimed that they were employed on work of equal value with male principal grade pharmacists and clinical psychologists employed in the NHS whose salaries exceeded theirs by about 60%. The Court of Appeal referred the case to the European Court of Justice[21]. This decided that the fact that differences in pay were mainly arrived at through collective bargaining is not sufficient objective justification for the difference in pay between the two jobs. It is for the national court to determine, whether and to what extent the shortage of candidates for a job and the need to attract them by higher pay constitutes an objectively justified economic ground for the difference in pay between the jobs in question. Subsequently the Court of Appeal held that the speech therapist was entitled to receive the same pay as a male comparator was currently earning[22].

Disability discrimination

The Disability Discrimination Act was passed in 1995. It is coming into force in stages and will, when fully implemented, give the disabled person certain rights in relation to employment, pensions and insurance, the provision of goods and services, and access to premises, education and public transport. The main provisions of the Act are set out below in Figure 22.6

Figure 22.6 **Disability Discrimination Act 1995.**

Part I   Definitions of disability and disabled person.

Part II   Employment: discrimination by employers, enforcement provisions, discrimination by other persons, occupational pension schemes and insurance services.

Part III   Discrimination in other areas: goods, facilities and services, premises, enforcement

Part IV   Education.

Part V   Public transport: taxis, public services vehicles, rail vehicles.

Part VI   National Disability Council.

Part VII   Supplemental: Codes of Practice, victimisation, help.

Part VIII   Miscellaneous.

Definition of disability

The Disability Discrimination Act 1995 defines a person as having a disability if

'he has a physical or mental impairment which has a substantial and long-term adverse effect on his ability to carry out normal day-to-day activities.'

Certain conditions are excluded from the definition of disability, including addiction to alcohol, nicotine or any other substance (unless the result of medical treatment), the tendency to set fires, steal, and to physically or sexually abuse other persons, exhibitionism and voyeurism, and seasonal allergic rhinitis[23].

Guidance has been issued by the Secretary of State about the matters which must be taken into account in the application of this definition together with a Code of Practice issued under section 53 of the Act[24].

Employment

In Part II, which covers discrimination in employment, it is made unlawful for an employer to discriminate against a disabled person (i.e. unjustifiably treat the disabled person less favourably) in arrangements for recruitment, and also in the terms of employment which are offered, including opportunities for promotion and training and other benefits. The disabled employee is also protected against dismissal or other detriment. Regulations have been made to cover these provisions and also to define further the duties of the employer in relation to physical arrangements[25].

The disabled person has the right to apply to an Employment Tribunal over any discrimination. There are also provisions covering discrimination of contract workers and discrimination by trade union organisations. Discrimination in the operation of occupational pension schemes and insurance services is also made illegal. The Department for Education and Employment (DfEE) has issued guidance for employers[26]. Annex B of this gives practical suggestions for avoiding discrimination in recruitment and employment. They include:

- Do not make assumptions
- Consider whether you need expert advice
- Plan ahead
- Consult
- Specify the job carefully
- Be able to justify any health requirement
- Think ahead for interviews
- Only ask about a disability if it is relevant
- Be fair

Generally employers should review recruitment, promotion and career development arrangements with the provisions of the Act in mind.

Goods, services and transport

Part III covers discrimination in the provision of goods, facilities and services. From 2004 it will be unlawful for a provider of services to discriminate against a disabled person by refusing to provide him with services, or in relation to the standard or terms of the service. There is a duty on service providers to take such steps as are reasonable to make alterations to buildings and the approach or access, and to provide auxiliary aids, such as audio tapes or sign language. Regulations determine what is reasonable and give guidance on the implementation of this duty.

Taxi accessibility regulations ensure that disabled persons and persons in wheel chairs can get into and out of taxis safely and also be carried in safety and in reasonable comfort. Taxi drivers also have a duty to carry the guide dogs and hearing dogs of passengers without making an additional charge. Regulations also cover public service vehicles and the access and carriage of disabled persons and wheelchairs.

The NDC and the Disability Rights Commission

Part VI establishes the National Disability Council (NDC). This Council, following consultation, advises the Secretary of State on relevant matters as requested, and prepares Codes of Practice. Unlike the Equal Opportunity Commission it will not have the power to take cases to an industrial tribunal. This role is taken by the Disability Rights Commission.

The Disability Rights Commission Act 1999 established the Disability Rights Commission in April 2000. The Commission employs 20 lawyers to assist those who claim that they have been discriminated against on account of their disabilities. The aim of the Commission is to attempt to resolve disputes through mediation, but it will bring cases to the courts and thus there will be established a body of case law on the rights of disabled people. The Commission will also provide information and advice to employers about how to meet their responsibilities under the 1995 Act.

It estimated that there are about 8.5 million disabled people in Britain, of whom about 2.6 million are unemployed or on benefits[27]. The Disability Rights Commission has been asked by the Government to draw up a Code of Practice to guide businesses on complying with the 2004 provisions on the Part III laws relating to the provision of goods and services.

Rehabilitation of Offenders Act 1974

The aim of this Act is to prevent discrimination against those who have had criminal convictions. It works by regarding certain offences as 'spent' after a certain length of time. This means that the person does not have to disclose the offence and to dismiss an employee on grounds that she failed to disclose a spent offence is automatically unfair. However the Act does not apply to serious crimes and many occupations are excluded from its effect including health service employment[28]. Under Schedule 1 to the Statutory Instrument, all members of any profession coming under the aegis of the Professions Supplementary to Medicine Act 1960 are excepted from the provisions of the 1974 Act and no convictions considered spent. All convictions will remain on the record. All radiographers and doctors are excluded from the provisions of the 1974 Act.

Trade unions

The protection and immunities which trade unions and their members enjoyed in the 1970s and 1980s have been eroded until they have very few rights in relation to protection as a result of industrial action. Industrial action itself is defined in narrow terms if it is to be construed as 'lawful'. Rules are laid down in relation to the holding of elections, and also for secret ballots before a strike can commence. Secondary industrial action is prohibited so that trade unions are not immune from liability for the effects of any secondary action. The individual citizen has been given a right to prevent disruption to his supply of any goods or services because of unlawful industrial action. If he can show that he has been or will be deprived of goods or services and that the industrial action is unlawful then he can apply to the court of an order to restrain the action.

The Employment Relations Act 1999, when fully implemented, will introduce a number of reforms to employment and trade union law as a result of the White Paper *Fairness at Work*[29]. There are new procedures for the recognition and derecognition of trade unions as being entitled to conduct collective bargaining on behalf of groups of workers. The Act also introduced new maternity rights, a right to leave for domestic reasons and the right to paternity leave (see above).

The reader is referred to one of the many specialist books on employment for further information on trade union rights and duties.

Whistle blowing

This is the term which refers to a person (usually an employee) who draws attention to concerns which have health and safety implications. Because of a fear that such persons, many of whom had a professional duty to draw attention to dangers and hazards, would be victimised as a result of their actions, the Department of Health issued a circular recommending that each Trust and authority should set up a procedure whereby an individual employee could draw these concerns to the management internally without being victimised and thus not needing to bring in the media or other external bodies.

The need to establish statutory protection for employees who raise concerns led to the passing of the Public Interest Disclosure Act 1998.

The Public Interest Disclosure Act 1998

The Public Interest Disclosure Act received the royal assent on 2 July 1998 and came into force on 2 July 1999 and introduces amendments to the Employment Rights Act 1996. The explanatory memorandum envisages that the Act will protect workers who disclose information about certain types of matters from being dismissed or penalised by their employers as a result. The Act applies to specific disclosures relating to:

- crimes
- breaches of any legal obligation
- miscarriages of justice
- dangers to health or safety
- environmental damage

and to concealing the evidence relating to any of these matters.

To qualify for protection, the worker making the disclosure must:

- make the disclosure to the employer or to another person to whom the failure relates or who has legal responsibility and
- be acting in good faith

Protected disclosures include:

- disclosures made to obtain legal advice
- disclosures to a Minister of the Crown (if the employee's employer is appointed by the Crown).

The Secretary of State has the power to make an order identifying other organisations or persons to whom a protected disclosure could be made provided that the employee makes it in good faith and reasonably believes that any allegations are substantially true.

Other disclosures are protected subject to specified conditions. These disclosures would include disclosures to the press, police, media and MPs. The specified conditions are that the worker:

- makes the disclosure in good faith
- reasonably believes that the information disclosed, and any allegation contained in it, are substantially true
- does not make it for personal gain and
- in all the circumstances of the case, it is reasonable for the worker to make the disclosure.

Such disclosure outside the employer's organisation can only be made if:

- the worker believes that she would be subjected to a detriment by the employer if she were to make the disclosure to the employer or the Secretary of State
- she fears that evidence will be concealed or destroyed or
- she has previously made a disclosure of substantially the same information to the employer.

The reasonableness of the employee's actions are judged in relation to:

- the person or body to whom the disclosure was made
- the seriousness of the relevant failure
- whether the disclosure was made in breach of a duty of confidentiality
- any action which the employer or other person could have taken when first notified
- whether the worker followed the procedure.

Any provision in an agreement between employer and worker is void if it purports to preclude the worker from making a protected disclosure.

Guidance[30] has been issued by the Department of Health which requires every NHS trust and Health Authority to have in place local policies and procedures which comply with the provisions of the Act.

In one of the first cases to be reported after the coming into force of the Act, compensation of more than a quarter of a £ million was awarded.

Case: Compensation for a whistle blower[31]

> An accountant who was dismissed after blowing the whistle on his managing director's expenses claims was awarded compensation (relating to his salary) of £293 441 by an employment tribunal. The Tribunal held that he was victimised by his employers for raising genuine concerns.

Criminal actions by health staff

Following the offences by Beverly Allit, the Clothier Inquiry made several recommendations

- to detect the possibility of personal disorder in applicants for nursing posts
- to set up procedures for management referrals to Occupational Health and
- to clarify the criteria for the triggering of such referrals.

There would therefore be a duty on any employee who suspects that a colleague is acting suspiciously to advise the appropriate manager.

The Clothier recommendations were reinforced by an Inquiry chaired by Richard Bullock following the case of Amanda Jenkinson, a Nottinghamshire nurse who was jailed for harming a patient. The Government have accepted the recommendations that all NHS staff will have a pre-employment health assessment. Information provided to Occupational Health staff will remain confidential unless disclosure is necessary because a member of staff is considered to be a danger to patients, other staff or themselves. In these circumstances there should be disclosure to the appropriate person or authority.

The Shipman case

An Inquiry has been established following the conviction of Dr Shipman for 15 murders of patients. At the time of writing, the report of the Inquiry is awaited.

On 1 June 2000 the NHS Executive issued a circular giving guidelines on the procedures to be followed in the appointment of hospital and community medical and dental staff[32]. Trusts are required to include in application forms by 31 July 2000 a declaration to be completed by all applicants (including locums) on whether or not they have been the subject of fitness to practise proceedings here or abroad and whether they have been the subject of a criminal investigation here or abroad. (The guidance was prompted by the discovery that a doctor who was guilty of professional misconduct in relation to a woman had been struck off the Register in Canada 15 years before.)

Grievance procedures

As stated above the Department of Health has recommended that each Trust should provide a procedure to ensure that an employee can raise any concerns to the awareness of senior management without suffering victimisation. The jurisdiction of the Health Service Commissioner does not extend to complaints and grievances of staff (see Chapter 19) but it may be that the Commission for Health Improvement set up under the White Paper proposals will be receptive to complaints from staff where these relate to deficiencies in the standards of care available to patients.

Future changes in employment law

Major changes have taken place in the law relating to employment as the result of the European Directives. The White Paper *Fairness at Work*[29] set out proposals for major changes in employment law most of which have now been implemented. However there is currently pressure upon the UK Government to implement wider employment rights which are set out in the European Community's Charter of Fundamental Social Rights.

The Employment Rights (Dispute Resolution) Act 1998 substituted the name employment tribunal for industrial tribunal and will when fully implemented introduce provisions designed to speed up the hearing of complaints. These include:

- cases which can be heard by a chairman alone
- certain matters being dealt with by a legal officer alone
- non-lawyers being able to enter into compromise agreements
- an alternative method for resolving disputes about employment rights by means of a new voluntary arbitration scheme.

ACAS is empowered to draw up an arbitration scheme.

Over the next few years there will continue to be significant changes in the laws relating to employment as workers' rights are expanded across the European Community and the Government's White Paper *Fairness at Work* is fully implemented. In implementing the NHS Plan[33], 'NHS Professionals' was introduced by the Department of Health in November 2000. It is a national scheme for managing and providing temporary staffing services. The key characteristics of

NHS Professionals is set out in a circular[34]. The initiative will be implemented nationally from 2001 to 2003 and is likely to have an impact on more flexible working and lead to greater uniformity in the payment of bank and agency staff. NHS Professionals is seen by the Government as being part of a whole systems approach modernising human resource systems in the NHS. It will link into the new NHS HR/Payroll system and with NHS Careers (a national service to provide information about careers in the NHS) and a new e-pensions service being developed by the NHS Pensions Agency. Such developments are likely to have a major impact on the human resources function of individual NHS trusts and health authorities.

 ## Questions and exercises

1   What rights do part-time employees have?
2   Look at the letter setting out your contract conditions and identify the source of each term, i.e. statutory, expressed as a result of personal agreement, expressed as a result of collective bargaining. What terms would be implied?
3   There are very few men who are employed as radiographers or assistants. What action do you consider your NHS trust could take to encourage the recruitment of more men, without breaking the law on sex discrimination?

References

1   *Johnstone* v. *Bloomsbury Health Authority* [1991] ICR 269
2   R v. *Secretary of State for Employment, ex parte Seymour-Smith and Perez* [1995] IRLR 464
3   EEC Equal Treatment Directive 76/207, Articles 1(1), 2(1) and 5(1) 1976
4   Unfair Dismissal and Statement of Reasons for Dismissal (Variation of Qualifying Period) Order 1999 SI No 1436 of 1999
5   Employment Protection Code of Practice (Disciplinary Practice and Procedures) Order 2000 SI No 2247 of 2000
6   Employment Relations Act 1999, Sections 10–15 (Commencement No 7 Order 2000)
7   Department of Health (1990) *Disciplinary proceedings for hospital and community medical and dental staff* Circular HC(90)9 DoH, London
8   *Saeed* v. *Royal Wolverhampton Hospitals NHS Trust* The Times Law Report, 17 January 2001
9   *Watling* v. *Gloucestershire County Council* Employment Tribunal EAT/868/94 17 March 1995; 23 November 1994, Lexis transcript
10   Employment Relations Act 1999, Schedule 4, Part I, paragraphs 76–80
11   Maternity and Parental Leave Regulations 1999 SI No 3312 of 1999
12   Employment Relations Act 1999, Schedule 4 Part II
13   Council Directive 93/104/EC; and Council Directive 94/33/EC
14   *Broadcasting, Entertainment, Cinematographic and Theatre Union (BECTU)* v. *Secretary of State for Trade and Industry* Case C-173/99, Opinion of Advocate General
15   B Dimond (1999) Working Time Regulations and the midwife *British Journal of Midwifery* (April 1999) **7**, 4, 232–4

16   Society of Radiographers *Working Time: A guide to the implementation of the Working Time Regulations in the NHS* (no date)

17   The Part-time workers (Prevention of Less Favourable Treatment) Regulations 2000 SI No 1551 of 2000

18   Directive 97/81/EC Part-time Work Directive, as extended to the UK by Directive 98/23/EC

19   *Marshall* v. *Southampton and SW Hampshire AHA* [1986] 2 All ER 584

20   *Enderby* v. *Frenchay Health Authority and the Secretary of State for Health* [1991] IRLR 44

21   *Enderby* v. *Frenchay Health Authority and Health Secretary* (C-127/92) October 1993 ECJ *Current Law* 1994, 4813

22   *Enderby* v. *Frenchay HA and the Secretary of State for Health (No 2)* [2000] IRLR 257 CA

23   Disability Discrimination (Meaning of Disability) Regulations 1996 SI No 1455 of 1996

24   Disability Discrimination (Guidance and Code of Practice) (Appointed Day) Order 1996 SI No 1996 of 1996; see website of the DDA and helpline:www.disability.gov.uk, 0345 622 622 or 0345 622 644

25   Department for Education and Employment *Code of Practice for the elimination of discrimination in the field of employment against disabled people or persons who have had a disability.* Stationery Office, London

26   DfEE (1999) *Disability Discrimination Act 1995: What employers need to know* Stationery Office, London

27   A. Frean (2000) Disabled rights group launched *The Times* 20 April 2000

28   Rehabilitation of Offenders Act 1974 (Exceptions) Order 1975 SI No 1023 of 1975

29   Department of Trade and Industry (1998) *Fairness at Work* (May 1998) Stationery Office, London

30   DoH (1999) *Public Interest Disclosure Act* HSC(99)198.

31   J. Booth (2000) Man who shopped boss wins £290,000 *The Times*, 11 July 2000

32   HSC 2000/019 *Appointment procedures for hospital and community medical and dental staff* (June 2000) DoH, London

33   DoH (2000) *The NHS Plan* Stationery Office, London

34   NHS Executive (HSC 2001/02) *NHS Professionals: Flexible organisations, Flexible staff* (February 2001) DH

Chapter 23
Departmental Management

Introduction

This chapter looks at the specific laws relating to departmental management. Other Sections of this book provide general information on the law relevant to departmental management and where necessary managers should be able to look for assistance from solicitors to the Trust and personnel officers or health and safety and other specialists employed within their organisation. Those clinicians who intend to take up a managerial role would find a book by Hugh Saxton[1], *Management in Imaging Departments*, of interest. Of more specific interest is the Audit Commission report on managing radiological services more effectively[2]. This is considered below.

Even though the internal market has, as such, been ended, much of the work undertaken at that time on specification for purchasers[3]; service level agreements[4]; writing a business case[5], contracting in clinical radiology[6] and advice on the private finance initiative[7] are still relevant to the successful development and resourcing of radiology departments.

Liability of a manager

A departmental manager will usually be a member of a registered profession and would therefore be personally accountable to the professional registration body for her professional conduct. The definition of professional conduct could also include her conduct as a departmental manager. In a recent case in Bristol, the Chief Executive of the Trust who was also a registered medical practitioner had to answer to the GMC for his conduct in managing the operations by paediatric cardiac surgeons (see below). In addition, of course, the manager will be personally liable for any criminal actions on her part and also may be guilty of a criminal offence if he or she has knowingly assisted in the criminal actions of others. Section 7 of the Health and Safety Act 1974 (see Chapter 15) enables an employee to be prosecuted in the criminal courts if he or she has failed to take reasonable care of his own or other employees' health and safety or has failed to co-operate in the implementation of the statutory functions placed upon the employer. A senior manager could be prosecuted for health and safety failings in his departmental management. Managers would also be contractually accountable to the employer if they have failed to obey reasonable instructions or failed to act with reasonable care and skill in the performance of their duties (see Chapter 22).

Situation: Liability of a manager

A senior radiographer who had charge of a department discovered that during her annual leave a basic grade radiographer had used defective equipment and as a consequence a patient was injured. Is the manager liable?

The principle of vicarious liability, which means that the employer is liable for the negligence of an employee whilst acting in the course of employment (see Chapter 14) does not apply to the relationship of senior to junior members of staff. Provided that work has been appropriately delegated and supervised, a senior is not liable for the negligence of a junior. In this situation the manager is not liable just because the basic grade practitioner has acted negligently. However the manager may be liable on her own account. How frequently was the equipment inspected? Who had the responsibility of maintaining it? Was she aware that the equipment was defective? If so, should she not have had it removed from the work place for repair and so that it could not be used inadvertently? If there is evidence that the manager has failed to follow a reasonable standard of care, then she would be personally and professional liable and the employer vicariously liable.

It follows too that any field of management which is the direct responsibility of the practitioner could, if she had failed in fulfilling her duties, result in her liability. Thus failure in ensuring a safe system of work, failure to draw the attention of senior management to any inadequacies in resources (including staffing and equipment) and failure to ensure that an appropriate system for determining priorities is established could all result in her personal liability and the employer would also be vicariously liable. A registered practitioner would also be held to account to the professional registration body for any professional misconduct indicated by the failures. In cases of gross misconduct there may be grounds for criminal prosecution as well.

Situation: Manager's responsibilities

A radiographer complains to the manager that she is receiving unwelcome attention from a patient. The manager tells her that this is an expected part of her work with patients and that she should try to ignore the problem. Unfortunately, the radiographer is assaulted by the patient when she is alone with him. She suffers significant injuries.

An inquiry would be undertaken into this incident. It is clear from the few facts given here that the manager acted entirely inappropriately and failed to take the situation seriously. The employee might well have grounds for suing the employer for compensation for the injuries which she suffered, because of the failure of the manager to take reasonable precautions to ensure the safety of the employee.

There will not always be a clear distinction between the role of the practitioner as manager and that person's role as a professional and the registered practitioner should be aware that she could be held to account in both roles.

Training and development as a manager

The fact that one has a professional qualification and is a state registered professional does not mean that one thereby has the personality, experience or skills necessary to be a successful manager. For example Tom Forbes and Neil James Paine[8] describe the role of radiographers as managers in the NHS. They examine how a group of radiographers developed management roles within the changing NHS and found that there was tension as a result of the role change from professional to manager. They noted that not all radiographers who have undertaken management roles are suited to this role and may be better placed to use their substantial clinical and organisational skills in clinical settings. They emphasised the importance of management development and training, which is essential if radiographer managers are to contribute to the performance of their NHS organisations. Exactly the same principles would apply to the work of a radiologist who moves from the clinical field to take on management responsibilities. It cannot be assumed that this move can be made without further training.

This kind of research undertaken by Forbes and Paine is essential in identifying the specific skills and post-registration training and development necessary before any practitioner could be expected to take on the legal responsibilities and liabilities of being a manager.

Managerial activities

Organisation and procedures

Ultimately the proper organisation of the department, the development of procedures and protocols, the audit and monitoring and implementation of recommendations from such audit are the responsibility of the manager.

C. Gunn and C.S. Jackson[9] provide advice to managers on the organisation of a department, the outlay and the minimum requirements, including information required for X-ray request forms and radiotherapy prescriptions.

Delegation and supervision

Central to the management of any department is the determination of who should be doing what, when and how. There can be primary liability on the part of a manager if inappropriate activities are given to staff who have not the experience or training to undertake them safely. The deployment of staff and decisions on the correct level of supervision necessary for those staff are therefore essential tasks for the manager.

Situation: Delegation and supervision

Lyn Roberts has been the manager of the radiography unit for two years. She asks a newly qualified radiographer to be responsible for a particular patient who needs a chest X-ray. She does not check that this radiographer is personally competent to perform this task.

The radiographer makes a mistake which no reasonable radiographer would have made. Who is liable?

In this situation, Lyn should be able to assume that a registered practitioner, even one who has recently qualified, should be competent to carry out basic tasks. If there are any doubts about a newly appointed member of staff's competence then clearly this should be checked out by the senior practitioners in the department. However there will be activities for which post-registration training and experience are necessary and before these are delegated the senior practitioner should make a personal assessment of the experience and knowledge of the radiographer for appropriate delegation. If no reasonable manager would have entrusted such an activity to that radiographer, then the employer would be vicariously liable for both the negligence of the manager and also the negligence of the radiographer which caused harm to the patient.

Advice has been provided by the RCR on *Delegation of tasks in Departments of Clinical Radiology*[10]. It gives examples of possible situations where delegation may be discussed:

- A referring doctor plans to delegate requests for radiological examinations to a nurse or nurses.
- A radiographer is to issue reports on imaging examinations.
- A clinical director, in the role of manager, is required by a more senior manager to implement a scheme which involves delegation but as a doctor cannot support the scheme for sound professional reasons.

The advice concludes:

> 'The interests of the patient are paramount. The risk and benefit analysis of a delegation policy must be clearly in favour of the initiative. The referring doctor and the responsible radiologist must retain responsibility throughout the delegation process. The Trust managers must be a party to any scheme involving delegation.'

Also of relevance is the RCR guide on *Medico Legal Aspects of Delegation*[11]. Standards of supervision go hand in hand with delegation. There will be some activities which cannot be delegated to a particular practitioner, there will be others where delegation would be permissible but only if a minimum level of supervision were provided (see Chapter 27 on the expanding role of the radiographer.) Health-care assistants, support workers and radiographic technicians are likely to have an expanding role within health-care. The consultation paper on the new Health Professions Council[12] stated that De Montfort University is conducting a study on behalf of the UK Health Departments into the role and function of support workers in health settings and those working in social care settings including the need for regulation to cover support workers. At the time of writing, its report is awaited.

Assistant practitioners in radiography

The use of assistant practitioners as part of a four tier career pathway in radiography was considered at a series of workshops held by the Society of Radiographers in March 2001[13]. It was envisaged that the assistant practitioner would undertake some radiographic tasks but different from those undertaken by a helper or radiography department assistant and would work under the supervision of a state registered practitioner who holds the responsibility for judgment and decision making. In this scenario the assistant practitioner would not therefore have the responsibility for justifying the exposure (see Chapter 16 and 27). Such a person would be an operator under the Ionising Radiation (Medicial Exposure)Regulations following procedures and protocols. The imaging role of an assistant would be limited to plain film radiography. It is envisaged that there would be a clear distinction between the operator and the registered practitioner.

Setting standards

If an activity is delegated then the standard which should be followed is the reasonable standard which should have been followed if the activity had not been delegated. The fact that the activity is carried out by a different professional or a less experienced member of staff or a person of a lower grade does not justify a lower standard of care. This was the principle laid down by the Court of Appeal in the case of *Wilsher* v. *Essex Area Health Authority*[14].

Managers have the responsibility in ensuring that standards within the departments are in keeping with the reasonable standard of care expected by the Bolam test (see Chapter 14). League tables across a wide range of specialties assist individual managers in analysing the quality provided in their departments in comparison with other hospitals. National Service Frameworks are also of assistance in setting standards.

Managerial liability

Whilst managers are not personally responsible for the professional misconduct of any individual staff member (unless they are personally at fault), the manager would be expected to take action if evidence came to light of professional misconduct. This would be required under her employment contract, and also in the civil law of negligence as part of the duty of care to patients.

It would also be required by the professional registration body. For example following the scandal of the deaths of children in Bristol following paediatric heart surgery, the manager was struck off the Register of the GMC for failing to take appropriate action to investigate the poor standards of care. This decision was upheld by the court in *Roylance* v. *General Medical Council*[15] when the Privy Council (the appellate court from professional body tribunal hearings) confirmed that serious professional misconduct could include failures by a Chief Executive, who was also a registered medical practitioner, because he did not respond to concerns about the professional standards of paediatric heart surgeons.

A&E reporting

The disgrace of A&E reporting is described by L.A. Williams[16]. He analyses a survey across the UK on the reporting of A&E films. He states that in 15 of the 250 hospitals, reporting was not done by a radiologist. In many of the other hospitals there was a wide variation in the type of reporting performed, e.g. only the chests, skulls and spines were reported. In others many days would pass between the time of the X-ray and the issuing of the report. He examines the reasons given for these facts – 'too much work and not enough staff', '95% are normal so what is the point?' or 'it is all rubbish anyway!'. The author describes his meetings with casualty staff to provide feedback from the cases to ensure that good practice can be maintained.

If harm were caused to patients as a result of defects in the reporting system, then there would probably be both vicarious liability by the employer for negligence of individual staff and also direct liability for failure to ensure that a safe effective reporting scheme was in existence.

Effective use of resources

The standards of the department which the manager must secure relate not only to high standards of clinical practice, but also to high standards of efficiency and effectiveness in utilising equipment and staff (see staffing and workloads below). Maximum use of expensive medical technology might require collaboration with other potential users of the equipment. Roger D.H. Ryall[17] writes of a management consultancy review of seven day working within a radiotherapy centre to make maximum use of a linear accelerator. He recommends the report to other centres[18].

Advice and guidance

Guidance provided by professional bodies

Organisations such as the Board of the Faculty of Clinical Radiology or the College of Radiography provide guidance to their members which would be incorporated into the Bolam test. If any practitioner failed to follow the guidance and harm were to occur, then the practitioner would have to show that there were exceptional circumstances why the guidance was not appropriate and that her actions would be supported by competent professional opinion. For example the *Good Practice Guide for Clinical Radiologists*[19] recognises the importance of self-regulation in the setting of standards, summarises for clinical radiologists existing RCR advice on good practice and the principles which underpin good practice in clinical radiology, and applies specific statements of the GMC to the particular working environment of clinical radiologists. The booklet covers national guidance, hospital and departmental responsibilities, individual responsibilities and maintaining good practice through audit, continuing professional development and education and revalidation.

Such publications as *The use of Computed Tomography in the initial investigation of common malignancies*[20], *The use of Imaging in the Follow-up of Patients with Breast Cancer*[21], *Guidance on Screening and Symptomatic Breast Imaging*[22] and a *Guide to the Practical use of MRI in Oncology*[23] would be quoted in court to provide evidence of the recommended practice. The latter document provides advice for the development of protocols but in the introduction states:

> 'The guidance deliberately avoids being too prescriptive since the flexibility of the MRI systems allows equally satisfactory results to be achieved using several different coils, sequences and imaging planes.'

Clinical governance and audit

Section 18 of the Health Act 1999 places upon each trust and health authority a duty to put and keep in place arrangements for the purpose of monitoring and improving the quality of health care which it provides to individuals (see Chapter 21). In practice, of course, the trust board will delegate the implementation of this duty to each director of clinical services who in turn will delegate certain responsibilities to departmental managers. The duty is two-fold:

● to make sure that monitoring arrangements are actually set up and
● to ensure that these are implemented and used effectively.

The Commission for Health Improvement (CHI) is taking on the responsibility for ensuring that the requisite standards are in place and has a programme of inspections for every Trust in the country, supplemented by additional inspections requested by the Secretary of State when areas of concern come to light (see Chapter 21). Failures in clinical governance can lead to a variety of sanctions including

● the removal of the Board, its chairman and chief executive
● sending in the CHI
● referral of a situation to the Director of Public Prosecutions or the Crown Prosecution Service
● referral to the registration body of any practitioner involved.

In addition the Secretary of State could set up an Independent Inquiry to investigate the circumstances and report.

Dr Ray Godwin[24], chairman of the clinical radiology audit sub-committee, identified the audit activities and processes which should be in place within departments of radiology. He refers to the College's clinical audit adviser[25] who can be contacted for advice and assistance.

The Audit Commission Report

In 1997 the Audit Commission reported on radiology services[2]. Amongst its recommendations it suggested that there should be:

● Negotiation and publication of agreed referral guidelines between clinicians and GPs.
● Proposals to secure good quality management information and to use it to modify departmental organisation.
● The provision of a better quality of service by establishing agreed standards to monitor performance.
● Institution of 'hot reporting' systems and other methods of achieving quality performance.
● More systematical planning of departmental business development and equipment replacement over periods of 5–10 years.
● Presentation of robust business cases for major investment.

It is probable that at present these recommendations have not been implemented in all hospitals. If a claimant could establish that harm has occurred because of such failures then he would have a *prima facie* case for obtaining compensation from the NHS trust. The Commission for Health Improvement on its visits to each hospital will have regard to national recommendations for good practice such as those published by the Audit Commission and the Royal Colleges.

Protocols, procedures and guidelines

In order to implement the duty of quality, protocols, procedures and guidelines may be drawn up for each department across a variety of clinical activities. The manager should ensure full consultation over the design of these guidelines since it is essential that they should conform to reasonable standards of care. Regular updating of these protocols would be required. Failure by the manager to ensure that protocols were in existence and that the department was organised effectively could lead to the liability of the manager, even when the latter is off duty. There are advantages in retaining obsolete guidelines, clearly marked as such and dated as to when they were in use. These old guidelines would be of assistance in the event of any litigation relating to incidents at the time these guidelines were operative. This is because the Bolam test (see Chapter 14) refers to the standards of care at the time of the alleged negligent actions, not those pertaining at the date the action is heard in court.

Areas where protocols or procedures would be advisable include some aspects of patient involvement identified by C. Gunn and C.S. Jackson. In their book on *Guidelines on Patient Care in Radiography*[9] they provide guidelines for departmental organisation and procedure, hygiene (including inflammation, infection and sterilisation instruments and dressings), management of patients and patient psychology, the care of the unconscious and anaesthetised patient, transportation of the patient, patient preparation, drugs and radiographic contrast agents, first aid, resuscitation, administration of oxygen, tracheostomy and suction, fractures, haemorrhage, and various conditions such as diabetes, colostomy and ileostomy, catheterisation and intubation, together with nursing procedures including temperature, pulse, respiration and blood pressure.

Risk management

Central to any health and safety strategy is risk management, both in clinical and non-clinical areas. The Department has provided advice on a risk management strategy in every area of hospital activity[26]. The Management of Health and Safety at Work Regulations[27] describe provisions for risk assessment and management in the workplace and are discussed in Chapter 15. It is the manager's responsibility to ensure that these regulations are implemented and that risk assessments are carried out in all the necessary areas of clinical and non-clinical practice. The manager would also have to ensure that documentation relating to the risk assessment and the action to be taken is completed and retained.

Reference should be made on the books on risk management including that edited by Charles Vincent[28]. In Chapter 3 of this book, James Reason[29] takes two radiological case studies to illustrate his theoretical framework for the stages of development of organisational accidents. One relates to a Therac-25 accident at East Texas Medical Centre which occurred in 1986 when a patient, as a result of a bug in the software, received a 25 000 rad blasts to his unprotected shoulder and saw a flash of blue light. He heard his flesh frying and felt an excruciating pain. He called out to the technician, but both voice and video intercom were switched off. The computer screen displayed a 'malfunction 54' error signal, which the technician took to mean that the beam had not fired, so she reset the machine and fired again and repeated this when the malfunction signal appeared again. The patient therefore had three 25 000 rad blasts to his neck and upper torso. He died four months later with gaping lesions on his upper body.

The second case study, which took place in Indiana Regional Cancer Centre in 1992, concerned an elderly patient with anal carcinoma who was treated with five catheters into each of which was inserted an iridium-192 source (4.3 curie, $1.6 E + 11$ becquerel). The iridium source was placed in four of the catheters without apparent difficulty but, after several unsuccessful attempts to insert the source wire into the fifth, the treatment was terminated. In fact a wire had been broken, leaving an iridium source inside one of the first four catheters. Four days later the catheter containing the source came loose, and eventually fell out of the patient. It was picked up and placed in a storage room by a member of staff of the nursing home who did not realise that it was radioactive. Five days later it was collected by a truck driver collecting the waste. After delay because of Thanksgiving it was then taken to a medical waste incinerator where the source was detected. This was nearly three weeks after the original treatment. The patient had died five days after the treatment session and over 90 people were irradiated in varying degrees by the iridium source.

The active and latent failures in these two case studies are examined by James Reason.

Every adverse incident, even where there have been no ill-effects, should be subjected to a review to establish the action which could reasonably be taken to ensure that such an incident does not reoccur. Risk assessment and management relates to resource management and staffing as well as health and safety issues which are considered below. The Government's introduction of a national system of reporting should lead to more effective risk management systems linked to identifiable risks[30]. This is further considered on pages 291–3.

Resource management

Increasingly budgets are devolved to managers to ensure effective expenditure. The manager would have a legal responsibility to stay within the budget or to notify the finance department and senior management if costs can only be contained at the expense of standards of care. It would be no defence to a claimant, who has been harmed as a result of a failure to follow the reasonable standard of care, that the resources were not sufficient to provide a suitable service. If funds are inadequate to provide a reasonable service, senior management would have to discuss with the funding body (health authority or department of health) a curtailment of the service.

Staffing issues

Workload

There are no staffing guidelines set by law, but the courts would require that staffing levels and skill mixes were such that a reasonable standard of care could be provided through out the department. Any research relating to the levels of staffing and workload would have to be brought into account in determining the reasonableness of particular staffing patterns. Levels of dependency and the complexity of the work are vital elements in the assessment of a reasonable workload.

Dave Nag[31] reports on a pilot survey to identify the nature and volume of work carried out in DGH hospitals in England. He provides statistics showing wide variations and warns of dangers of both under and over counting. He concludes that a DGH radiology department serving a population of 200 000 that finds its workload figures at the top end of the spectrum in all categories is likely to require at least two more consultants.

The RCR has published guidance on workload and manpower in Clinical Radiology[32]. It does not claim to provide a definitive or prescriptive statement on workload levels – it recognises that individuals work at different rates, but it does review methodologies which have been used in the past and it suggests a practical means of linking radiologists' workplans to workloads. Appendix B explains the Addenbrooke's Formula. It makes recommendations to ensure that a suitable balance between workload and manpower is achieved and can be maintained.

It is essential when determining workloads that all factors are taken into account. For example an open letter from the Executive Committee of the British Paediatric Radiology and Imaging Group[33] points out that where a radiologist has a major interest in paediatric radiology then her performance is likely to be much lower than that of other colleagues due to the extra length of time it takes to perform paediatric ultrasound, screening, CT, MR etc. The writers ask whether 'Is it not now time for such sub-speciality groups (in vascular, obstetric, geriatric or other intensive specialities) to agree their norms for average cases per session for specialist radiologists.'

Many radiologists may feel that they are working at levels in excess of the official recommendations and therefore they are practising unsafely. In such circumstances, they should make use of the whistle blowing circular to raise their concerns with senior management. There is a duty under the principle of clinical governance to set in place standards for quality assurance and monitor them and this applies to resources and workloads (see Chapter 21). In addition one of the lessons from the Bristol Report[34] relating to paediatric heart surgery is that staff should be prepared to make known their concerns about unsafe practice. If a practitioner, because of a workload in excess of official recommendations, was negligent and caused harm to a patient it would not be a defence to assert that there was too much work for a reasonable standard to be followed. The practitioner could be questioned by any inquiry, disciplinary hearing or professional conduct committee to ascertain what action she had taken to draw her concerns about workload to senior management.

Skill mix

Any review of appropriate staffing levels must consider the skills mix in any department. Advice has been provided by the RCR on skill mix[35]. It follows on the document published jointly by the RCR and the ScoR *Inter-professional roles and responsibilities in a Radiology Service*[36]. The advice on skill mix assesses the principles of proper delegation, the requirements for appropriate skill mix and the medico-legal responsibilities. It also warns of the pitfalls to be avoided:

- Inadequately defined lines of responsibility
- Compromised quality of training
- Insufficient numbers of trainers and trainees
- Fragmentation of care
- Failure to incorporate into consultant radiologists' job plans, extra time for review and reporting of delegated work
- Failure to extend services or techniques because of lack of knowledge or experience by the delegated operator
- Lack of resources
- Inter-professional rivalry
- Skill mix being seen as a substitute for the appropriate establishment of clinical radiologists
- Loss of flexibility

Out of hours working

Advice has been provided to Clinical Radiologists with regard to out of hours working by the Board of Faculty of Clinical Radiology and the Royal College of Radiologists[37]. It recommends that there should be a clear policy in each department on out of hours working which includes guidance on which examinations influence the immediate medical management of the patient. There should be an agreed portfolio of examinations which can be offered safely and reliably out of hours and consideration could be given to extending the normal working day with flexible hours (NB the significance of the Working Time Directive (see Chapter 22)). Increasing the number of consultant radiologists available might also be an option. The advice also recommends that consideration be given to the installation of a facility to review images or completed examinations in the home of the on-call clinical radiologist. It recommends:

> 'Careful monitoring, or audit, of out of hours work should be carried out on a regular basis in order to confirm the appropriateness of the work that has been carried out.'

The Society of Radiographers has also published guidelines on emergency duties out of hours[38]. It gives advice to members on renegotiating the rota for out of hours duties in the light of the removal of the contractual obligations to work out of hours (see also Chapter 22).

There appears to be no immediate solution to the shortage of registered practitioners in radiography and radiology although hopefully managing the recruitment, retention and coverage of staff in a department is likely to have been facilitated by the establishment of NHS Professionals in November 2000[39]. This national scheme for managing and providing temporary staffing services is mentioned in Chapter 22.

Safety issues

Whistle blowing and the Public Interest Disclosure Act 1998

It is a requirement under DoH guidance[40] following the Public Interest Disclosure Act 1998 that each NHS organisation has in existence a procedure which enables an employee who has concerns to bring these concerns to the attention of the appropriate officer. The departmental manager should ensure that this procedure is implemented in the department and is known by all staff. (See Chapter 22 for further consideration of this Act.)

Health and safety responsibilities and reporting

Statutory health and safety responsibilities which are placed upon the employer may be delegated to a departmental manager for implementation. It follows therefore that one of the most important activities of the manager would be the undertaking of a risk assessment (see above) in accordance with the Management of Health and Safety in the Workplace Regulations 1999. In addition the manager should be aware of any unreasonable stress being suffered by individual employees, should ensure that there is no bullying, and that the appropriate procedures are in place for staff to raise any grievances (see Chapter 15). The Medical Devices Regulations are considered in Chapter 17. The Departmental manager has clear responsibilities in relation to the implementation of these regulations and ensuring that all relevant adverse incidents are reported to the Medical Devices Agency. The responsibilities of ensuring that the RIDDOR reports are notified to the appropriate authorities will also fall upon the manager.

Cross infection – AIDS, HIV and hepatitis

In Chapter 15 a recent report by the National Audit Office[41] on hospital acquired infection (HAI) is considered. The Report suggested that HAI could be the main or a contributory cause in 20 000 or 4% of deaths a year in the UK and that there are at least about 100 000 cases of HAI with an estimated cost to the NHS of £1 billion. Clearly the departmental manager will have responsibilities in identifying the risks of cross infection and in ensuring policies on standards of sterility and infection control are implemented and monitored. This will include establishing procedures for health checks for staff and ensuring that any of their concerns about the risk of cross infections are speedily resolved.

Medicines

The proper storage, transport and supply of medicines which are used within the Department would be the manager's responsibility. The oversight of prescribing arrangements following the Crown recommendations will become a major managerial task (see Chapter 20).

Staff management

Giving instructions

The manager would have line responsibility for those who work in her department. An employer is entitled to expect that reasonable instructions given to an employee will be obeyed. However there may be issues relating to what is reasonable in the light of the professional practice of individual employees. If conflicts arise over what is or is not a reasonable instruction given by a manager, it is essential that this is resolved early, before it becomes a major concern within the department. Each organisation should have a grievance procedure where disputes over what is or not a reasonable instruction could be determined speedily.

Employment law

The departmental manager would be expected to have a basic understanding of the principles of employment law, employees' rights and discrimination rules in managing the department (see Chapter 22). In addition the manager should know where to obtain further advice and assistance. Good links with human resource directors within the organisation can significantly support the manager's role. This is particularly so where the manager is facing a problem of discipline or professional misconduct. There should be an organisational disciplinary procedure, and the manager should be familiar with this and be aware of those situations when a manager has the right to dismiss a member of staff instantly for gross misconduct. The manager would be required to give evidence in the event of a disciplinary hearing of any member of staff. It is also essential that the manager follows the correct procedures when dealing with misconduct, since early failures in this field could make an ultimate dismissal unfair.

References
If a reference is written negligently then liability can arise both to the recipient of the reference, if in reliance upon that reference he has suffered harm[42] and also to the person who is the subject of the reference[43]. Every care should be taken to ensure that it is written accurately in the light of the facts available.

Property
The manager will also be responsible for ensuring that procedures in relation to staff and patient's property are implemented. There may be occasions where patients or staff wish to entrust property to the safe care of the manager who would then be accountable for its loss or damage. If there are no local safe-keeping facilities, access to those in the General Office should be made available.

Multi-disciplinary working

Although multi-disciplinary working is the recommended practice within health care, the law does not recognise a concept of team liability. Each individual team member is personally and professionally accountable for her actions and could not use orders from the team as a successful defence to any action. The manager of any department would have significant responsibilities in ensuring that there were effective communications across different departments and clinical groups.

This issue has been discussed in a guest editorial in *Radiology* by Hazel Colyer[44] and Susan Dilly[45].

Inter-professional roles and responsibilities in a radiology service are recognised in a joint publication[46] of the RCR and the College of Radiographers which recognises that:

- The proper care of a patient within a radiology service depends on a multi-disciplinary team.
- Each member of the team must work within the law and comply with regulations imposed by their own statutory body and each should take account of advice from their professional organisations.
- The roles and responsibilities of each member of the team may not always be distinct and will vary from team to team.
- A good working relationship between team members will help to ensure that they take good care of the patient.

It is one of the main functions of the manager to ensure that there is effective team working and that roles and responsibilities are clarified.

In an editorial for *Clinical Radiology* R.W. Blamey[47] discusses the role of the radiologist in breast cancer from the perspective of a surgeon. He shows the developments following the Forrest Report[48] (which led to the introduction of the NHS Breast Screening Programme) led to major changes of practice, especially the introduction of specialist multi-disciplinary expertise. He concludes that team working stimulates other members to learn from each other and also encourages good communication. He sees multi-disciplinary working in this field as having improved diagnosis and standards of service delivery; it is also leading the way and setting the standards for workers in other cancers to follow.

The development of clinical networks in specific specialities such as cardiac care and cancer care present interesting challenges for management and accountability. These clinical networks cross organisation and professional boundaries and, to ensure that they can work effectively, careful consideration and planning of the delegation of responsibilities and decision making will be required.

Patients' rights

In addition to the above topics, a manager must ensure that all those rights of the patient considered in Chapter 3, in particular the Human Rights Act 1998, are protected and protocols and procedures relating to them are regularly audited and updated. Provisions for special groups such as children and mentally incapacitated adults and pregnant women must also be made. The printing of forms and information leaflets for patients and their regular updating will also be the manager's responsibility.

Handling complaints

Each department should have a complaints procedure which accords with the Government guidelines (see Chapter 19). It would be the manager's responsibility to audit the implementation of the complaints procedure and ensure that any corrective action was taken as a result of complaints being made. Most managers would also ensure that any informal issues are recorded and dealt with in an appropriate way even though the complainant did not wish to make a formal complaint.

Conclusions

A well run department will not only benefit the patients but also raise the morale of staff, who are more likely to be attracted to work there and also less likely to leave. The manager must be mindful that the potential for litigation increases the pressures and stress upon clinicians. Stuart Field, Chairman of the RCR Breast Group, reported[49] on a survey carried out by the RCR Breast Group on the workforce and morale within breast screening units. The findings were disturbing. For example 70% of respondents stated that they were concerned about litigation. Under 'morale' the comment was made that in a number of responses colleagues showed evidence of severe stress. The overall conclusion was that most of the concerns are related to lack of resources, both human and financial, and if these can be resolved then morale and fears of litigation would improve.

The manager undoubtedly has major challenges to overcome.

 Questions and exercises

1 You have just been appointed as a senior manager within your department. How does the law impact upon your new responsibilities?
2 A member of your staff has told you that she feels extremely pressured within the department, cannot sleep at night and feels that she is close to breaking point. What action would you take and how could you prevent a successful action for breach of the employer's duty to take reasonable care of the health and safety of an employee being brought by that member of staff (see also Chapter 15).
3 A student informs a member of staff (not yourself) that she has seen one of the radiologists helping himself to drugs kept in the department. She is threatening to blow the whistle. What action would you take as manager?
4 You are concerned about the standards of care provided in your department and have heard that an inspection from the Commission for Health Improvement is to take place next month. What action would you take to prepare for the visit and what powers could you expect the Commission to use? (see also Chapter 21)

References

1   H. Saxton (1998) *Management in Imaging Departments* Schering, Germany
2   Audit Commission (1997) *Improving your image, How to Manage Radiology Services More Effectively* The Audit Commission, London
3   Board of Faculty of Clinical Radiology (1995) *Clinical Radiology Quality Specification for Purchasers* (BFCR(95)7) RCR, London
4   Board of Faculty of Clinical Radiology (1998) *Service Level Agreements* (BFCR(98)4) RCR, London
5   Board of Faculty of Clinical Radiology (1997) *Clinical Radiology: Writing a Good Business Case* (BFCR(96)7) RCR, London
6   Board of Faculty of Clinical Radiology (1995) *Contracting in Clinical Radiology* (BFCR(95)5) RCR, London
7   Board of Faculty of Clinical Radiology (1996) *Advice on the Private Finance Initiative* (BFCR(96)5) RCR, London
8   T. Forbes and N.J. Paine (2000) Moving domains: radiographers as managers in the NHS *Radiography* (May 2000) Vol 6, pages 101–110
9   C. Gunn and C.S. Jackson (1991) *Guidelines on Patient Care in Radiography* Churchill Livingstone, Edinburgh
10 Board of Faculty of Clinical Radiology (1996) *Advice on Delegation of tasks in Departments of Clinical Radiology* (BFCR(96)4) RCR, London
11 Royal College of Radiologists (1993) *Medico Legal Aspects of Delegation* RCR, London
12 NHS Executive (2000) *Modernising Regulation The New Health Professions Council: A consultation document* (August 2000) Department of Health, London
13 News item (2000) Workshop explores role of Assistant Practitioner *Synergy* (June 2001)
14 *Wilsher* v. *Essex Area Health Authority* [1986] 3 All ER 801 CA
15 *Roylance* v. *General Medical Council* [1999] Lloyd's Rep. Med. 139 (PC)
16 L.A. Williams (1994) The disgrace of A&E reporting *RCR Issue No 39* (Summer 1994) page 19
17 R.D.H. Ryall (1994) Seven day Working in Radiotherapy Centres *RCR Issue No 39* (Summer 1994) page 19
18 Salter Baker and Associates Ltd *A review of linear accelerator capacity/cancer care* Botley Mill, Botley, Southampton SO3 2GB
19 Board of Faculty of Clinical Radiology (1999) *Good Practice Guide for Clinical Radiologists* (BFCR(99)11) RCR, London
20 Council The Royal College of Radiology (1995) *The use of Computed Tomography in the initial investigation of common malignancies* (RCR(95)1) RCR, London
21 Council of the Royal College of Radiology (1995) *The use of Imaging in the Follow-up of Patients with Breast Cancer* (RCR(95)3), RCR London
22 Board of Faculty of Clinical Radiology (1999) *Guidance on Screening and Symptomatic Breast Imaging* (BFCR(99)12) RCR, London
23 Board of Faculty of Clinical Radiology (1999) *A Guide to the Practical use of MRI in Oncology* (BFCR(99)6) RCR, London
24 R. Godwin (1995) Audit in clinical radiology: where should we be? *RCR Issue No 42* (Spring 1995) page 18
25 CJ Squire, 0207 436 4251/38 Portland Place London WIN 4JQ
26 Department of Health Risk Management in the NHS London NHS Executive (EL(93)111) 1993
27 Management of Health and Safety at Work Regulations 1999 (SI No 3242 of 1999)
28 C. Vincent (Ed) (1996) *Clinical Risk Management* BMJ Publications, London

29 J. Reason (1996) 'Understanding Adverse Events: Human Factors' Chapter 3 in: *Clinical Risk Management* BMJ Publications, London

30 Department of Health (2001) *Building a Safer NHS for Patients* (April 2001) DoH, London

31 D. Nag (1995) Radiological workloads in District General Hospitals *RCR Issue No 41* (Winter 1995) page 12

32 Board of Faculty of Clinical Radiology (1999) *Workload and manpower in Clinical Radiology* (BFCR(99)5) RCR, London

33 A. Hollman and others *RCoR Radiology Issue No 59* (Autumn 1999) letter to the editor from the Executive Committee of the British Paediatric Radiology and Imaging Group, Page 12

34 Bristol Royal Infirmary Inquiry (2001) *Learning from Bristol: the report of the public inquiry into children's heart surgery at the Bristol Royal Infirmary* 1984–1995 Command paper CM 5207

35 Board of Faculty of Clinical Radiology (1999) *Skills Mix in Clinical Radiology* (BFCR(99)3) RCR, London

36 RCR and the ScoR (1998) *Inter-professional roles and responsibilities in a Radiology Service* RCR, London

37 The Board of Faculty of Clinical Radiology (1996) *Advice to Clinical Radiology Members and Fellows with Regard to out of hours working* (BFCR(96)3) RCR, London

38 Society of Radiographers *Emergency Duties Out of Hours* (No date)

39 NHS Executive HSC 2001/02 *NHS Professionals: Flexible organisations, Flexible staff* (February 2001) DH, London

40 DoH (1999) *Public Interest Disclosure Act* (HSC 1999/198) DoH, London

41 National Audit Office (2000) *The Management and Control of Hospital Acquired Infection in Acute NHS Trusts in England* Stationery Office, London

42 *Hedley Byrne* v. *Heller & Partners Ltd* [1963] 2 All ER 575

43 *Spring* v. *Guardian Assurance PLC* and others Times Law Report, 8 July 1994

44 H. Colyer (1999) Interprofessional teams in cancer care *Radiography* (November 1999) Vol 5, pages 187–189

45 S. Dilly (1999) The multidisciplinary approach for health education, research and practice *Radiography* (November 1999) Vol 5, 191–2

46 Board of Faculty of Clinical Radiology and the College of Radiographers (1998) *Interprofessional roles and responsibilities in a Radiology Service* (BFCR(98)) RCR, London

47 R.W. Blamey (1998) The role of the Radiologist in Breast Diagnosis: a Surgeon's Personal View *Clinical Radiology* (June 1998) Vol 53, pages 393–395

48 'Forrest Report' (1986) *Breast Cancer Screening: A report to the Health Ministers of England, Scotland and Northern Ireland* HMSO, London

49 S. Field (1998) Breast Screening issues *RCR Issue No 52* (Summer 1998) page 12

Section F
Specialist Areas

Chapter 24
PACS and Teleradiology

Introduction

The 1997 White Paper on the NHS[1] envisaged a vast investment in information technology within the NHS which would ultimately link GP surgeries and hospitals to an NHS wide information network. The Government published an information strategy[2] in September 1998 with a commitment to invest at least £1billion over the lifetime of the strategy. By June 2000 £139 million from the 'Modernisation Fund' had been provided for information technology investment in 2000/01. Investment is also being made in IT access by patients to the NHS – on 14 July 2000 the Department of Health announced that all local NHS organisations would be required to publish information on the Internet about the performance of their local health and social care services. They will also be required to provide user-friendly information on accessing local GPs, pharmacists, dentists, opticians, social services and key voluntary services[3].

In January 2001[4] the Department of Health announced that it was to fund a telemedicine information service with a telemedicine website[5] which would be run by the British Library in association with Portsmouth University, at a cost of £90 000 over three years. The aim is to improve the take-up of telemedicine technology in the UK. The medical profession, patients and carers will have access to top quality information on the latest products and developments. It is the intention that, through the electronic patient records system, by 2005 all local health services are to have facilities for telemedicine allowing patients to connect with staff electronically for advice, to book appointments and to see their test results. In February 2001 a press release by the Department of Health announced the development of its plans to ensure that every patient had an electronic health record (EHR) by March 2005[6].

Early feedback

The potential of telemedicine is gradually being appreciated and, although exaggerated claims are being made for its role within health-care and there are many hurdles to be overcome, some of the benefits are emerging. Keith Clough, Ian Jardine and John Navein[7] describe some of the studies which have been undertaken on the subject of telemedicine. For example in a study in Hillingdon in the speciality of coronary heart disease it was found that the staff interviewed considered that the most important applications for telemedicine were:

- Using remote monitoring of physiological symptoms and virtual visiting to support home-based rehabilitation and continuing care packages for the chronically ill
- Transmitting ECGs, clinical details and other communications from ambulances to hospitals
- Using 'store and forward' techniques and transmitting test results between primary and secondary care and between secondary and tertiary care
- Using decision support systems (on laptops) to improve the assessment of care for patients in their own homes.

Further reading

An excellent book on the legal and ethical aspects of telemedicine by Ben Stanberry is recommended for a more detailed review of the law covered in this chapter[8]. He defines telemedicine as including the provision of any of the following services.

- The data transfer of medical, health care, research and/or educational materials in electronic form
- Audiovisual or multimedia communication between health care providers
- Audiovisual or multimedia communication between health care providers and their patients.

Ben Stanberry includes within the term telemedicine many different activities, but this chapter will concentrate on the legal issues arising in teleradiology. Chapter 18 considers the legal implications of record keeping and the use of X-rays in evidence, here we consider the use of computerisation facilities in X-ray and radiotherapy departments and the issues which relate to this.

Picture Archiving and Communication Systems (PACS)

The filmless hospital has not yet arrived but there are major developments in the implementation of PACS in new and existing departments. (The recently completed Royal Glamorgan Hospital in South Wales is possibly closest to a filmless situation.) It is recommended that to ensure maximum efficiency PACS should be on a hospital-wide basis and be founded upon the hospital information system. The PACS can be based upon a central element (hub and spoke) or it can be a distributed (with multiple local archives). Each linked cluster has its own short-term storage units (usually a small Redundant Array of Inexpensive Devices (RAID)).

A PACS and Teleradiology Special Interest Group has been set up[9] by the Society of Radiographers.

Many advantages have been claimed for PACS including:

- Financial savings
  - ○ Reduced cost of film and chemistry
  - ○ Savings on equipment and maintenance associated with conventional processing

○ The end of the 'lost film' which can be as much as 22%
○ Minimal storage and transport costs
- Enhanced patient care
  ○ Improved access to information and availability of images
  ○ Multiple users are able to review an image at the same time (It is possible to obtain a second opinion from someone in a different part of the hospital – or a different hospital – without having to transport the film physically)
  ○ Fewer retakes of X-ray because of the ability to manipulate images (With conventional films it would be necessary to retake the film, but CR/PACS enables the image to be controlled and there is therefore less radiation for the patient)
  ○ Fewer unreported films
- Streamlined working practices
  ○ Saving on storage costs faciliates compliance with protocols requiring images to be stored in case of litigation
  ○ Educational benefits (Radiology images can be easily imported into powerpoint and so slides are not necessary)

PACS as a new approach to working

Martin Hill considers the implications of the development of PACS in the NHS[10]. He points out that the installation of PACS is not simply a new piece of equipment but it should be seen as a catalyst that creates new ways of working. He describes how by the end of 2000 it was planned that the Royal Brompton Hospital should be film free. The process of introducing PACS began in 1997 when the Siemens Sienet PACS was bought. The equipment included:

- four units for digital luminescence radiography and associated post-processing workstations
- three reporting stations
- a central archive
- connection to the RIS
- interface to an Imatron CT scanner
- viewing facilities in both adult and paediatric intensive care.

A PACS check list provided by Martin Hill asks the following questions:

- Has a business plan been prepared, assessing benefits inside and outside radiology?
- Have all staff affected by PACS been consulted and brought 'on board'?
- Does the modality image quality meet your requirements and the expectations of your users?
- Does the system have a track record of successful use in A&E or a similar high demand location?
- Is the system fully scaleable to meet future demand/expansion?
- Will the IT network cope with initial and future demands?
- Is the system intuitive and easy to use?
- Have new ways of working been considered?
- Would web browser technology create additional benefits?

Teleradiology

Teleradiology is the point-to-point communication of radiological images for the purpose of primary reporting or specialist advice. The RCR has published a guide[11] to information technology in radiology covering teleradiology and PACS. It offers guidance on the minimum required standards for the equipment and its operation to enable safe radiological practice. It emphasises that

> 'As in all other areas of radiology, it is the responsibility of the reporting radiologist to ensure that the images are fit for use.'

It follows from this that the reporting radiologists should have an input into the selection of any PACS system which is installed.

The RCR guide notes the significant impact which the development of teleradiology could have on staffing and structure. Smaller X-ray departments may lose their radiologists as images are sent to a central location for reporting. Teleradiology includes: image capture; image compression; image transmission and image review. Quality assurance audit is necessary on a regular basis, with the results recorded. Although teleradiology does not in itself require a link to the hospital information system (HIS) or to the radiology information system (RIS), such links are highly desirable.

Teleradiology is reviewed by G.W. Boland (writing from an American perspective) in terms of its impact on the delivery of health care[12]. He analyses the historical and current technological developments of teleradiology and its potential future implementation into mainstream radiology. He concludes that, for any teleradiology system to be ultimately effective, it must be implemented as part of a comprehensive and strategic plan not only at hospital level, but also at regional, country and federal levels.

> 'If a comprehensive teleradiology system can be implemented as a part of an integrated health care delivery system to a region or country, then issues of licensing, malpractice and protectionism could be organised at a governmental level.'

He also points out that these developments may increase the requirement for subspecialty radiologists.

Areas of concern identified by the RCR

Some of the areas identified as matters of concern by the RCR[11] are given below. The RCR emphasises how important is regular review and update of these guidelines as relevant recommendations become available. (Since the guidelines were published the Data Protection Act 1998 been implemented. This is discussed in Chapter 6.)

- **Security of computer data** The RCR states that no hospital electronic-record system should be in use without complying with the NHS IM&T Manual[13], supplemented by Appendix A of the 1998 Health Circular *Using Electronic Patient Records in Hospital*[14].
- **Teleradiology and the Internet** Patient recognition and demographic data has to be removed prior to transmission.

- **Teleradiology from overseas**. All parties must ensure that they are legally protected.
- **Retention of records** The RCR states that it is the report which is the primary document for retention in medical records, whilst radiographs are to be retained in accordance with local guidelines and policies. In future, if not electronically initiated, X-ray requests on paper may be scanned into a PACS system. (This is considered in chapter 18 and new advice from the Department of Health is awaited.)
- **Service level agreements** The RCR recommends that written protocols required under the service level agreement for teleradiology should cover the following issues:
  - Availability of the radiologist at the receive station, speed of despatch of reports and to whom the result will be sent
  - Accuracy of data received, including degree of compression and/or resolution of data compared to original
  - Speed of communication between send and receive station
  - Responsibility for retention/archiving of records and report, and duration of retention of records
  - Consistency and frequency of quality assurance auditing of teleradiology service
  - Security of information trail, and compliance with legislation relevant to security and confidentiality
  - Presence of a maintenance contract and a specified call-out time
  - Appropriate change in consultant radiology job plans and resources to reflect extra levels of activity as a consequence of teleradiology
- **Acceptance of teleradiology systems into practice** RCR has set out acceptance criteria and stresses that they should be as stringent as the acceptance criteria for any other medical device and should be clearly related to the manner in which the system is being operated with frequent quality assurance tests to ensure continuing safe practice.

Failure to comply with this guidance from the RCR may, if harm has occurred as a result, give rise to an action for negligence in the civil courts on the grounds that the reasonable standard of care as recommended by the Royal College has not been followed.

Legal issues in using teleradiology and PACS

There are many legal issues which arise from these developments, the most important of which are considered below.

Standards

Determining the standard of care in a new area of expertise
In its guidance[11] the RCR points out that there is at present effectively no legal framework within which to develop teleradiology and PACS, and gives as an example the issue of who is responsible for selecting the distant opinion – the health board, the Trust or the clinician? (The answer may depend upon contracts

which may not be clinician-led.) In practice, however, the law does not recognise a legal vacuum. In the absence of specific statutory provisions, judges in determining cases rely upon principles established by common law, or, in the case of the House of Lords, set the principles themselves. If, therefore, an issue arises over accountability or standards of care and comes before the courts, these questions would be answered by reliance upon the basic principles discussed in Chapter 14:

- Is there a duty of care?
- How would the standard of care be defined in accordance with the Bolam test?
- What would reasonable competent professional practice have laid down?
- Is there any causal link between a breach of the reasonable standard of care and any harm which has occurred?

In Chapter 14 the duty of care which arises in the law of negligence is considered together with how the required standard of care is determined in the civil courts. These same principles would apply to any cases of negligence which arise from the use of teleradiology. Expert evidence would be required to define what standards would have been expected in the individual circumstances which arose. Clearly in a new field such as this, where a professional body under the aegis of one of the Royal Colleges has still to be recognised, standards will constantly rise as technology and training improves. Under the Bolam test, the courts apply to the alleged negligence, the standards which should have applied at the time of the incident which caused the harm.

Ben Stanberry in *Legal and Ethical Aspects of Telemedicine*[8] notes that, at the time he was writing, there had been no litigation. He advises a pro-active policy in identifying the risks of harm as the best form of prevention. He lists the likely risks as follows (chapter numbers indicate where these topics are to be found in the book):

- Teleconsultant acting beyond his ability (Chapter 27)
- Quality of reproduction of pathology slides and radiographs (Chapter 14 on standards of care)
- Improper or negligent delegation (Chapter 27)
- Poor training of teleconsultants (Chapter 13)
- Unclear delineation of responsibility (Chapter 27)
- Lack of telemedical equipment (Chapters 3, 17 and 21)
- Communication problems – (including protocols for 'live' teleconsultancy Chapter 4) and post-incident management (Chapter 19)
- Telecomplacency (Chapter 14 on standards of care)
- Malfunctioning of telemedical equipment (Chapter 17)

Other concerns about standards
Could radiographers in isolated primary care units use PACS, only referring to a radiologist when there are concerns? There is no reason, provided the appropriate education and training was given, why radiographers could not make use of PACS. In fact the opportunity to consult a radiologist through computer contact, might facilitate the use of X-rays in community hospitals and health centres. The expanded role is discussed in Chapter 27.

Should professionals expect NHS trusts to provide the necessary equipment in their own homes? Clearly if telemedicine is introduced and consultants are required to report on images when on-call from their homes, all the necessary equipment would have to be provided and maintained by the employer at an acceptable standard. If the consultant makes private use of this equipment, then this could be the subject of an agreement between Trust and consultant.

Are there any dangers in complete reliance on the image? For example, if instead of giving an opinion at a distance, the consultant comes into hospital to see the patient, would not other factors be taken into account in treatment and diagnosis? The answer to this is 'probably', but it does not follow that an opinion given on an image at a distance would necessarily be below the reasonable standard of care. There will of course be circumstances where a definitive opinion is withheld until there has been an actual physical examination of the patient.

Conclusions on standards

Since this is such a new area of development we can expect over the next few years the GMC, the Royal Colleges and the Professional Associations to publish standards of practice, procedures and protocols setting out what they would expect. It is possible too that the field of telemedicine may receive the attention of the National Institute of Clinical Excellence and even, if things go wrong, the Commission for Health Improvement (see Chapter 21). As these standards emerge and are supported by research on clinically effective practice they will become merged within the Bolam test of approved acceptable practice.

Telemedicine applications and equipment should be subject to the same quality assurance and risk management processes as other areas of clinical practice. Adam Darkins in his analysis of the management of clinical risk in telemedicine applications[15] suggests that:

'Although there are risks associated with the widespread introduction of telemedicine, these should be viewed in their proper perspective and managed in the context of a risk management approach, not evoked as a spectre to haunt and inhibit the growth and reputation of telemedicine.'

He is quoted by the NHS Estates of the Department of Health in its *Health Guidance Note* on telemedicine[16].

Accountability

Disputes may arise if, for example, a GP is present with a patient during a video conference with a consultant or the consultant recommends that minor surgery is carried out by the GP under the televised supervision of the consultant. If harm occurs to the patient who is liable? Both doctors are subject to the Bolam test in determining the extent to which a reasonable standard of care was followed. In determining liability it will be a question of deciding, on the actual facts, whose negligence caused the harm. If, for example, the consultant gave incorrect advice to the GP, who reasonably relied upon that advice, then the consultant would be accountable. Failure by a GP to provide the correct or sufficient information to the consultant about the patient's history, medication and condition, as a result of which the consultant makes an incorrect diagnosis, could lead to liability on the part of the GP. Diana Brahams[17] points out that additional skills may be required from doctors practising from a distance with the aid of tele-communications.

Consent to telemedicine

Trespass to the person
The principles relating to consent and giving information to the patient are considered in Chapter 4 and obviously apply to the practice of telemedicine. In Chapter 4 it was pointed out that there are two aspects of consent:

- the actual consent to what would otherwise be a trespass to the person; and
- negligence in the failure to fulfil the duty of care in informing the patient of risks pertaining to the treatment.

It is submitted that since a trespass to the person requires an actual or intended touching of the person, there can be no such trespass by a doctor who is pro-viding an opinion from a distance, whether on the radio, the internet or other tele-methods. No touching of the body is possible and looking at a screen and commenting on it could not therefore be actionable as a trespass to the person. On the other hand, there could be a trespass to the person action against the person present with the patient, if the patient's consent to the X-raying and physical contact to obtain various pictures or other examinations were not obtained. One of the significant differences between an action for trespass to the person and negligence is that the former is actionable without proof of any harm (i.e. actionable *per se*) and the other is only actionable on proof that reasonably foreseeable harm resulted from the breach of the duty of care.

There may, however, be a breach of Article 8 of the European Convention on Human Rights and the right to respect for privacy if telemedicine is used without the patient's consent (see Chapter 3).

Failure in the duty of care to inform
The law would require that the patient is informed according to the Bolam test of all the significant risks of substantial harm which could arise from the use of telemedicine. Consent does not include consent to the risk of practitioners being negligent, but the information to be given would include risks of harm which could occur even if all reasonable care were taken. The patient's consent to the disclosure of information would also be required under the laws relating to confidentiality (see below).

Where the use of telemedicine is contemplated there are considerable advantages in ensuring that documentation for securing the patient's consent spells out exactly what is proposed and also provides written information about any significant risks which may arise. The consent form is not the actual consent, but evidence that consent was given. The form should be accompanied by an explanation by word of mouth as to how the system will work, to ensure that the patient has reasonable information on which to give a valid consent. If there are doubts about the patient's mental competence to give a valid consent, an independent person could be asked to give an opinion on the patient's mental capacity.

Acting in an emergency or for the mentally incapacitated

Where the patient is unconscious or lacks the mental capacity to give consent by reason of mental disability, then the common law permits the health professional to act in the best interests of the patient, providing care according to the standard required by the Bolam test. This was held by the House of Lords in the case of *Re F*[18]. There has not yet been a decided case where telemedicine has been used in an emergency, but the following situation shows the possibilities.

Situation

> A patient is involved in a very severe road accident in a rural part of the country. The patient is transferred to the nearest Accident and Emergency Department, but this hospital does not have neurosurgical facilities. The patient has a head injury and is unconscious. Treatment at a hospital with neurosurgical facilities would involve either a long ambulance journey or a helicopter flight, both of which would not be without risk to the patient. There are telemedical facilities at the first hospital and they are able to communicate with specialists in the neurosurgical department at the DGH and obtain an opinion on whether the first hospital can treat the patient or whether the patient should be transferred. Can treatment decisions be lawfully made on the basis of a teleconsultation without the patient's consent?

One would hope that any decided case would answer the question raised in the situation with a categorical 'yes'. Since the doctors have a duty to treat the patient according to the reasonable standards at that time, then the use of whatever facilities are available to ensure an accurate diagnosis and correct treatment is required. The decision in the case of *Re F* enables action to be taken out of necessity in the best interests of the patient and would be a defence against any potential litigation by the patient or his relatives. Indeed it could be argued that failure to make use of telemedical facilities in such a situation could be seen as negligence. (The right of the mentally competent patient to refuse even life saving care is covered in Chapter 4.)

Confidentiality

One of the most significant concerns with telemedicine and PACS is in ensuring a secure system so that no unauthorised persons are able to access the information. Security is necessary not only to meet the duty of confidentiality owed in respect of information obtained from the patient (see Chapter 5) but also under the European Directive and the Data Protection Act 1998. The provisions of this legislation are discussed in detail in Chapter 6. Here only their particular impact upon PACS and teleradiology will be considered.

Article 8 of the European Convention of Human Rights which recognises the right to respect for a person's privacy also applies. The Convention is set out in Schedule 1 to the Human Rights Act 1998 which is discussed in Chapter 3.

Before a computerised system which includes patient records is established it is vital:

- that the system is robust in term of pass words and the level of access;
- that regular monitoring of its security takes place; and
- that all reasonable means are taken to prevent hackers entering into the data.

Article 1 of the European Directive[19] requires member states to:

'protect the fundamental rights and freedoms of natural persons and in particular their right to privacy with respect to the processing of personal data.'

Under the 1998 Act it is an offence to transmit data to a third country with inadequate levels of protection. A patient who considered his rights have been breached would be able to claim damages from the culprit.

Situation 24.2

A patient in this country is suffering from a severe kidney complaint. Without his knowledge, X-rays and other clinical information is transmitted to America to a renal specialist. The American specialist without authority shows the information to a journalist who writes up the story for an American publication. The patient eventually discovers what has happened. What are his rights?

In this situation, not only would the patient be able to obtain compensation from the doctor in this country, who allowed the information to be transmitted without the patient's consent, the patient would also have a right of action against both the American doctor and the journalist, though there would be problems relating to the different jurisdictions (see below) and the patient would have to show that they were both aware that the information was held in confidence and they knew that he had not given his consent. In addition the doctor or controller may be technically guilty of a criminal offence in permitting the cross-border transmission of data to a country which does not ensure an adequate level of data protection. It would however be a defence for the defendant to establish that the patient had given his consent to the transmission or that it was made to protect the vital interests of the data subject[20].

Principle 8 of the Data Protection Act 1998 (see Chapter 6) prohibits the passing of personal data to a country outside the European Economic Area unless that country ensures an adequate level of protection for the rights and freedoms of data subjects in relation to the processing of personal data. Schedule 4 to the Act however sets out cases where this eighth principle does not apply. These include situations were the data subject has given his consent to the transfer or the transfer is necessary to protect the vital interests of the data subject.

If possible practitioners should discuss the issue with the patient, fully explaining the risk of unauthorised disclosure, and obtain his consent to the transfer (preferably evidenced in writing). If the patient is unable to give a valid consent (for reasons of incapacity or in an emergency) then the fact that the practitioners were acting to protect the vital interests of the patient (the data subject) should be a defence. Practitioners should, however, consider these issues, e.g. whether there is not an appropriate specialist in the EEA, and this fact should be recorded in the patient's notes.

Clearly if international transfer of patient sensitive information is to take place, it is essential for the parties to clarify the level of data protection and try to ensure by contractual arrangements that comparable standards to those required in this country are stipulated.

Criminal offences

In addition to the criminal offences under the Data Protection Act 1998 (see Chapter 6) there are also specific statutes which create offences in relation to the interception of information held in computers or communicated by wireless. Thus the Computer Misuse Act 1990 makes it a criminal offence for a person deliberately to hack into computer system where records are stored. The offence takes place if:

- a person causes a computer to perform any function with intent to secure access to any programme or data held in any computer;
- the access he intends to secure is unauthorised; and
- he knows at the time when he causes the computer to perform the function that this is the case.

The Wireless Telegraphy Act 1949 and the Interception of Communications Act 1985 also create criminal offences for unauthorised interception of data being transmitted. These offences would also apply to staff who were making unauthorised access to personal sensitive data held by their employer and NHS organisations should therefore make it clear through policies that disciplinary and possibly criminal action will be taken against staff who disobey the rules.

Rights of access

Exactly the same provisions apply to access to information transmitted through teleradiology as to the personal health records of the patient. These rights of access together with exclusions to the right are set out in Chapter 6.

Telemedicine equipment

The standards of the initial installation, its maintenance, inspection and upkeep of telemedicine equipment are vital if the clinical standards of reporting are to comply with the Bolam test. In Chapter 17 the role of the Medical Devices Agency is considered together with the laws relating to Consumer Protection. These also apply to equipment which is used in telemedicine.

Documentation

Where videos of telemedicine are retained, these could be accessed by patients under Data Protection legislation. Disputes could arise where videos have been edited, possibly to reduce the need for storage space. Where however a video of the teleconsultation is retained it could be used in court, providing evidence of what was taken into account by the consultant in her recommendations on diagnosis and treatment and what was stated by the patient and any other person present.

Jurisdictional problems

Where telemedicine takes place within one country there are unlikely to be problems over jurisdiction. In contrast with the United States of America, where individual states have their own laws relating to confidentiality, consent and other topics, subject of course to the overriding Bill of Rights and Federal laws, the United Kingdom, with the exception of Scotland and Northern Ireland, shares for the most part a common legal system.

As international telemedicine is likely to develop further in the future, jurisdictional issues could arise as the situation below shows.

Situation

> A doctor in Gibraltar asks for the expert opinion of a radiologist living in England. The radiographs are transmitted and an opinion obtained and the treatment provided accordingly. It then transpires that as a result of a completely negligent opinion, the patient has been given the wrong treatment and has suffered harm. Who is liable?

International contacts across the world, with the means of communication now available, could lead to practitioners in many different countries sharing medical knowledge and requesting opinions. Issues arise not only of liability, but of indemnity cover: would a Trust accept vicarious liability for the negligence of a radiologist providing a report on a radiograph of a patient living in another country? Whether in law the Trust is vicariously liable would depend upon the definition of 'in the course of employment' (see Chapter 14). In which country would the claimant sue the defendant? These and other issues are considered by Ben Stanberry in his work cited above[8]. It is likely that as telemedicine across international boundaries expands statute and case law will develop to cover some of the many legal issues. The parties can, prior to any international consultation, negotiate the terms of the contract which apply to the activity and specifically define which country's laws should apply to the agreement.

Educational use of PACS

Information systems can also assist in training programmes for clinical staff. For example Omair Rauf and Richard Whitehouse[21] used the Radiology Departmental management system to produce a logbook for specialist registrars. It also provided the RCR Tutor with consistent data on registrar training experience. The GMC has provided guidance on making and using visual and audio recordings of patients[22]. It emphasises the importance of obtaining the patients' consent to the recording and its use for any other purpose than that originally agreed. It provides a check list for action to be taken before, during and after the recording. The GMC guidance on confidentiality also applies to video recordings and therefore implicitly to the recordings from telemedicine.

The future

This is a rapidly expanding field and there are many areas for the law to be refined and clarified. The European Commission will probably eventually legislate to ensure that the legal issues arising from telemedicine are covered across the Community, but international agreements will be required to cover other countries. In addition professional standards in training and competence are still in the process of development. It may be that in the future failure to make use of the opportunities afforded by telemedicine could itself be grounds for negligent practice. As Diana Brahams[17] pointed out 'ultimately many of the questions raised here about the medico-legal implications of such telemedicine will be determined by litigation'.

However it must not be assumed that plain film reporting will soon become a thing of the past. Plain film reporting is likely to remain a significant part of the work of the radiologist. Dennis Stoker[23] points out that plain film radiology still accounts for the bulk of the work of a department of radiology and outlines the dangers of forgetting this in terms of standards. Plain film is significant in many diagnostic situations and serious miscarriages of diagnosis can occur if MRI is used as a diagnostic method without reference to a prior radiograph. Most medico-legal cases in respect of radiological problems relate to errors in plan film reporting by radiologists or others. He shows the dangers of leaving plain film reporting to junior staff, since 'if consultants to not continue the practice of allocating time to looking at plain films, who will teach the radiologists in training?'

 ## Questions and exercises

1 What additional precautions, if any, do you consider should be taken to protect the rights of the patient if telemedicine is used?
2 What contribution could telemedicine make to continuing professional development and training?
3 What legal concerns do you have with the introduction of teleradiology and how could these be resolved?

References

1 DoH (1997) White Paper on the NHS *The New NHS – Modern Dependable* Stationery Office, London
2 NHSE (1998) *Information for Health* NHSE, Leeds
3 Department of Health (2000) Press Release (2000/0427) 14 July 2000
4 Department of Health (2000) Press Release (2001/0031) 16 January 2001
5 www.tis.bl.uk
6 Department of Health (2001) *Patients to gain access to new at-a-glance Electronic Health Records* 4 February 2001
7 K. Clough, I. Jardine & J. Navein (2001) Virtual Consultations *Health Management* (February 2001) pages 22–24
8 B.A. Stanberry (1998) *The Legal and Ethical aspects of Telemedicine* Royal Society of Medicine Press, London

9   *RCR Newsletter* Issue No 54 (Summer 1998) and previous issue. (Interest invited and contact with nicola.strickland@btinternet.com)
10   M. Hill (2000) PACS: incremental or big bang? *Synergy* (July 2000) pages 10–13
11   Board of Faculty of Clinical Radiology (1999) *Guide to information Technology in Radiology: Teleradiology and PACS* (BFCR(99)1) RCR, London
12   G.W. Boland (1998) Review Teleradiology: Another Revolution in Radiology? *Clinical Radiology* (August 1998) Vol 53, pages 547–553
13   Department of Health (1996) *NHS IM&T Security Manual* (HSG(96)15) HMSO, London
14   Department of Health (1998) *Using Electronic Patient Records in Hospital: Legal Requirements and Good Practice* Health Service Circular (HSC 1998/153) DoH
15   A. Darkins (1996) The management of clinical risk in Telemedicine applications *Journal of Telemedicine and Telecare* **2**, 4, 179–84
16   NHS Estates *Telemedicine Health Guidance Note* DoH (No date)
17   D. Brahams (1995) The medicolegal implications of teleconsulting in the UK *Journal of Telemedicine and Telecare* **1**, 4, 196–201
18   *Re F* [1990] 2 AC 1
19   European Data Protection Directive (formally adopted on 24 October 1995)
20   Article 26 Derogations
21   O. Rauf & R.W. Whitehouse (2000) Using the Departmental Radiology Information System to replace specialist registrars' Log books *Clinical Radiology* Vol 55, No 1 (January 2000) pages 62–66
22   General Medical Council (1997) *Making and using Visual and Audio Recordings of Patients* (September 1997) GMC, London
23   D. Stoker (1994) The Report of the Death of the Plain Film was an exaggeration *RCR* Issue No 40 (Autumn 1994) page 11

Chapter 25
Dental X-rays[1]

Although exposure levels to ionizing radiation are very low in dentistry, legal problems can arise. In the distant past there was a failure to recognise that exposure to X-ray and a failure to take proper protection could lead to biologically damaging effects such as skin cancer, leukaemia or congenital abnormalities in the off spring. More recently these harmful effects have been recognised and there has been increasing public concern. However this extremely low risk should be put into perspective.

Guidance for dental X-rays

Guidelines on radiology standards for primary dental care is provided by the Royal College of Radiologists and the National Radiological Protection Board[2]. The guidelines were produced by a joint working party of the RCR and the NRPB and note that, although the individual risks from dental radiology are low, there is a significant potential for reduction in the collective dose and for improvements in the diagnostic quality of radiographs. The working party recommendations cover all aspects of dental radiology:

- training and examination regimes for dentists and staff
- patient selection and clinical justification for radiography
- diagnostic interpretation
- equipment
- procedural aspects
- quality assurance.

The guidelines also assess the economic implications of their recommendations, providing a cost and benefit analysis for each recommendation, from which they conclude that there is strong economic justification for the implementation of the full package of recommendations. Guidance is also provided by the Department of Health for Dental Practitioners on the use of X-ray equipment. This covers the 1999 and 2000 Regulations[3].

Guidance on selection criteria in dental radiography has been prepared by the Faculty of General Dental Practitioners (UK) and the Royal College of Surgeons[4]. The advice recommends that one of the main criteria for dental radiography should be where the result (positive or negative) will alter the management or add confidence to the clinician's diagnosis and/or treatment planning. There is also a need to ensure that any exposure is likely to be of benefit to the patient and this outweighs the risk. Dentists are subject to the Ionising Radiation (Medical

Exposure) Regulations 2000[5] and must ensure that justification for and the level of the exposure complies with those regulations (see Chapter 16). Their documentation must also be in compliance with the regulations. It is possible that as the workload for the National Institute for Clinical Excellence develops and the National Service Frameworks are developed that there might be guidelines laid down for dentistry practice including dental radiography. In this case, failure to follow these guidelines might raise a presumption that the reasonable standard has not been followed and evidence would have to be given of specific reasons why the national guidance was not appropriate in the special circumstances of the case (see Chapter 14 on standards of care).

Health and safety issues arising from dental X-rays

Dentists have a responsibility for the health and safety of both themselves and their staff, and also for the patient. It is recommended that they should follow the selection criteria on doses and exposures set out by the Faculty of the General Dental Practitioners[6]. The selection criteria also identifies the gaps in the research evidence for several areas of practice including aspects of periodontology, prevalence of hidden dentine caries and symptom-free teeth which are restored – how often do they need radiographs? The advice points out the uselessness of keeping national guidelines on a dusty shelf and emphasises the importance of the use of clinical audit to maintain good practice and of developing local guidelines for effective practice. Each dentist would be required to appoint a radiological protection adviser (RPA).

Control of Substances Hazardous to Health (COSHH)

These regulations are considered in Chapter 15 and practitioners have the responsibility of ensuring that their staff are instructed in the safe handling of substances and what action to take in the event of an emergency. Documentation should record the hazardous materials stored in the practice.

Medical devices warnings and dentistry

Much of the equipment used by dentists will be defined as a medical device and come under the Medical Devices Regulations. These are considered in Chapter 17. Advice on equipment is also provided in guidance notes issued by the Department of Health and professional bodies[7].

Risk assessments

Dentists must comply with the regulations on the Management of Health and Safety in the Workplace (see Chapter 15) and carry out regular risk assessment exercises. Records should be kept of the assessment and the management plans. Contingency plans are required for the disposal of chemicals and developing solutions.

Specific statutory provision in relation to dental radiography

Dentists are required to ensure that their room plan, installation and specification of X-ray equipment is approved by the Radiation Protection Adviser. Manufactures and suppliers should provide clear guidance on the minimum requirements for routine maintenance. A radiation survey should be undertaken immediately following any major service and in any case at intervals not exceeding three years[8].

Liabilities in law

Liability to the patient arising from the use of X-rays

The National Radiological Protection Board reported that there had been a 50% increase in dental radiology examinations since 1983[9]. The dentist would be liable in the laws of negligence both for taking X-rays negligently or unnecessarily or overprescribing or underprescribing and causing harm to the patient. The burden would be on the patient (or in the case of a child or mentally incompetent adult, the representative of the patient) to establish on a balance of probabilities that the dentist failed to follow the reasonable standard of a dentist practising radiography and radiology. One difficulty faced by the potential claimant in such an action is the considerable time which may elapse before harm is shown and in proving that it was negligence by the dentist which caused that harm (i.e. causation) (see Chapter 14).

The time limit for bringing an action for negligence does not commence until the claimant has knowledge or constructive knowledge that he has suffered harm as the result of negligence (see Chapter 14). This would allow a claim to be brought many years after negligent exposure. However, clearly the longer the gap between the exposure and harm being shown, the more difficult it is to prove that it was the exposure in the dental surgery which caused the harm from which the patient is suffering. The Faculty of General Practitioners (UK) Selection Criteria Guidance[10] states that:

> 'Radiation detriment can be considered as the total harm experienced by an irradiated individual. This includes the risk of fatal cancer, non-fatal cancer and benign tumours, hereditary effects and the length of life lost. Risk is age-dependent, being highest for the young and least for the elderly.'

Liability to the patient arising from failure to take X-rays

Dentists could be liable if allegations are made that they have failed to provide a reasonable standard of dental diagnosis and treatment which might be the case if they failed to take X-rays when it would be reasonable for a practitioner to have done so.

Consent and information giving

It would be rare for dentists to obtain written consent from the patient for X-rays to be taken. Usually the dentist would rely upon consent by word of mouth. However there may be cases where the dentist does not ask the patient if he consents to X-rays being taken, but simply goes ahead with the X-ray, perhaps relying upon non-verbal behaviour of the patient in not refusing. This is known as implied consent. It is unsatisfactory since the dentist should establish that the patient has not had an X-ray recently elsewhere. There are also considerable advantages in giving the patient information about any risks of harm (without alarming the patient) and obtaining clear consent either in writing or by word of mouth. The law on consent is discussed in Chapter 4. Where there are possible risks or the chance that a patient could subsequently deny that consent was given, there are advantages in ensuring that the consent is expressed in writing. Prior to any X-rays being taken the dentist should ask the patient for any relevant information which may affect the decision to take X-rays.

Pregnancy and dental X-rays

The selection criteria of the Faculty of General Dental Practitioners (UK)[4] states that:

> 'It is unusual for an X-ray beam to be pointed at the abdomen (only for vertex occlusal radiographs which are rarely indicated) and in those cases where this may happen, it is an official guideline to use abdominal lead protection when a foetus lies in the primary beam. While a foetus is at risk of harm if exposed to X-rays, the evidence indicates that foetal doses from scattered radiation during dental radiography of pregnant women approach an unmeasurably low level. Consequently, normal selection criteria for dental radiography do not need to be influenced by the possibility of a female patient being at any stage of a pregnancy.'

In spite of this advice and the negligible risk of harm from dental X-rays to the foetus, many dentists would avoid taking X-rays of known pregnant patients and, if a radiograph was essential to the patient's treatment, ensure that abdominal lead protection was used. There would appear to be no justification for the routine use of lead aprons for patients in dental radiography. Dentists would tend to follow the general guidance for the treatment of pregnant patients considered in Chapter 9. If dentists follow this practice, it has a psychological effect on the patient and demonstrates that the dentist is exercising her duty of care. This in itself can be reassuring to the apprehensive patient.

Liability for students

The guidelines on radiology standards for primary dental care of the RCR and the NRPB[11] has noted that 'there is a significant number of dental practices which do not yet meet the requirements of current legislation and there are reports that the quality of radiography is also unsatisfactory in a proportion of practices'. There is an association between low standards and defects in education and training. In dental schools there was found to be considerable variation in the amount of time allocated to the teaching of dental radiology during undergraduate years. The working party of the RCR and NRPB therefore recommended that there should be a specific examination in dental radiology in every dental school and in its guidelines it recommended a 'core curriculum' in dental radiography and radiology for undergraduate dental schools, suggesting the time required for lectures, practical radiography and diagnostic seminars. The General Dental Council emphasises that students should receive instruction, practical experience and appropriate testing in X-rays[12].

Any student who considered on reasonable grounds that there had been a failure by the dental school to provide a reasonable standard of training as a dentist, would (in addition to the possibility of an action in negligence for breach of its duty to provide a reasonable standard of tuition if harm were to be caused as a reasonably foreseeable result) also have the possibility of an action for breach of contract. Where students have clinical placements in dental surgeries and other locations, they will be under the supervision of a registered dentist. If there are failures in delegating to the student activities which are outside her competence or in failing to provide an adequate level of supervision to ensure safe practice, then the supervisor will be liable for such negligence.

There may also be liability on the part of the student for acting outside her competence. In the latter situation, the dental school which arranged the location will be responsible for the negligence of the student. There would normally be a memorandum of agreement between the dental school and the dentist providing the clinical placement over the liability for the negligent acts of the student and also for any harm suffered by the student.

Professional and practical issues

Post-graduate professional development

To remain a registered practitioner, each dentist must undertake recognised post-graduate training every five years. In addition, under the Ionising Radiations Regulations 1999, clinical staff directly engaged in any aspect of radiography must have appropriate and adequate training commensurate with their duties.

Expanded role of the dental nurse

In some dental surgeries, the dental nurse may take on the expanded role of taking radiographs. In such a situation her employer is directly responsible for ensuring that she has the necessary training for undertaking such work and operates only within her competence. The employer is also vicariously liable for any negligence by the dental nurse or assistant which causes harm to the patient. A course in dental radiography for dental nurses is offered at the University of Wales Dental Hospital. This course covers radiation protection, radiographic technique, imaging and quality assurance, together with the relevant health and safety laws and statutory instruments. In the future it may be possible to develop the scope of professional practice of the dental nurse further with training in the interpretation of some of the more simple X-rays. However any such development, like that of dental radiography, must accord with the laws relating to delegation and supervision and the scope of professional practice which are considered in Chapter 27.

The introduction of PACS and teleradiology into dentistry

The high costs of introducing PACS and Teleradiology in individual surgeries in general dental practice will prevent a widespread take up of this new technology. However in the larger practices, and dental schools and hospitals, the advantages of PACS and teleradiology will be seen. The legal issues arising from these developments are discussed in Chapter 24. Clearly where these facilities exist, general dental practitioners can seek the opinions of consultant dental radiologists on diagnostic issues by means of teleradiology, enabling rapid interpretation of results to be made available. The potential medico-legal implications of computed radiography in dentistry are considered by K Horner, D.S. Brettle and V.E. Rushton[13]. They are concerned at the possibility that, unlike films, clinical images produced by computed radiography can be altered to give an untrue picture. They suggest that manufacturers of digital radiographic equipment should incorporate means of uniquely identifying original image data or ensuring that a permanent record of all images is maintained.

Record keeping

The clear implications of the Ionising Radiation (Medical Exposure) Regulations 2000[14] are that record keeping must ensure that the justification for the exposure, the level of exposure and the evaluation of the X-ray are carefully documented. Chapter 18 covers the legal issues relating to records. Unlike General Practitioner NHS records, which must be returned to the health authority when a patient leaves the practice or dies, there is no such requirement on NHS general dental practitioners. However under the 2000 regulations, justification for a new exposure cannot properly be undertaken without a knowledge of previous exposures, so dentists should ensure that they obtain documentation relating to a patient's previous exposures from the earlier dentists and transfer their records to the patient's new dentist if he moves on.

References

1   I am extremely grateful for the assistance of Dr E.G. Absi University of Wales Dental Hospital with this chapter
2   Royal College of Radiologists and the National Radiological Protection Board (1994) Documents of the NRPB **5**:3 *Guidelines on Radiology Standards for Primary Care NRPB; Guidance notes for dentists* NRPB http://www.org.uk/dentalgn.htm
3   NRPB (2001) *Guidance notes for dental practitioners* http://www.org..uk/dentalgn.htm
4   Faculty of the General Dental Practitioners (UK) and the Royal College of Surgeons of England (1998) *Selection Criteria for Dental Radiography*
5   The Ionising Radiation (Medical Exposure) Regulations 2000 Statutory Instrument No. 1059 of 2000
6   Faculty of the General Dental Practitioners (UK) and the Royal College of Surgeons of England (1998) *Selection Criteria for Dental Radiography*
7   DH Guidance Note PM77 (1992) *Fitness of equipment used for medical exposure to ionising radiation* London HMSO
8   Royal College of Radiologists and the National Radiological Protection Board (1994)

Documents of the NRPB **5**: 3 *Guidelines on Radiology Standards for Primary Care* NRPB

9   R.J. Tanner *et al.* (2001) *Frequency of Medical and Dental X-ray Examinations in the UK* NRPB R-320 NRPB

10 Faculty of the General Dental Practitioners (UK) and the Royal College of Surgeons of England (1998) *Selection Criteria for Dental Radiography*

11 Royal College of Radiologists and the National Radiological Protection Board Documents of the NRPB **5** 3 1994: *Guidelines on Radiology Standards for Primary Care NRPB*

12 General Dental Council (1990) *Dental Curriculum 1990*

13 K. Horner, D.S. Brettle and V.E. Rushton (1996) The potential medico-legal implications of computed radiography in dentistry *British Dental Journal* **180**: 7 April 6 1996

14 The Ionising Radiation (Medical Exposure) Regulations SI No 1059 of 2000

Chapter 26
Complementary Therapies

Introduction

Access to complementary therapies has increased dramatically over recent years both within and outside the NHS. Whilst the use of complementary therapy has so far had little role in diagnostic radiography (though there is potential for development as relaxants and some would argue diagnostic capabilities), there is a growing use of complementary therapies within radiotherapy centres. This chapter briefly sets out the law relating to complementary therapy practice.

More detailed analysis of the law for the individual practitioner in a complementary therapy and the legal implications of many different therapies are to be found in a book by this author[1].

Practitioners are affected by the increase in the popularity of complementary therapies development in two ways:

- Some are undertaking training in a therapy regarded as complementary to conventional medicine.
- Others are aware that their patients are consulting practitioners in complementary medicine therapies and may be taking homeopathic or herbal remedies or other treatment for the same conditions for which the practitioner is giving advice.

Definition of complementary therapies

'Complementary is defined as: completing: together making up a whole, ... of medical treatment, therapies, etc ... (1. Complementum – com-, intents, and plere to fill)' (Pamphlet[2] of the British Complementary Medicine Association (BCMA)). It is thus seen to work in parallel with orthodox medicine. The BCMA therefore states that therapy groups which are represented by the BCMA advise and encourage patients to see their doctor wherever appropriate. The House of Lords Select Committee on Science and Technology held an inquiry into complementary medicine. It reported[3] in November 2000 and recommended that there should be regulation of complementary and alternative medicines and there should be further research to evaluate their effectiveness. It divided such therapies into three groups:

- Professionally organised therapies, where there is some scientific evidence of their success, though seldom of the highest quality, and there are recognised systems for treatment and training of practitioners. This group includes acupuncture, chiropractic, herbal medicine, homeopathy and osteopathy.

- Complementary medicines where evidence that they work is generally lacking but which are used as an adjunct to rather than a replacement for conventional therapies, so that lack of evidence may not matter so much. Included in this group are the Alexander Technique, aromatherapy, nutritional medicine, hypnotherapy and Bach and other flower remedies.
- Techniques that offer diagnosis as well as treatment, but for which scientific evidence is almost completely lacking. This group cannot be supported and includes Naturopathy, crystal therapy, kinesiology, radionics, dowsing and iridology

The House of Lords Committee considered that some remedies such as acupuncture and aromatherapy should be available on the NHS and NHS patients should have wider access to osteopathy and chiropractics. The implementation of these recommendations will lead to fundamental changes in how complementary and alternative therapies are viewed in relation to orthodox medicine and within the NHS.

The client in complementary therapy

Disclosure to the practitioner

When a patient is referred to a practitioner in the NHS, then information relating to that person's care within the NHS would also be given. Thus the practitioner should have basic information about the patient in order to determine the care which is required by him. In addition the practitioner would usually have access to health records kept on the patient, to ensure that her care is compatible with other treatment the patient is receiving.

In contrast where the patient is receiving treatment from a complementary therapist, there is usually no official way in which this information can be made known to the practitioner other than through the patient. The practitioner therefore relies upon the openness of the patient in disclosing information which may be relevant to the treatment and care which the practitioner is offering.

Clearly the importance of this communication between patient and practitioner will depend upon the relevance of the complementary therapy to the treatment and care which the practitioner provides. Some therapies may have little effect, others such as acupuncture and homeopathy, may have a significant effect on the recommendations the practitioner may make. If there is a conflict between the two treatments, then the practitioner and therapist need to discuss this with the patient who should be given the choice over which course to pursue, with a reassurance that they can return to the other, when that course has ended.

Ignorance on the part of the practitioner

Does it matter that the practitioner has no knowledge of the complementary therapy which the patient is undergoing? The answer is that it may have an important effect and had the practitioner been aware of certain information about the therapy she may have advised the patient differently. Where harm has occurred, expert evidence on causation would be required to show if anything the practitioner had done could have caused that harm. It is hoped that, in reviewing the practice of the practitioner, it would be revealed that the patient had been receiving treatment from other persons. In the light of this, any liability on the part of each of these persons could be analysed.

This might appear to suggest that those who only practise in conventional medicine should be expected to know the implications of a patient receiving treatment from a complementary or alternative therapy, but this is probably not what is required. What reasonable practice would require, however, is that once a practitioner ascertains that the patient is receiving alternative or complementary therapies then she should make all reasonable inquiries e.g. from the complementary therapist or from others who could be reasonably be expected to point out any contra-indications, so that the patient is reasonably safe.

The practitioner as complementary therapist

Agreement of employer

It is recognised that many practitioners are considering the use of complementary therapies in the treatment of clients. If a therapeutic radiographer obtains a training in a complementary therapy, she should ensure that she obtains the agreement of the employer before she uses this skill as part of her practice. If the NHS trust gives expressed or implied consent to complementary therapies being used by a practitioner then her work in this field could be seen as being in the course of employment, in which case the NHS trust would be vicariously liable for any harm which has been caused. On the other hand if the NHS trust were unaware of the complementary therapy work, then it may refuse to accept vicarious liability for any harm caused by her complementary therapy, arguing that the work was not performed in the course of her employment as a practitioner (see Chapter 14 on vicarious liability). In this case the practitioner would have to accept personal liability.

It is also essential for the practitioner to obtain the consent of the employer if she intends to practice privately during working hours. In the case of *Watling* v. *Gloucester County Council*[4] an occupational therapist was dismissed when he saw private patients for alternative therapy during working hours. His application for unfair dismissal failed. He had been warned by his employers not to conduct his private business during his working hours and lunch times were for a break, not for private work (see page 301).

Consent of the patient

It is also essential that the patient should explicitly give consent before the practitioner uses any complementary therapies on him. The basic principles of obtaining consent apply (see Chapter 4) but since a patient would not normally expect a practitioner to be providing complementary therapies, it is imperative that the practitioner gives full details of all that is involved and makes it absolutely clear that the patient is fully entitled to receive the conventional treatment usually provided by the practitioner even though he refuses the complementary medicine treatment and care. It is preferable to obtain the consent in writing and to put in a leaflet the information which the patient should be told about the treatment.

Defining standards

One of the difficulties of some complementary therapies is that there may not be a clear definition of the expected standard of care. If harm were to occur to a patient and the patient wished to claim compensation, the patient would have to establish that the therapist failed to use the reasonable standard of care which he was entitled to expect from her. This may not be easy to prove. Reference must be made to the various bodies providing accreditation for individual therapies on what would be regarded as the reasonable standards of their specific therapy in those particular circumstances.

The issue of the standards within Chinese medicine arose in a recent case:

Case: Standard of care of a complementary therapist[5]

Mr Shakoor who was suffering from a skin condition consulted a practitioner of traditional Chinese herbal medicine. After taking nine doses of the herbal remedy he became ill and later died of acute liver failure, which was attributable to a rare and unpredictable reaction to the remedy. His widow brought proceedings against the practitioner but failed. The High Court held that, on the evidence before it, the actions of the practitioner had been consistent with the standard of care appropriate to traditional Chinese herbal medicine in accordance with established requirements.

Use of complementary therapies in radiotherapy

Carolyn Featherstone and M. Hemmick reported the findings of a survey on the provision of complementary therapies at UK radiotherapy centres[6]. They found that the provision of complementary therapies may occur as a result of a response to patient demand or initiatives by cancer care practitioners or the managerial change agent. It tended to be associated with a supportive organisational culture, although this is not universally the case. The ten most common therapies (in order of popularity) are:

(1) Acupuncture
(2) Aromatherapy
(3) Art therapy
(4) Alexander
(5) Chiropractic
(6) Drama therapy
(7) Aromatherapy
(8) Massage
(9) Meditation
(10) Hypnotherapy

The authors conclude that the extension of education to embrace complementary therapies for medical professions and professions allied to medicine would ensure a low cost solution to patient demand and give greater confidence in professional judgment.

National developments

There is no doubt about the interest which now exists in complementary or alternative therapies. It is estimated that a third of the population have tried its remedies or visited its practitioners[7]. The Health Education Authority has published an A to Z guide which covers 60 therapies[8]. Much research needs to be done on the efficacy of these therapies and the Health Authority Council has approved a research project to be undertaken by the National Association of Health Authorities and Trusts into the prevalence of complementary therapies and their services for patients, purchasers and providers.

The Prince of Wales suggested the setting up of a group to consider the current positions of orthodox, complementary and alternative medicine in the UK and how far it would be appropriate and possible for them to work more closely together. Four working groups looking at

- research and development;
- education and training;
- regulation; and
- delivery mechanisms

were established under a steering group chaired by Dr Manon Williams, Assistant Private Secretary to HRH the Prince of Wales. It reported in 1997 and made extensive recommendations[9]. These include

- encouraging more research and the dissemination of its results;
- emphasising the common elements in the core curriculum of all health-care workers, both orthodox and in complementary and alternative medicine;
- establishing statutory self-regulatory bodies for those professions which could endanger patient safety;
- identifying areas of conventional medicine and nursing which are not meeting patients' needs at present.

It also recommended the establishment of an Independent Standards Commission for Complementary and Alternative Medicine.

An information pack for primary care on complementary medicine has been sponsored by the Department of Health[10]. The pack was initiated after a survey found that one in four adults would use alternative therapies at some point in their lives.

Conclusions

There is every likelihood that the interest and demand for complementary therapy will continue to grow and patients will demand that these therapies should be provided within the NHS. In the past some GP fund holders have used their purchasing power to buy such therapies for their patients. In remains to be seen what effect the abolition of GP fundholding and the establishment of Primary Care Groups and Primary Care Trusts will have on the availability of complementary therapies within the NHS. The BMA at its conference in 2000 pressed the Government to make acupuncture available on the NHS. Following the recommendations of the House of Lords Select Committee on Science and

Technology (see above) there will be more requirements for research based evidence of the clinical effectiveness of many complementary therapists so practitioners are likely to become involved in this area.

✎ Questions and exercises _____

1 You have decided that you would like to undertake a training in aromatherapy and eventually use it as part of your practice as a therapeutic radiographer. What actions would you take to ensure that your plans are compatible with your role as a therapeutic radiographer?

2 Identify the ways in which the knowledge that a patient was receiving complementary therapy treatment could affect the tests, care or treatment which you give that person.

3 Do you consider that those complementary therapists who so wish, should be permitted to have registered status under the Health Professions Council? (Refer also to chapter 11). If not, what criteria would you lay down for a profession to receive registered status?

References

1 B. Dimond (1998) *The Legal Aspects of Complementary Therapy Practice* Churchill Livingstone, Edinburgh

2 Further information can be obtained from the BCMA at Exmoor Street, London W10 6DZ; Tel 020 8964 1205, Fax 020 8964 1207

3 House of Lords Select Committee on Science and Technology, 6th Report *Complementary and Alternative Medicine* (21 November 2000) Session 1999–2000

4 *Watling* v. *Gloucester County Council* Employment Appeal Tribunal EAT/868/94 17 March 1995; 23 November 1994, Lexis transcript

5 *Shakoor (Administratrix of the Estate of Shakoor (Deceased))* v. *Situ (T/A Eternal Health Co)* (2000) *The Independent* 25 May 2000

6 C. Featherstone & M. Hemmick (1999) Provision of complementary therapies at UK radiotherapy centres *Radiography* Vol 5, 147–153

7 J. Laurance (1996) Alternative Health: An honest alternative or just magic? *The Times* 5 February 1996

8 Health Education Authority (1995) *A-Z guide on complementary therapies*

9 Foundation for Integrated Medicine (1997) *Integrated Healthcare: A Way Forward for the Next Five Years*

10 Complementary Medicine Information Pack for Primary Care (www.doh.gov.uk)

Chapter 27
Scope of Professional Practice and the Expanded Role

Introduction

The past decade has seen major changes taking place in professional development. Whilst in the past, basic training and advanced practice diverged very slightly, more recently many health professions have developed their practice, often taking on activities which had previously been the monopoly of the medical profession. Nurses have possibly been the group most influenced by this development – the role of the clinical nurse specialist, the new post of consultant nurse and the general changes in the scope of professional practice of the basic grade staff nurse have irrevocably revolutionised the role of the nurse.

However other health professionals are also taking part in this advance which is being encouraged by the Government. Pragmatic reasons such as the reduction of junior doctors' hours are only a part of the explanation. Other reasons relate to the need to introduce into the NHS more flexible ways of working, with defined national standards of practice set by NICE and enforced through CHI. The White Paper *The New NHS*[1] set out the vision and the Health Act 1999 saw its implementation (see Chapter 21 for further discussion on these initiatives). The NHS Plan[2] envisages further role expansion and flexible ways of working.

The Ionising Radiation (Medical Exposure) Regulations 2000 (see Chapter 16) can be seen as an example of the Government recognising the value of flexibility in who does what in the health services. The regulations focus on the responsibilities to be assumed by any competent health care professional who undertakes the duties, rather than on the professional background of the person. Thus the definitions of referrer, practitioner and operator all emphasise the competence of the individual to perform that function rather than on a particular professional background. For example a 'practitioner' is defined as

> 'a registered medical practitioner, dental practitioner or other health professional who is entitled in accordance with the employer's procedures to take responsibility for an individual medical exposure.'

'Other health professional' does not limit the activity to those trained in radiography, although in practice they are the most likely group to be undertaking this work. Some may take a more restrictive view of the width of these definitions and there are concerns that in some areas radiographers might not be identified as practitioners under the Regulations. However it is clear that since the practitioner has the duty to justify the exposure, all those, including on-call radiographers or reporting radiographers, should have that responsibility.

Protocols and procedures drafted within each department or Trust to implement the Regulations should ensure that there is clarity over the allocation of responsibilities and the training requirements. The RCR has issued guidance[3] on justification for clinical radiologists which examines the different roles identified within the Ionising Regulations. It emphasises that decisions on who is entitled to act as a practitioner should be taken at local level by agreement between employer and health care professionals involved in medical exposure. This principle will apply to all the areas where the scope of professional practice of individual health professionals is expanding.

Diagnostic radiographers are expanding their role by reporting on X-rays and undertaking many activities formerly undertaken by radiologists. Therapeutic radiographers are also concerned to develop their skills and knowledge in cancer care and their strategy for such development is considered below.

Areas within which role expansion could take place

Obtaining consent

Obtaining the consent of the patient and his signature on the consent form may be delegated to a person other than the practitioner who will be carrying out the treatment. In such a case the RCR recommends[4]:

'2.6.1 If you delegate this responsibility [i.e. obtaining consent], you must do so under the GMC Guidelines on referral and delegation[5].

2.6.3 You must ensure that those members of your team are trained and qualified, understand the risks and benefits of the procedure and will act in accordance with the GMC Guidelines exactly as you would do yourself.'

As in all professional activities, it is essential that practitioners taking on this role understand the limitations of their knowledge and, if questions are asked by the patient to which they do not know the answers, it is arranged for the patient to be seen by the doctor. Obtaining consent is not simply a question of obtaining a signature on a form. Consent is the voluntary agreement of a mentally capacitated person, based on the necessary information, to what is being proposed. Therefore the signature must be preceded by a clear explanation to the patient. The person talking to the patient must be able to answer the patient's questions fully and honestly and know the limits of their competence and when they need to bring in someone else to talk to the patient. If things go wrong and the patient claims he was not properly informed, the adequacy of the explanation might have to be justified in court.

Breast clinics

Specialist breast nurses have begun to take on diagnostic responsibilities in breast clinics. If they are to undertake Fine Needle Aspiration for Cytology (FNAC), then they must have the training to satisfy the BASO guidelines for the management of symptomatic breast cancer[6].

Ultrasound

The extent to which radiographers performed general diagnostic ultrasound (excluding obstetric and cardiac ultrasound) was investigated by G.A. McKenzie and others[7]. They found that, of 150 hospitals randomly selected, in 72.2% radiographers carried out general diagnostic ultrasound. Procedural guidelines existed in half of the departments. In 55.1% of cases radiologists reported images in conjunction with the radiographer. Radiographer enthusiasm was cited as the main reason for selecting radiographers to train. The authors recommend that 'radiologists and radiographer should co-operate further to establish ultrasound services which provide a level of service which is acceptable to referring clinicians and patients'.

The personal experience of a sonographer expanding her role from working within the NHS to working in industry is described by Karen Middlehurst[8]. Sonographers have expanded their role over recent years and have increased their input into abdominal and vascular applications both scanning and reporting their findings. They may expand in the new areas of ultrasound including 3D and 4D techniques.

3D ultrasound is considered in an article by Paul Baines[9]. The four main advantages claimed for 3D ultrasound are:

● time saving
● availability of new planes
● volume analysis
● visualisation of spatial relationships in 3D.

There is evidence that it can be particularly useful in echocardiography, obstetrics, urology and vascular work. In a two part article Neil Prime, Regina Fernando and other colleagues discuss the development of occupational standards for the practice of diagnostic ultrasound. Part 1 gives the background[10] and Part 2 discusses the process and outcomes. The project, which was commissioned by the NHS Executive South and West and the College of Radiographers, was prompted by the recognition that the application of ultrasound was escalating and being used by a wide variety of practitioners. These included medical practitioners from a variety of specialities of radiology, obstetrics, gynaecology, paediatrics, urology, gastroenterology, cardiology, vascular surgery endocrinology and general practice, and health-care workers from radiography, nursing, midwifery, cardiac technology, vascular technology and medical physics. The aim was to develop occupational standards to specify benchmarks of good practice common to all practitioners who use ultrasound in their work with patients. The background paper described the standards developed by professional bodies and associations and how they can be used in clinical governance to help in the definition and measurement of quality by providing a framework for continued assessment of individual practice. The second paper sets out the process of designing the occupational standards. Information from acknowledged experts in the field led to the development of draft standards which were used for a nationwide consultation. The standards were then completed and finalised. The authors conclude that it remains to be seen whether the standards are used by all those who practice diagnostic ultrasound. They state

'The standards document is designed to be a resource, a tool to encourage managers and practitioners to improve the quality of service, a tool for persuasion rather than coercion.'

GPs and ultrasound

There are considerable advantages for ultrasound use to be developed in primary care, but the role of the GP and the necessary ultrasound training are controversial issues. The College of Radiologists has produced a document *Basic ultrasound training for General Practitioners* which lead to some heated discussion[11]. The document was criticised on the grounds that there was inadequate consultation prior to publication and there was insufficient theoretical and practical training in the scheme. More specific concerns are given by Paul Dubbins[12] who states that in the scheme:

- GPs have no training in cross-sectional imaging.
- They have no experience of other contributory imaging investigations.
- The availability of high quality ultrasound equipment to GPs is limited.

Financial pressures within the health service may well provide the stimulus for such investigations by GPs rather than a balanced consideration of clinical need.

'We do not advocate a role for general practitioners in the performance and interpretation of X-rays yet lend the College's support to their performance of ultrasound after minimal training.'

Keith Dewsbury[13] in the same journal is concerned at the lack of statutory regulation for ultrasound, but sees the setting down of agreed standards of training as a 'small step in the right direction'. Even though the training is limited (a five day course and one session of practical work every week over a year) he sees this as a considerable commitment for a busy GP, who would still be able to perform only a limited number of examinations. GM Baxter[14] in a letter to the editor suggests that the solution may be the appointment of more radiologists or to employ more ultrasonic radiographers under the auspices of the Radiology Department where high ultrasonic standards can be maintained. George McInnes[15] warns of the dangers of giving a financial incentive to GPs in this field. RJ Peck and MC Collins[16] report on their experience of ultrasound outreach clinics. They concluded that the scanning quality is compromised in favour of patient convenience and was expensive in terms of equipment usage and radiologists' time. For example an ultrasound machine that is capable of doing 3000 scans a year probably does no more than 300 scans in total per year. Their conclusions support a joint RCR and GP document[17] that the cost of radiological equipment was an argument in favour of the centralisation of such equipment. These considerations must clearly be taken into account in determining the justification for any investment in scanning facilities for GPs. The establishment of Primary Health Groups and Primary Health Trusts may facilitate the development of a strategy in relation to ultrasound use in primary care, so that the capital costs are justified by the usage and that the appropriate training is provided for those GPs who use it.

Reporting of X-rays by radiographers

The GMC's guidance on delegation by doctors requires the doctor to ensure that the delegate is competent to undertake the procedure or therapy involved. It emphasises that the doctor will still be responsible for managing the patient's care[18]. In its statement on *Reporting in Departments of Clinical Radiology*[19] the Faculty of Clinical Radiologists within the Royal College of Radiologists has said that

'After suitable training there may be no statutory impediment to a non-medically trained person reporting a radiological examination and making technical observations, but a person without a medical training cannot reasonably be expected to provide a medical interpretation.'

The College of Radiographers in its vision paper states that 'reporting by radiographers is not an option for the future, it is a requirement'[20]. In the joint paper published by the RCR and the ScoR[21], in defining the two elements of reporting – the descriptive report and the medical report – it is stated that the descriptive report may be provided by those members of the team who are competent to do so, in accordance with a protocol agreed by the medical members of the team. The author of the descriptive report bears responsibility for its content. The medical report provides a report and opinion on the further medical management of the patient and this can be provided only by an appropriately trained registered medical practitioner, normally a radiologist.

The need for radiographer reporting in A&E is considered in a guest editorial in *Radiology* by N. Brayley[22]. He notes that in his own hospital at Colchester a red dot system was in existence, the missed error rate is of the order of 2% and the majority of the missed abnormalities are of a trivial nature, usually avulsion flake fractures around the ankle. Clearly the speedier the examination by the radiologist, and the shorter the time before the abnormality is detected, the less likelihood of litigation. Brayley points out that there are an insufficient number of radiologists to meet the increased demands upon them and therefore further delegation to radiographers will be necessary.

There are many justifications for radiographers to have the additional training, supervision and experience which enables them to develop an expertise in identifying abnormalities in certain X-Rays. However it is extremely important to define the parameters within which this expanded activity can take place. It may be that only certain X-Rays, such as chest X-Rays or X-Rays to ascertain if there have been fractures, would come within the scope of the expanded role of the radiographer. It may be, too, that within that restricted sphere there would be only specific abnormalities on which they would be expected to comment and other more complex or more subtle indicators would remain the province of the radiologist alone. It may also be that the radiographer would be expected only to identify an anomaly and not to interpret it in terms of the clinical condition. In addition, any comment by radiographers would, in all cases, be followed up by the radiologist. These detailed points for role expansion must be debated and agreed between the Royal College of Radiologists and the College of Radiographers. At the same time the necessary training to equip the radiographer with the skills for this limited role expansion must be defined and accredited by the appropriate bodies and agreed with the employers.

N J Prime and others analysed the content of the curricula of radiographic reporting courses in six established sites[23]. The study identified some key pointers:

- Programmes should explicitly link clinical and academic learning
- They should demonstrate the fundamental importance of the inter-relationship of the roles of radiologists and radiographers in reporting
- They should contain considerable experiential learning and emphasise that reporting is a skill which must be developed in the workplace
- Assessment of competence is a vital component of programmes.

The monitoring of performance in reporting is also essential. Susan Carter and David Manning considered, by means of a case study, the performance monitoring during postgraduate radiography training in reporting[24]. They concluded that improvement in performance was attributable to a number of factors such as familiarisation with normal variants, tutorial support on search strategies and increased sophistication in report writing. They recommend the practice of monitoring radiographer performance over time in similar training programmes in order to accelerate performance. They also considered that monitoring could predict the level of diagnostic performance for patient populations with various levels of medical disorder.

Gastro-intestinal imaging

Radiographic managed gastro-intestinal imaging is an emerging specialty within radiography, in particular the double-contrast barium enema (DCBE). The implication of this development was considered by Julie Nightingale at a Gastrointestinal Radiographers Special Interest Group Conference in September 2000[25]. She pointed out the value of GI radiographers being involved in gastrointestinal clinical meetings or case conferences, and felt that those centres which did not provide this opportunity were not following practices which served the best interests of the patient 'and as such they are likely to be identified and eradicated through quality audit procedures'. She identified three areas for GI radiographer development:

- developing the GI imaging role;
- formalising radiographic reporting of the GI examination; and
- raising awareness of the GI radiographer's role.

She concluded

'It is likely that the service offered by GI radiographers will continue to increase as more responsibilities are explored and education and training courses meet the service demand for competent practitioners.'

Clearly the positive encouragement by the Government for flexible working (see the NHS Plan) will accelerate the identification of other areas where the professional practice of the non-doctors can develop.

Standards of practice

No team liability

The Court of Appeal has held that the courts do not recognise the existence of team liability[26]. Each individual practitioner is personally and professionally accountable for his or her own actions and cannot blame the team or team instructions for negligence which has led to harm.

The Bolam test

At the heart of any determination of the scope of professional practice is the concept of competence: is the individual practitioner competent to do the activity? Where negligence is alleged against a professional, then the claimant would have to show that there has been a failure to follow the reasonable standard expected of a competent practitioner according to the Bolam test[27] (see Chapter 14).

No defence of inexperience

The Court of Appeal has also held that the patient is entitled to the reasonable standard of care who ever provides the treatment. A junior practitioner will be expected to provide the same reasonable standard of care which a more senior person would provide. It is no defence to argue that a young or inexperienced person carried out a particular activity and that it why it was performed negligently[28]. In practice, of course, the junior member of staff, even though a registered practitioner, should receive supervision from more senior practitioners, who should ensure that she has some support for responsibilities which require more experience than she has obtained.

It follows from what has been said that, where a practitioner takes on responsibilities which would normally be undertaken by another professional, then the same standard of care would be expected of that practitioner as would have been provided by the other. Thus it would be no defence to argue that a therapeutic radiographer, carrying out the addition of drugs to an intravenous transfusion, could follow a lower standard of care than would have been provided by the doctor who in the past normally performed that activity. It would therefore follow that if a radiographer reported upon an X-Ray instead of a radiologist a lower standard of reporting would not apply. If reliance is placed upon that radiographer's report then the standard should be that of the radiologist.

Nevertheless, in areas where 100% success is not usually the norm and there can be a failure rate even if the best practice is followed, it is difficult to define what is a reasonable standard of care. For example if there is a 5% failure to identify problems in the ordinary reasonable standard of the competent radiologist, should not a radiographer, when taking on the reporting activity, be 'entitled' to that same 5% mis-diagnosis?

Circumstances where the Bolam test was not applied

In a case which involved determining the standards of care to be followed by those involved in reading cervical smear slides, the High Court held that the Kent and Canterbury Hospital were liable for the failure by cytoscreeners to refer the slides of three women for review by a more senior screener. This case is causing considerable concern[29] and is considered in more detail in Chapter 14. The principle that the Bolam test did not apply to the work of screeners because there was no use of professional discretion is open to debate on both the law and the facts. The decision will have serious implications not just for cytology screening but also for the work of the commenting and reporting on X-Rays and other diagnostic tests.

Ironically there is a danger that where activities are delegated to less senior practitioners, higher standards of care will be expected.

Standards of care following delegation to other professionals

R.L. Law and colleagues carried out a retrospective five-year study on the accuracy of the Barium Enema Examination (BaE) performed by radiographers[30]. The authors' conclusion was that radiographer performed barium enemas with double reporting produces a very high standard of examination with detection rates for significant lesions comparable with published data. In an invited commentary on the study Clive Bartram[31] states that:

'This practice [of radiographer performed barium enemas] is becoming widespread, and with appropriate quality control, is to be commended. The benefits of this in radiologist's time and in controlling examination costs are obvious. The efficacy demonstrated in this paper also provides a strong argument for the radiographer performed BaE being part of colorectal cancer screening.'

Determination of competence

One of the most difficult areas for individual practitioners in expanding their role is to know whether they are competent. In the past competency in an individual task was evidenced by a certificate following a training course. Now, however, the tendency is to move away from such task-based professional development and certificates are not relied upon. Other forms of competence determination are required.

Patricia Williams and Judith Berry in a two part article on competence[32] consider whether a new model is required for diagnostic radiographers. Part 1 describes the background to the study, its methods and the results; Part 2 discusses the findings and the implications for professional practice and research. They developed a model of competence which incorporated a range of knowledge, skills and attributes which could be used as a starting point for making judgments on the scope of practice. More than 50% of the competencies could be classified as multi-professional. The research also showed that there were unclear boundaries around the areas of qualification. The findings on the primary role of radiographers pointed to a greater emphasis on patient care. This had important significance for the development of the scope of professional practice for the radiographer. The authors suggest that

> 'Building on the findings of this study the profession needs to redefine the scope of practice, so the stage can be set for radiographers to develop a unique combination of professional and transferable skills which would better equip them for their expanded professional role in the future NHS.'

One interesting approach to the determination of competence, setting standards and ultimately delegation of activities is the 'think aloud' technique considered by Nick Prime and S.B. Le Masurier[33]. Clinical scenarios were designed in the form of scripts which were videotaped using actors. The video tapes were then shown to a series of radiographers and the thought processes generated were audio-taped for compilation into a verbal protocol. Fifty two such protocols were compiled. There are clear implications for CPD and standard setting.

Education and training for the expanded role

Continuing Professional Development (CPD) has become a requirement of reregistration for radiologists and for radiographers. It is essential that there should be approved courses by which practitioners can develop their professional practice. The legal issues of education and training are considered in Chapter 13.

Legal principles of delegating and supervision

The role expansion of the radiographer is likely to be accompanied by increasing delegation to imaging technicians or technicians for therapeutic radiography or to assistant practitioners and other health-care support workers. The legal implications of delegation and supervision are considered in Chapter 23.

Sometimes of course the role expansion is not from a doctor to a radiographer but from a radiologist to a General Practitioner as the RCR report on *Diagnostic Imaging and the Primary Care Sector*[34] shows. This postulates that outreach services should be considered where appropriate for limited services in rural areas, but should be under the management of a Department of Clinical Radiology. It also suggested that imaging services within general practice may be appropriate in a limited service but should be carefully evaluated in terms of quality of the imaging and radiological opinion, and also for value for money. The Report concluded that:

> 'Clinical radiologists should remain the key personnel for the provision of radiological opinions in both the secondary and primary care sectors. Clinical radiologists have the breadth of training and depth of knowledge to provide a flexible, high quality clinical service. If other medical professions undertake reporting they should undergo appropriate training and be prepared to take legal responsibility for their opinions.'

Dispute between professionals

As role expansion develops there may be disputes between radiographers and doctors over what is the reasonable standard of care, as the following situation illustrates.

Situation What is appropriate?

A radiographer decided that a request by a doctor for an X-ray was inappropriate and would lead to unnecessary exposure. The doctor insisted that the X-ray should be taken. What is the law?

In this situation the radiographer must have good evidence to show that the X-ray was inappropriate. If there are good grounds for that belief, then the radiographer would be justified in refusing to perform the X-ray. The radiographer is personally and professionally accountable for her actions, and it would be no defence for the radiographer, when facing professional conduct proceedings for serious professional misconduct, to say 'I was obeying the instructions of the doctor'. However this kind of dispute should not just be a question of personalities and personal battles. There should be a procedure within the department for such differences of opinion to be discussed and resolved. Evidence would be required of both points of view. Under the new Ionising Radiation Regulations, more emphasis is placed on individual patient exposure, and this should lead to greater vigour in determining the appropriateness of each and every individual exposure of the patient.

Accountability and the red dot system

Situation Reporting on X-rays in A&E[35]

Patients are seen by a doctor (or possibly by a nurse practitioner exercising her expanded role) and referred for X-Ray. The X-Ray is taken by the radiographer. The patient waits for the X-Ray to be checked and commented upon by the radiographer and then returns to the junior doctor (or nurse) for further examination in the light of the X-Ray. There is no red dot or comment by the radiographer. The doctor assumes therefore that there is no abnormality and suggests to the nurse that the patient should be strapped up and then can go home. Subsequently when the X-ray is reported upon by the radiologist, a fracture is identified. What, if any is the liability of the radiographer?

From the doctor's point of view, the absence of a red dot is misleading. Does it mean that there is, on an immediate assessment of the X-Ray, no obvious abnormality, i.e. Nothing Abnormal Discovered (NAD) or does it mean that the radiographer has negligently failed to spot an evident abnormality, but will not be held accountable for this omission, since the junior doctor or nurse will be the accountable professional? If the doctor can place no reliance upon a reasonable standard of care by the radiographer then it may be wiser to have no red dot system in use.

From the perspective of junior doctors, they need to be assured that, if a red dot system is operating, then those undertaking it will follow the reasonable standard of care of a qualified and trained radiographer in making an assessment. There should be in place a safe system to ensure that the radiologist reports on all X-rays, including those reported upon by a radiographer using the red dot system, so that the patient can be speedily recalled, if necessary.

Prescribing drugs and the Crown Report

In Chapter 20 the recommendations of the Final Crown Report are discussed. When implemented these will have a significant effect on the role of radiographers, whether therapeutic or diagnostic. Those taking on the responsibility as dependent or independent prescribers must ensure that they obtain the requisite training, that the necessary protocols are in place and that there are full discussions with all those staff and patients and carers who are likely to be affected by their new roles. From August 2000 radiographers are amongst those professionals who may be recognised as competent to prescribe according to patient group directions. These are considered in Chapter 20 where the requirements for a valid patient group direction are set out.

Expanding the role of the therapeutic radiographer

The Calman-Hine Report on cancer services could have far reaching consequences for all practitioners working in this field. A joint strategy group set up by the Radiotherapy Vision Group, the Radiotherapy Advisory Group and a working group appointed by the Council of Radiographers has published a strategy for consultation[36]. Underlying the strategy is the assumption that therapeutic radiographers could develop their skills and knowledge in cancer care and become specialists at higher levels of professional practice, both in primary and palliative care.

The key features of the strategy are:

- Public protection and safe working practices will be secured through state registration.
- New entrants to the profession will be supported through a structured pre-ceptorship to ensure that they develop into confident practitioners.
- Supportive clinical supervision will be introduced at all levels of practice to give practitioners the chance to develop and reflect on practice.
- Inter-professional teamwork and cross boundary working will be enabled at higher levels.
- A four tier structure will be introduced encompassing assistant, registered, specialist (senior) and consultant roles
- A new kind of cancer therapist which better reflects professional skills and makes the professional more visible to patients and other professionals.

At the time of writing funding is being sought to pilot the strategy and roadshows will be set up to support the consultation process. The National Cancer Plan[37] was published by the Government in October 2000.

The potential for role extension in the work of the radiotherapy treatment review radiographer is noted by H Colyer[38] who emphasises the importance of the therapeutic radiographer having proper education and clinical support and strong professional leadership. The opportunity for role extension by therapeutic radiographers is also considered by B Suter and others[39] in relation to machine verification radiographers. Their research showed that radiographers demonstrated sufficient parity with the clinicians to warrant a change to the departmental protocol so that responsibility for verification film assessment was transferred from clinicians to therapy radiographers. As a result of the research, radiographers were responsible for film assessment for up to five radiotherapy treatment fractions before the films were viewed by clinicians.

Expanded role by other professionals

The developments in the roles of other health professionals could have a major impact upon the future role of the radiographer. For example at a conference of nurses who work in radiography departments, participants were asked in which areas they saw their scope of professional practice developing and the results were published[40].

Main concerns about safe role expansion

The main concerns which they had about developing competence for the roles fall under the following categories:

- How the decision is made over the appropriateness of a nurse undertaking the activity and the setting up of the protocol and training.
- Difficulties in obtaining the training, being assessed and continuing assessment, and maintaining competence.
- Reactions of others:
  - radiographers
  - other nurses
  - doctors
  - patients
- Increase in legal liability, stress etc.

A similar exercise was conducted with clinical nurse specialists, consultant nurses and other nursing staff a few years later[41]. Similar concerns were identified but many more quoted management attitudes as being a hurdle to their expanding their scope of professional practice.

Conclusion

The expansion in the scope of professional practice cannot be seen in isolated terms of an individual profession. It has major implications for the whole multi-disciplinary team, for managers and for patients and carers. Each directorate, division, unit or department must consider the scope for development in its area, the impact this will have on the functions of all staff and the measures which must be put in place (training, resources, protocols, guidelines, etc.) in order to ensure the protection of the patient and the safe development of the individual practitioner. The significant legal principle is that the reasonable standard of care for the patient must be secured whoever undertakes the activity.

Questions and exercises

1 Identify the activities which you consider could be delegated to therapeutic or diagnostic radiographers and the necessary preparation to secure the competence of the radiographer to perform the activity safely.

2 What are the main obstacles to role enhancement and how could these be overcome?

3 In what circumstances would a delegating doctor be held to be accountable if harm occurred as the result of negligence by the radiographer undertaking an activity normally undertaken by medical staff?

4 In what circumstances could a radiographer undertake the prescribing of medications or contrast agents? (Refer also to Chapter 20.)

References

1 DoH (1997) *The New NHS – Modern Dependable* Stationery Office, London
2 DoH (2000) *The NHS Plan* Stationery Office, London
3 Board of Faculty of Clinical Radiology (2001) *A Guide to Justification for Clinical Radiologists* Royal College of Radiologists, London (1999)
4 Royal College of Radiologists *Guidance on Consent by patients to examination or treatment in Departments of Clinical Radiology* (BFCR(99)8) RCR, London
5 General Medical Council (1998) *Good Medical Practice* GMC, London
6 *European Journal of Surgical Oncology* 1995; 21 Suppl A: 1–13. 1998; 24; 464–76
7 G.A. McKenzie, S.A. Mathers, S.T. Graham & R.A. Chesson (2000) Radiographer performed general diagnostic ultrasound *Radiography* (August 2000)
8 K. Middlehurst (1999) Clinical applications in ultrasound: a personal experience *Synergy* (May 1999) pages 20–22
9 P. Baines (2000) 3D ultrasound: how does it work and what is it used for? *Synergy* (March 2000) pages 12–17
10 N. Prime, R. Fernando, L. Miller & L. Mitchell (1999) The development of occupational standards for the practice of diagnositc ultrasound: Part 1, background, *Radiography* (November 1999) **5**, pages 215–20; Part 2, the process and the outcomes, *Radiography* (February 2000) **6**, pages 43–50
11 Letter to editor (1993) J.K. Hussey and many others *RCR* Issue 36 (Augumn 1993) page 20
12 Paul Dubbins (1993) *RCR* Issue 36 (Autumn 1993) page 13
13 Keith Dewsbury (1993) *RCR* Issue 36 (Autumn 1993) page 13
14 G.M. Baxter (1994) letter to editor *RCR* Issue 40 (Autumn 1994) page 20
15 G. McInnes (1995) letter to editor *RCR* Issue 41 (Winter 1995) page 20
16 R.J. Peck & M.O. Collins (1995) General practice ultrasound *RCR* Issue 42 (Spring 1995) page 16
17 RCR (1993) Radiology and the patients of GPs *RCGP Connection* (February 1993) Hillprint Ltd, Bishop Auckland
18 General Medical Council (1995) *Good Medical Practice* GMC, London
19 Board of the Faculty of Clinical Radiology (1995) *Statement on Reporting in Departments of Clinical Radiology* The Royal College of Radiologists, London
20 College of Radiographers *Reporting by Radiographers: A vision paper* (March 1997)
21 RCR and the ScoR (1998) *Inter-professional roles and responsibilities in a Radiology Service* RCR, London

22 N. Brayley (2000) The need for radiographer reporting: An accident and Emergency Department (A&E) perspective *Radiography* Vol 6 Issue 4(November 2000) pages 227–9

23 N.J. Prime, A.M. Paterson & P.I. Henderson (1999) The development of a curriculum – a case study of six centres providing courses in radiographic reporting *Radiography* Vol 5, pages 63–70

24 S. Carter & D. Manning (1999) Performance monitoring during postgraduate radiography training in reporting a case study *Radiography* Vol 5, pages 71–78

25 J. Nightingale (2000) Gastro-intestinal imaging for radiographers: current practice and future possibilities *Synergy* (December 2000) pages 16–19

26 *Wilsher* v. *Essex Area Health Authority* [1986] 3 All ER 801 (CA)

27 *Bolam* v. *Friern Hospital Management Committee* [1957] 1 WLR 582

28 *Nettleship* v. *Weston* [1971] 2 QB 691

29 D. Owens & M. Corcoran (1999) Great Expectations: an end to the Bolam Test *British Journal of Health Care Management* (April 1999) **5**, 4, 139–41

30 R.L. Law *et al* (1999) A Retrospective 5-year Study on the Accuracy of the Barium Enema Examination Performed by Radiographers *Clinical Radiology* (February 1999) Vol 54, pages 80–84

31 C. Bartram (1999) Invited Commentary *Clinical Radiology* (February 1999) Vol 54, pages 83–84

32 P. Williams & J. Berry (1999) What is competence? A new model for diagnostic radiographers Part 1 *Radiography* (November 1999) Vol 5, pages 221–235, Part 2 (February 2000) Vol 6, pages 35–42

33 N. Prime & S.B. Le Masurier (2000) Defining how we think: an investigation of decision making processes in diagnostic radiographers using the 'think aloud' technique *Radiography* (August 2000) **6**, 3, 169–178

34 Board of Faculty of Clinical Radiology (1996) *Diagnostic Imaging and the Primary Care Sector* (BFCR(96)6) RCR, London

35 B. Dimond (2000) Red Dots and Radiographers' Liability *Health Care Risk Report* (October 2000) **6**, 10 10–12

36 *Radiography* (November 2000) Vol 6, Issue 4, pages 245–51

37 www.doh.gov.uk/cancer

38 H. Colyer (2000) The role of the radiotherapy treatment review *Radiography* (November 2000) **6**, 4, 253–60

39 R.B. Suter, B. Shoulders, M. Mclean & Balyeki (2000) Machine Verification radiographs: an opportunity for role extension *Radiography* (November 2000) vol **6**, 4, 245–51

40 B. Dimond (1998) Radiology Nursing: Legal issues surrounding the expanded role *British Journal of Nursing* **7**, 13, 793–6

41 B. Dimond (2001) The scope of professional practice. *Health Risk Report* March 2001, **7**, Issue 4, pages 16–17

Chapter 28
Legal Aspects of Research

Introduction

Whilst there are clear statutory regulations for the carrying out of research on animals (Animals (Scientific Procedures) Act 1986) and for the testing of medicinal products (the Medicines Act 1968), and for testing on embryos (the Human Fertilisation and Embryology Act 1990) most of the law on research relating to clinical work derives from common law principles, supported by declarations from International Conventions and guidelines from professional registration bodies or associations. These declarations and guidelines, whilst they are frequently incorporated into the standards of professional practice, are not in themselves directly enforceable in the courts in this country, unless they echo an existing common law principle or statute. In contrast the incorporation of the European Convention on Human Rights into the law of this country (see Chapter 3) gives statutory protection to those who consider that they have been treated in an inhuman or degrading way, and this can be applied to participation in research. As the need for research based, clinically effective practice increases, there is a greater likelihood that most health professionals will become involved in research either directly as participants in research projects or indirectly as the provider of services to patients who are research subjects. This chapter looks at both the protection of patients who are asked to take part in research projects and also the laws which apply to the setting up, carrying out and publication of research work.

Protection of patients and volunteers

International conventions

Nuremberg code
At the end of the Second World War, military trials were held in Nuremberg where members of the Nazi party, some of the worst perpetrators of crimes against humanity, were prosecuted. In its judgment, the Court set out 10 basic principles for research which should be observed in order to satisfy moral, ethical and legal concepts. These have become known as the Nuremberg Code[1]. The 10 principles are summarised in Figure 28.1.

Figure 28.1 **Principles for research from Nuremberg Code.**

(1)   The voluntary consent of the human subject is absolutely essential.

(2)   The experiment should be such as to yield fruitful results for the good of society, unprocurable by other methods.

(3)   The experiment should be based on results of animal experiments and a knowledge of the natural history of the disease or other problem so that the anticipated results should justify the performance of the experiment.

(4)   The experiment should be so conducted as to avoid all unnecessary physical and mental suffering and injury.

(5)   No experiment should be conducted where there is an *a priori* reason to believe that death or disabling injury will occur; except, perhaps, in those circumstances where the experimental physicians also serve as subjects.

(6)   The degree of risk to be taken should never exceed that determined by the humanitarian importance of the problem to be solved by the experiment.

(7)   Proper preparations should be made and adequate facilities provided to protect the experimental subject against even remote possibilities of injury, disability or death.

(8)   The experiment should be conducted only by a scientifically qualified person. The highest degree of skill and care should be required, through all stages of the experiment, of those who conduct or engage in the experiment.

(9)   During the course of the experiment the human subject should be at liberty to bring the experiment to an end if he has reached the physical or mental state where continuation of the experiment seems to him to be impossible.

(10) During the course of the experiment the scientist in charge must be prepared to terminate the experiment at any stage, if he has probable cause to believe, in the exercise of the good faith, superior skill and careful judgment required of him, that a continuation of the experiment is likely to result in injury, disability, or death to the experimental subject.

Declaration of Helsinki

The World Medical Association published a Declaration of Helsinki in 1964 which set out principles for the carrying out of research on human subjects. Amendments were made in 2000 following a conference in Edinburgh[2]. Details of the Declaration of Helsinki can be found on the internet.

United Nations Convention on the Rights of the Child

The United Nations Convention on the Rights of the Child was drawn up in 1989[3] and represents clear guidance for the development of rights-based and child-centred health care. The UK ratified the Convention in 1991.

The European Convention on Human Rights and Biomedicine

This Convention[4] also applies to research practice and Article 17 gives guidance on research on patients lacking the mental capacity to give a valid consent.

Professional guidelines on research

Most health professional organisations have produced guidelines in respect of different aspects of research along the lines of the international conventions. Thus the Royal College of Paediatrics and Childhealth (in its previous identity of the British Paediatric Association) provided a guide to the UN Convention[5]. Subsequently the Royal College has published guidelines on clinical research involving new-born babies and infants[6], and children[7]. In 1996 the Royal College of Physicians published guidelines on the practice of ethics committees[8]. Guidance has also been provided by the Royal College of Radiology[9].

Guidance from the General Medical Council
The Standards Committee of the GMC issued draft guidance on *Medical Research: The role and responsibilities of doctors*[10]. The GMC states that:

> 'Previously our advice on medical research has been published within our other guidance documents. Conduct in medical research has been of growing interest and concern to the profession, patients, the pharmaceutical industry, and others for some years now. We have therefore decided that we need a guidance document that sets out the core values and principles that we expect doctors to adhere to when they are involved in medical research projects.
>
> This draft document sets out these standards and principles and also indicates other information sources that need to be consulted.'

The GMC draft guidance covers the following topics:

- The duties of a doctor registered with the GMC
- Good Practice in Medical Research
- Principles governing research practice
- Putting the principles into practice
- Protecting the autonomy and interests of participants
- Conflicts of interest
- Funding and payments
- Research Design
- Recording and reporting research results
- Involving vulnerable adults in research
- Involving children and young people in research
- Including participants in the research process
- Valid consent
- Seeking consent: the competent adult
- Adults with learning difficulties
- Adults with mental disorder
- Children
- Consent for research into treatment in emergencies
- Seeking consent to retain organs and tissues
- Advance Statements
- Establishing capacity
- Fluctuating capacity
- Confidentiality
- Teaching, training and management

- Teaching and supervision
- Keeping up to date
- Managerial responsibilities for research

The GMC emphasises that the principles set out in its guidance *Good Medical Practice, Seeking Patients' Consent: The Ethical Considerations* and *Confidentiality: Protecting and Providing information* must be followed when undertaking research.

Research Governance Framework

As part of the clinical governance initiative, the Department of Health has published a Research Governance Framework[11]. This sets out the responsibilities of a research sponsor and requires that organisations willing to take on these duties to be included on a list of recognised sponsors and complete a base line assessment. The framework seeks to establish standards for all those involved in research in health and social care. Standards are set and the appropriate legislation identified together with other sources of guidance in the areas of:

- Ethics,
- Science,
- Information,
- Health, safety and employment
- Finance and intellectual property

Consent

The basic principle from all the international declarations and from professional guidance is that the consent of a mentally competent adult is the fundamental requirement in any research. Special procedures must be established for children and mentally incapacitated adults. Failure to obtain consent from a mentally competent patient/volunteer or the Gillick competent child (see Chapter 8) or from parents of children before research is carried out could lead to an action for trespass to the person (see Chapter 4). It is also essential that all relevant information should be given about any risks of harm from the research. Failure to provide sufficient information could lead to an action for breach of the duty of care to inform. This is on the basis that all researchers have a duty to ensure that a reasonable standard of professional practice is complied with in providing information before the patient gives consent (see Chapter 4). The rights of parents to give consent on behalf of their children to research projects is restricted to situations where there is no undue risk to the child. Further discussion of this difficult area is considered in a BMA publication[12].

A distinction was made in the Helsinki Declaration between therapeutic and non-therapeutic research in the discussion of consent in relation to research. Research which is linked with the treatment of the patient would be described as 'therapeutic', whereas research which has no immediate benefit to that particular patient is described as 'non-therapeutic'. In the discussions which took place between 1998 and 2000 on revisions to the Declaration of Helsinki it was agreed that the distinction should be dropped from the Declaration. However in practice there is likely to be a distinction since where the patient/client stands to benefit personally from the research, it could be argued that the research on adults incapable of giving consent could be conducted as part of their treatment plan, even though that person lacks the mental capacity to give a valid consent. However if the individual has no personal benefit from the research, research to which any risks were attached would not be justified. This would also apply to research on children.

The information which is given to the patient/client and the consent form to be signed should be approved by the Local Research Ethics Committee (see below) before the research commences.

Confidentiality

Exactly the same principles of confidentiality apply in relation to the personal information obtained from undertaking research as do to any other personal data or patient information. It is probable that the exceptions to the duty to maintain confidentiality recognised by the law in relation to personal information obtained in the course of caring for patients (see Chapter 5) would apply to information obtained through research. For example if information relating to the health or safety of the patient or of other people were obtained during the research, there may be justification in passing this to the appropriate authorities.

In 1996 three doctors were brought before professional conduct proceedings of the General Medical Council as a result of the publication of a case study on a patient which she claimed to have recognised as being about herself and she alleged it to have been published without her consent. The doctors were not struck off the Register. It was emphasised however that the rules were now that it is necessary to get the specific consent of the patient to the publication of a case study or the details should be anonymised and changed to make it impossible for the patient to be identified.

Compensation

At present if people suffer harm as a result of involvement in a research project, they could sue in the tort of negligence, but would have to prove that the researcher failed to follow a reasonable standard of care (this could also include the disclosure of information to the patient prior to consent to the research being obtained) and as a consequence they suffered harm.

The Pearson Report[13] in 1978 recommended that both volunteers and patients who take part in medical research and clinical trials and who suffer severe damage as a result should receive compensation on the basis of strict liability. This recommendation has never been implemented in law, though the Association of the British Pharmaceutical Industry has recommended that such persons should obtain compensation without proof of negligence if harm arose as a result of the research project. Research Ethics Committees are required to establish that there has been an agreement to pay compensation before any research on medicinal products takes place.

Research based practice

The Bolam test which is discussed in Chapter 14 is the accepted test for defining reasonable acceptable professional practice. As was discussed, what a reasonable body of responsible practitioners would accept as appropriate practice will change as standards of care improve and develop. The findings from substantiated research will therefore eventually become integrated into accepted practice and it is essential that the professional keeps abreast of changes in recommended practice.

A *Guide to Radiological Research*[14] has been published by the RCR which provides a useful navigator to the funding of research, the sources of grants and how to write a grant application. It also explains the basic steps to be followed in undertaking research:

- obtaining ethical approval;
- using radiation and radionuclides in the research;
- dealing with people;
- handling statistics; and
- using computers and the internet.

Finally it provides advice on presentation of the research findings and publication.

An example of a project to identity research needs within radiography is provided by the work of Susan Nixon. She undertook a study to determine what the research needs of the radiography profession are and to discover how radiography education centres are equipping graduates to meet those needs[15]. She concluded that research skills were necessary for reflection and Continuing Professional Development (CPD) activity, and vital to the future of the profession. Research by undergraduates was also seen to benefit departments since it made clinical staff more aware of their own practices and encouraged an evidence-based approach to practice. The knowledge base of radiography was seen to be so diverse that a variety of research methods were required in order to add to that knowledge base and thus inform practice.

Local Research Ethics Committees

The Department of Health has requested each health authority ensure that an LREC[16] is set up to examine research proposals. Any NHS body asked to agree a research proposal falling within its sphere of responsibility should ensure that it has been submitted to the appropriate LREC for research ethics approval. A manual for research ethics committees provides guidance on every aspect of their work, including the special procedure for multi-centre research[17]. In certain cases Multi-Centre Research Ethics Committees (MRECs), established by the Department of Health, oversee research which is carried on across several LREC catchment areas. Where less than five LRECs are involved, one LREC can act on behalf of the others.

The role of the LREC is defined as being 'to consider the ethics of proposed research projects which will involve human subjects' and to advise the NHS body concerned. It is the NHS body which has the responsibility of deciding whether

or not the project should go ahead, taking into account the ethical advice of the
LREC. They are not 'in any sense management arms of the District Health
Authority'[12]. The LREC is comprised of multi-disciplinary members including lay
persons.

The guidelines require the LREC to be consulted for any proposal which
involves:

- NHS patients including those private sector patients treated under contract
- Fetal material and IVF involving NHS patients
- The recently dead in NHS premises
- Access to the records of past or present NHS patients
- The use of, or potential access to, NHS premises or facilities.

The LREC *must* be consulted, but the NHS body must also give permission
before the project can proceed.

Obtaining the approval of an LREC should ensure that the patient/client is
reasonably protected from zealous researchers. However particular difficulties
can arise where the researcher is also the health professional concerned with the
treatment of the patient. In such cases, it is not easy to ensure that treatment
concerns remain paramount and patients are assured that they can opt out of the
research at any time without suffering any sanction from the health professional.

Research issues

Publication

It is extremely wise for researchers to discuss and agree arrangements for possible publication of the research before it is undertaken in order to prevent
disputes arising over censorship and control once the outcome is known. Some
funding bodies sponsoring research may require that they see the findings before
they permit publication. This may be seen, however, as an unjustified restraint on
the dissemination of the results. Clearly if major concerns are unearthed during a
research investigation and the researcher is an employee of the organisation
concerned, the employee would have the protection of the Public Interest Disclosure Act 1998 in bringing these concerns to the attention of the appropriate
senior management (see Chapter 22).

Research results may be publicised at conferences by way of poster displays.
An extremely useful article[18] gives guidance on the preparation of posters for
display.

Accuracy

If research is published which contains errors of design and interpretation and
persons suffer harm as a result of dependence upon the conclusions drawn, then
there could be liability in negligence. A centre for cancer treatment in women in
Bristol suffered financial loss as the result of a research report which suggested
that the Centre achieved worse results than other treatment centres. It was later
learnt that the researchers had failed to take account of the fact that the Bristol
Centre took patients at a much later stage in their illness compared with other

centres and therefore like was not being compared with like. Practitioners who knowingly take part in research which is not sound could face professional conduct proceedings.

In addition there may be liability on the part of LREC members if the committee has failed to fulfil its functions appropriately and, as a consequence, someone has suffered harm. The LREC is not itself a statutory body, but the action would lie against the health authority on whose behalf the LREC has acted. Where it is claimed that financial loss has occurred, it would have to be established that there was justifiable and known clear reliance upon statements by the LREC as a consequence of which harm has been caused. Causation would however be difficult to establish. The LREC does not necessarily guarantee the scientific validity of research for which it gives its consent. In this case the researchers themselves could be personally liable and, if employees, their employer vicariously liable.

Fraud in research

Research misconduct unfortunately takes place and inevitably receives considerable publicity. The BMA has published a book[19] on fraud and misconduct in medical research. A national Committee on Publication Ethics (COPE) has been set up to prevent plagiarism, redundant publication and fraudulent manipulation of data.

Intellectual property and copyright

Sometimes research projects can lead to lucrative rewards, e.g. the design of a new piece of equipment or an innovative idea for supporting disabled persons. The right of ownership of any such inventions or innovations depends upon the nature of the contract between employer and employee. If the practitioner is undertaking research and development as part of her work as a full-time employee, then the employer would be seen as the owner of the research, though a generous employer may well develop an income sharing scheme with the employee. If, on the other hand, the research has been developed by the practitioner entirely on her own, with no involvement from the employer or its resources, she would be the owner of the intellectual property. Advice should be taken on patenting the design so that ownership is legally recognised[20].

Conclusions

Practice must be based on knowledge obtained through research. Evidence-based practice is essential in the 21st century. Ultimately the Bolam test (see Chapter 14) as to what is the accepted approved practice of the reasonable practitioner should be supported by clinical evidence. The European Convention on Human Rights as published in Schedule 1 to the Human Rights Act 1998 must be respected in the conduct of research. The initiatives set out in the 1997 White Paper[21] – the National Institute of Clinical Excellence, National Service Frameworks Standards and the Commission for Health Improvement should lead to standards being developed across all health specialities and professions.

Research should be encouraged to underpin practice. There is therefore considerable pressure to ensure that the rights of patients and volunteers are protected and that the research complies with the standards set by International Declarations and professional guidance.

✎ Questions and exercises

1   You are wishing to carry out a research project. Draw up a schedule setting out the initial tasks you should undertake before you actually begin the data collection.
2   How do the requirements in relation to consent to participation in a research project apply to mentally competent and mentally incompetent adults and children.
3   Obtain a copy of the local procedure for obtaining the approval of the LREC to a research project and consider the extent to which it protects the interests of patients and volunteers.

References

1   I. Kennedy & A. Grubb (2000) *Medical Law* (3rd edn.) Butterworths, London
2   European Forum for Good Clinical Practice *Bulletin of Medical Ethics: Revising the Declaration of Helsinki – a Fresh Start* London 3–4 September 1999
3   United Nations Convention on the Rights of the Child, (20. xi. 1989); TS 44; Cm 1976
4   Convention for the Protection of Human Rights and Dignity of the Human Being with regard to the application of Biology and Medicine: Convention on Human Rights and Biomedicine (4.iv. 1997)
5   British Paediatric Association (1996) *A paediatrician's brief guide to the UN Convention on the Rights of the child* BPA, London
6   Royal College of Paediatrics and Child Health (1999) *Safeguarding informed parental involvement in clinical research involving newborn babies and infants* RCPCH, London
7   Royal College of Paediatrics and Child Health (2000) *Guidelines for the ethical conduct of medical research involving children* RCPCH, London; *Archives of Disease in Childhood* 2000, Vol 82, 1777–82
8   Royal College of Physicians (1996) *Guidelines on the Practice of Ethics Committees in Medical Research Involving Human Subjects* (3rd edn) RCP London
9   Board of Faculty of Clinical Radiology (1997) *A guide to Radiological Research* (BFCR(97)3) RCR, London
10   GMC (2001) *Medical Research: The role and responsibilities of doctors* GMC, London
11   Department of Health (2001) *Research Governance Framework* DoH, London; www.doh.gov.uk/research/rd3/nhsrandd/researchgovernance.htm
12   British Medical Association (2001) *Consent, Rights and Choices in Health Care for Children and Young People* BMJ Publications, London
13   Royal Commission on Civil Liability and Compensation for Personal Injury (chaired by Lord Pearson) Cmnd 7054 1978 HMSO, London
14   Board of Faculty of Clinical Radiology (1997) *A guide to Radiological Research* (BFCR(97)3) RCR, London
15   S. Nixon (1999) Undergraduate research: theory or practice *Radiography* (November 1999) Volume 5, pages 237–249

16 HSG(91)5

17 Centre for Medical Law and Ethics King's College, (1997) *King's College Manual for Research Ethics Committee* Kings College, London

18 R. Murray, M. Thaw & R. Strachan (1998) Visual Literacy: Designing and Presenting a Poster *Physiotherapy* (July 1998) **84**, 7, 319–27

19 S.J. Lock & F. Wells (1999) *Fraud and Misconduct in Medical Research* (2nd edn) British Medical Association, London

20 J. McKeough (1996) Intellectual Property and scientific research *Australian Journal of Physiotherapy* 42/3 (235–242)

21 Department of Health (1997) *The New NHS: Modern – Dependable* Command Paper 3807, HMSO, London

Chapter 29
The Future

Significant changes are taking place in the technology and the organisation of health care. Present government plans to ensure that by March 2005 every patient will have their own individual electronic health record will, if the investment is made available, enable major changes to take place in the development of picture archiving and communication systems including teleradiology. The development of intermediate care facilities, greater use of community hospitals, emphasis on primary care services and the establishment of Care Trusts with significant powers under the Health and Social Care Act 2001 will lead to new arrangements for the delivery and management of health care, including significant changes in the scope of professional practice of individual health professionals. The concept of clinical governance, the work of NICE, the National Service Frameworks and the inspections by the CHI will place curbs upon professional discretion and increase the demands upon clinicians.

The appropriateness of the new machinery for professional registration and regulation under the Health Professions Council and the expanded powers of the General Medical Council are still to be evaluated. There is no evidence that litigation is decreasing. On the contrary the conclusions of the National Audit Office in May 2001 that almost £4 billion would be required to meet the costs of known and anticipated claims in the NHS[1] suggests that unless there are radical changes in how liabilities in health care are to be met and administered, the bill will continue to grow. It is possible that the Woolf reforms, by speeding up the process of cases and facilitating the progress of claims, will encourage others to seek compensation. The possibility of a new scheme introduced in the NHS for compensation for clinical negligence could have a major impact on complaints and litigation.

Inevitably there will be new legislation, much emanating from the European Economic Community and new precedents set by the courts. The impact of the Inquiry Report on the heart surgery for children in Bristol[2] is, at the time of writing, still to be felt. The challenges and, hopefully, the opportunities ahead are formidable. It is my hope that the legal framework set out within this book will assist the practitioner in taking on these challenges and opportunities.

References

1   National Audit Office (2000) *Handling Clinical negligence claims in England: Report by the Comptroller and Auditor General* (HC 403) Session 2000–2001 (3 May 2001) Stationery Office, London

2   Bristol Royal Infirmary Inquiry *Learning from Bristol: the report of the public inquiry into children's heart surgery at the Bristol Royal Infirmary 1984–1995* Command Paper CM 5207

Table of Cases

Table of Statutes

Glossary

accusatorial	a system of court proceedings where the two sides contest the issues (contrast with *inquisitorial*)
Act	of Parliament, statute
Actionable *per se*	a court action where the claimant does not have to show loss, damage or harm to obtain compensation e.g. an action for trespass to the person.
actus reus	the essential element of a crime which must be proved to secure a conviction, as opposed to the mental state of the accused (*mens rea*)
adversarial	the approach adopted in an *accusatorial* system
advocate	a person who pleads for another – it could be paid and professional (such as a barrister or solicitor), or it could be a lay advocate, either paid or unpaid
Arrestable offence	an offence defined in section 24 of the Police and Criminal Evidence Act 1984 which gives to the citizen the power of arrest in certain circumstances without a warrant
assault	a threat of unlawful contact (see *trespass to the person*)
balance of probabilities	the standard of proof in civil proceedings
barrister (counsel)	a lawyer qualified to take a case in court and who also gives specialist advice
battery	an unlawful touching (see *trespass to the person*)
Bench	the magistrates, Justices of the Peace
Bolam test	the test applied by the Courts (taking its name from the case of *Bolam* v. *Friern HMC*) on the standard of care expected of a professional in cases of alleged negligence (i.e. that of 'the ordinary skilled man exercising and professing to have that special skill')
burden of proof	the duty of a party to litigation to establish the facts (or in criminal proceedings the duty of the prosecution to establish both the *actus reus* and the *mens rea*)
cause of action	the facts that entitle a person to sue
civil action	proceedings brought in the civil courts
civil wrong	an act or omission which can be pursued in the civil courts by the person who has suffered the wrong (see *torts*)
committal proceedings	hearings before the magistrates to decide if a person should be sent for trial in the Crown Court
common law	law derived from the decisions of judges (case law, judge-made law)

conditional fee system	a system whereby client and lawyer can agree that payment of his fees is dependent upon the outcome of the court action
constructive knowledge	knowledge which can be obtained from the circumstances
continuous service	the length of service which an employee must have worked with the employer in order to be entitled to receive certain statutory or contractual rights
contract	an agreement enforceable in law
contract **for** services	an agreement, enforceable in law whereby one party provides services, not being employment, in return for payment or other consideration from the other
contract **of** service	a contract for employment
coroner	a person appointed to hold an inquiry (inquest) into a death in unexpected or unusual circumstances
criminal wrong	an act or omission which can be pursued in the criminal courts
damages	a sum of money awarded by a court as compensation for a *tort* or breach of *contract*
declaration	a ruling by the court, setting out the legal situation
dissenting judgment	a judge who disagrees with the decision of the majority of his or her fellow judges hearing the case
distinguished (of cases)	the rules of *precedent* require judges to follow decisions of judges in previous cases. However in some circumstances it is possible to come to a different decision because the facts of the earlier case are not comparable to the case now being heard, and therefore the earlier decision can be 'distinguished'
ex gratia	of payment offered to a claimant – as a matter of favour i.e. without admission of liability
expert witness	evidence given by a person whose general opinion based on training or experience is relevant to some of the issues in dispute
frustration (of contracts)	the ending of a contract by operation of law, because of the existence of an event not contemplated by the parties when they made the contract e.g. imprisonment, death, blindness
Re F ruling	a professional who acts in the best interests of an incompetent person who is incapable of giving consent, does not act unlawfully if he follows the accepted standard of care according to the *Bolam test*
guardian ad litem	a person with a social work and child care background who is appointed to ensure that the court is fully informed of the relevant facts which relate to a child and that the wishes and feelings of the child are clearly established. The appointment is made from a panel set up by the local authority
hearsay	evidence of facts which has been learnt from another person rather than observed directly
hierarchy (of courts)	the recognised status of courts which results in lower courts following the decisions of higher courts (see *precedent*). Thus decisions of the House of Lords must

be followed by all lower courts unless, they can be *distinguished* (see above)

indictment	a written accusation against a person, charging him with a serious crime, triable by jury
injunction	an order of the court restraining a person
inquisitorial	a system of justice whereby the truth is revealed by an inquiry into the facts conducted by the judge e.g. coroner's court
judicial review	an application to the High Court for a judicial or administrative decision to be reviewed and an appropriate order made: e.g. declaration
Justice of the Peace	a lay magistrate, i.e. not legally qualified, who hears offences in the Magistrates Court in a group of three (*bench*)
limitation period	time within which proceedings can be brought, calculated from the date of the wrong doing, or the claimant's knowledge (actual or deemed) of it
litigation	civil proceedings
magistrate	a person (see *JP* and *stipendiary*) who hears summary (minor) offences or those triable either way which can be heard in the magistrates court
mens rea	the mental element in a crime (contrasted with *actus reus*)
next friend	a person who brings a court action on behalf of a minor
ombudsman	a Commissioner (eg health, Local Government) appointed by the Government to hear complaints
part 36 offers	formal offers to settle an action with costs consequences if refused and the ultimate outcome is no better
plaintiff	term formerly used to describe one who brings an action in the civil courts (now the term claimant is used)
plea in mitigation	a formal statement to the court aimed at reducing the sentence to be pronounced by the judge
practice direction	guidance issued by the head of the court to which they relate on the procedure to be followed, guidance notes in the CPR
precedent	a decision which may have to be followed in a subsequent court hearing (see also *hierarchy*)
prima facie	at first sight, or sufficient evidence brought by one party to require the other party to provide a defence
privilege	in relation to evidence, being able to refuse to disclose it to the court
professional misconduct	conduct unworthy of a health practitioner
proof	evidence which secures the establishment of a claimant's or prosecution's or defendant's case
prosecution	the pursuing of criminal offences in court
quantum	the amount of compensation, or the monetary value of a claim
reasonable doubt	to secure a conviction in criminal proceedings the prosecution must establish beyond reasonable doubt the guilt of the accused
solicitor	a lawyer who is qualified on the register held by the Law Society

statute law (statutory)	law made by Acts of Parliament or Statutory Instruments
stipendiary magistrate	a legally qualified magistrate who is paid (i.e. has a stipend)
strict liability	liability for a criminal act where the mental element (*mens rea*) does not have to be proved and in civil proceedings liability without establishing negligence
subpoena	an order of the court requiring a person to appear as a witness (*subpoena ad testificandum*) or to bring records/documents (*subpoena duces tecum*)
summary offence	a lesser offence which can only be heard by magistrates
summary judgment	a procedure whereby the claimant can obtain judgment without the defendant being permitted to defend the action
tort	a civil wrong excluding breach of contract. It covers negligence, trespass (to the person, goods or land), nuisance, breach of statutory duty and defamation
trespass to the person	a wrongful direct interference with another person. Harm does not have to be proved
ultra vires	outside the powers given by law (e.g. of a statutory body or company)
vicarious liability	the liability of an employer for the wrongful acts of an employee committed whilst in the course of employment
volenti non fit injuria	'to the willing there is no wrong' – the voluntary assumption of risk
ward of court	a minor placed under the protection of the High Court, which assumes responsibility for him or her and all decisions relating to his or her care must be made in accordance with the directions of the court
without prejudice	'without detracting from or without disadvantage to' – the use of the phrase prevents the other party using the information to the prejudice of the one providing it
writ	a form of written command, formerly the document which used to commence civil proceedings in the High Court – now a claim form is served

Further Reading

Appelbe, G.E. & Wingfield, J. (eds)(1993) *Dale and Appelbe's Pharmacy: Law and Ethics* 5th edn, The Pharmaceutical Press.

Brazier, M. (1992) *Medicine, Patients and the Law*, Penguin Books.

Brazier, M. & Murphy, J. (eds) (1999) *Street on Torts*, Butterworths.

British Medical Association (1998) *Medical Ethics Today*, BMJ Publishing.

Card, R. (2001) *Card, Cross and Jones: Criminal Law* 15th edn, Butterworths.

Committee of Expert Advisory Group on AIDS (1994) *Guidance for health care workers' protection against infection with HIV and hepatitis*, HMSO.

Department of Health (1993) *AIDS/HIV Infected Health Care Workers*, April 1993.

Denis, I.H. (1999) *The Law of Evidence* Sweet and Maxwell.

Dimond, B.C. (1994) *Legal Aspects of Midwifery*, Books for Midwives Press.

Dimond, B.C. (1996) *Legal Aspects of Child Health Care*, Mosby.

Dimond, B.C. (1997) *Legal Aspects of Occupational Therapy*, Blackwell Science.

Dimond, B.C. (1997) *Legal Aspects of Care in the Community*, Macmillan.

Dimond, B.C. (1997) *Mental Health (Patients in the Community) Act 1995: An Introductory Text*, Mark Allen Publications.

Dimond, B.C. (1998) *Legal Aspects of Complementary Therapy Practice*, Churchill Livingstone.

Dimond, B.C. (1999) *Legal Aspects of Physiotherapy*, Blackwell Science.

Dimond, B.C. (1999) *Patients' Rights, Responsibilities and the Nurse*, 2nd edn, Central Health Studies, Quay Publishing.

Dimond, B.C. & Barker, F. (1996) *Mental Health Law for Nurses*, Blackwell Science.

Ellis, N. (1994) *Employing Staff*, 5th edn, British Medical Journal.

Faulder, C. (1985) *Whose Body Is It?* Virago.

Finch, J. (ed.) (1994) *Speller's Law Relating to Hospitals*, 7th edn, Chapman and Hall.

Gann, R. (1993) *The NHS A to Z*, 2nd edn, The Help for Health Trust.

Glover, J. (1984) *Causing Death and Saving Lives*, Penguin.

Glover, J. (1984) *What Sort of People Should There Be?* Penguin.

Gunn, C. & Jackson, C.S. (1991) *Guidelines on Patient Care in Radiography*, Churchill Livingstone, Edinburgh.

Harris, P. (1997) *An Introduction to Law*, 5th edn, Butterworths.

Health and Safety Commission (1992) *Management of Health and Safety at Work Regulations: Approved Code of Practice*, HMSO.

Health and Safety Commission (1992) *Manual Handling Regulations and Approved Code of Practice*, HMSO.

Health and Safety Commission (1992) *Guidelines on Manual Handling in the Health Services*, HMSO.

Hepple, R.A., Matthews, M.H. & Howarth, D. (1999) *Tort Cases and Materials*, 5th edn, Butterworths.

Heywood Jones, I. (ed.) (1999) *The UKCC Code of Conduct: A Critical Guide*, Nursing Times Books.

Hoggett, B.& Hale, J. (1996) *Mental Health Law* 4th edn, Sweet & Maxwell.

Howells,G. & Weatherill, S. (1995) *Consumer Protection Law*, Dartmouth Publishing.

Hunt, G. & Wainwright, P. (eds) (1994) *Expanding the Role of the Nurse.* Blackwell Science.

Hurwitz, B. (1998) *Clinical Guidelines and the Law,* Oxford Radcliffe Medical Press.

Ingman, T. (1998) *The English Legal Process,* 7th edn, Blackstone Press.

Jones, R. (2001) *Mental Health Act Manual,* 7th edn, Sweet and Maxwell.

Keenan, D. (1998) *Smith and Keenan's English Law,* 12th edn, Pitman Publishing.

Kennedy, I. & Grubb, A. (2000) *Medical Law – Text with Materials* 3rd edn, Butterworths.

Kennedy, T. (1998) *Learning EU Law,* Sweet and Maxwell.

Kidner, R. (1998/9) *Blackstone's Statutes on Employment Law,* 8th edn, Blackstone Press.

Kloss, D. (2000) *Occupational Health Law,* 3rd edn, Blackwell Science.

Knight, B. (1992) *Legal Aspects of Medical Practice* , 5th edn, Churchill Livingstone.

Mandelstam, M. (1998) *An A-Z of Community Care Law* Jessica Kingsley Publishers.

Markesinis, B.S. & Deaking, S.F. (1999*) Tort Law* 4th edn Oxford University Press.

Mason D. & Edwards, P. (1993) *Litigation: A Risk Management Guide for Midwives,* Royal College of Midwives.

Mason, J.K. & McCall-Smith, A. (1999) *Law and Medical Ethics,* 5th edn, Butterworths.

McHale, J. & Fox, M. with Murphy, J. (1997) *Health Care Law,* Sweet and Maxwell.

McHale, J. & Tingle, J. (1998) *Law and Nursing* Butterworth Heinemann.

Miers,D. & Page, A. (1990) *Legislation* 2nd edn, Sweet and Maxwell.

Morgan, D. & Lee, R.G. (1991) *Human Fertilisation and Embryology Act 1990,* Blackstone Press.

Montgomery, J. (1997) *Health Care Law,* Oxford University Press.

National Association of Theatre Nurses (1993) *The Role of the Nurse as First Assistant in the Operating Department.*

Pearse, P. *et al.* (1988) *Personal Data Protection in Health and Social Services,* Croom Helm.

Pitt, G. (2000) *Employment Law* 4th edn, Sweet and Maxwell.

Pyne, R.H. (1991) *Professional Discipline in Nursing, Midwifery and Health Visiting,* 2nd edn, Blackwell Science.

Richards, P. (1999) *Law of Contract,* Pitman Publishing.

Royal College of Midwives, (1993) *Examples of Effective Midwifery Management.*

Royal College of Midwives, (1993) *The Midwife: Her Legal Status and Accountability.*

Royal College of Nursing, (1992) *Focus on Restraint,* 2nd edn.

Rowson, R. (1990) *An Introduction to Ethics for Nurses,* Scutari Press.

Rumbold, G. (1993) *Ethics in Nursing Practice* 2nd edn, Ballière Tindall.

Salvage, J. (1988) *Nurses at Risk: Guide to Health and Safety at Work,* Heinemann.

Salvage, J. & Rogers, R. (1988) *Health and Safety and the Nurse,* Heinemann.

Saxton, H. (1998) *Management in Imaging Departments,* Schering, Germany.

Selwyn, N. (1999) *Law of Health and Safety at Work,* Croom Helm.

Selwyn, N. (2000) *Selwyn's Law of Employment,* 11th edn, Butterworth.

Sime, S. A. (2000) *A Practical Approach to Civil Procedure,* 4th edn, Blackstone Press.

Skegg, P.D.G. (1998) *Law, Ethics and Medicine,* 2nd edn, Oxford University Press.

Stanberry, B.A. (1998) *The Legal and Ethical Aspects of Telemedicine* Royal Society of Medicine Press, London.

Steiner, J. & Woods, L. (1998) *Textbook on EC Law,* 6th edn, Blackstone Press.

Stone, J. & Mathews, J. (1996) *Complementary Medicine and the Law,* Oxford University Press.

Tingle, J. & Cribb, A. (eds) (1995) *Nursing Law and Ethics,* Blackwell Science.

Tschudin, V. & Marks-Maran, D. (1993) *Ethics: A Primer for Nurses,* Ballière Tindall.

Vincent, C. (ed.) (1996) *Clinical Risk Management,* BMJ Publications.

Vincent, C., *et al.* (1993) *Medical Accidents,* Oxford University Press.

White, R. Carr, P. & Lowe, N. (2001) *Children Act in Practice,* 3rd edn, Butterworth.

Wilkinson, R. & Caulfield, H. (2000) *The Human Rights Act: A Practical Guide for Nurses,* Whurr Publishers.

Young, A.P. (1994) *Law and Professional Conduct in Nursing,* 2nd edn, Scutari Press.

Zander, M. (1995) *Police and Criminal Evidence Act 1984,* 3rd edn, Sweet and Maxwell.

Index